Nutritional and Health Aspects of Food in South Asian Countries

Nutritional and Health Aspects of Traditional and Ethnic Foods

Nutritional and Health Aspects of Food in South Asian Countries

Volume editors:

JAMUNA PRAKASH
Visiting Professor, Zheziang Gongshang University, P.R. China;
Ambassador for India, Global Harmonisation Initiative, Vienna, Austria

VIDURANGA WAISUNDARA
Australian College of Business & Technology - Kandy Campus,
Sri Lanka

VISHWESHWARAIAH PRAKASH
Ramaiah University of Applied Sciences, Bangalore, India
IFRIFANS, Mysore, India

Series editors:

HUUB LELIEVELD

VESLEMØY ANDERSEN

VISHWESHWARAIAH PRAKASH

JAMUNA PRAKASH

BERND VAN DER MEULEN

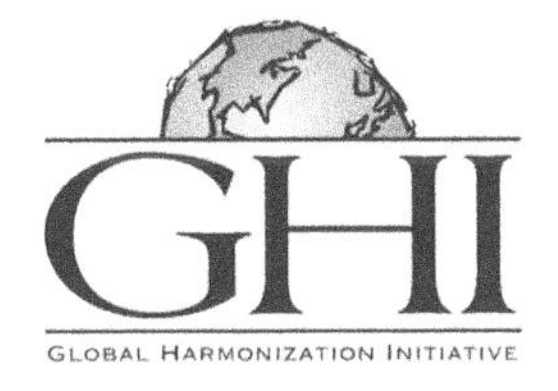

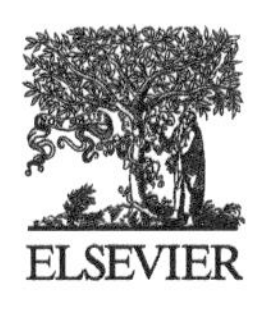

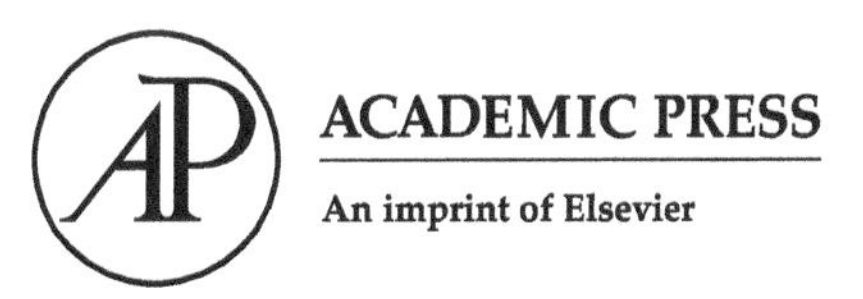

Academic Press is an imprint of Elsevier
125 London Wall, London EC2Y 5AS, United Kingdom
525 B Street, Suite 1650, San Diego, CA 92101, United States
50 Hampshire Street, 5th Floor, Cambridge, MA 02139, United States
The Boulevard, Langford Lane, Kidlington, Oxford OX5 1GB, United Kingdom

Notices
Knowledge and best practice in this field are constantly changing. As new research and experience broaden our understanding, changes in research methods, professional practices, or medical treatment may become necessary.

Practitioners and researchers must always rely on their own experience and knowledge in evaluating and using any information, methods, compounds, or experiments described herein. In using such information or methods they should be mindful of their own safety and the safety of others, including parties for whom they have a professional responsibility.

To the fullest extent of the law, neither the Publisher nor the authors, contributors, or editors, assume any liability for any injury and/or damage to persons or property as a matter of products liability, negligence or otherwise, or from any use or operation of any methods, products, instructions, or ideas contained in the material herein.

British Library Cataloguing-in-Publication Data
A catalogue record for this book is available from the British Library

Library of Congress Cataloging-in-Publication Data
A catalog record for this book is available from the Library of Congress

ISBN: 978-0-12-820011-7

For Information on all Academic Press publications
visit our website at https://www.elsevier.com/books-and-journals

Publisher: Charlotte Cockle
Acquisitions Editor: Megan R. Ball
Editorial Project Manager: Sara Valentino
Production Project Manager: Omer Mukthar
Cover Designer: Greg Harris

Typeset by MPS Limited, Chennai, India

Transferred to Digital Printing in 2020

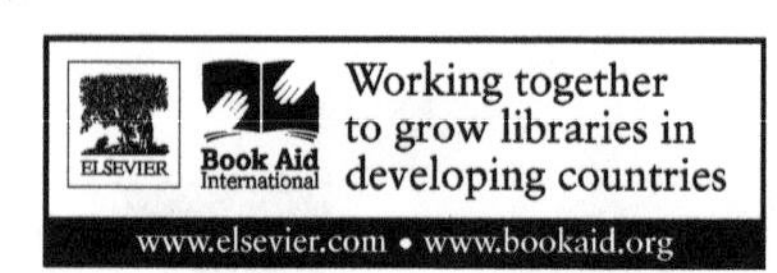

Contents

List of Contributors

Anwaar Ahmed
Institute of Food and Nutritional Sciences, PMAS-Arid Agriculture University, Rawalpindi, Punjab, Pakistan

S. M. Nazmul Alam
Department of Social Sciences, Faculty of Humanities, Curtin University, Perth, WA, Australia

Rai Muhammad Amir
Institute of Food and Nutritional Sciences, PMAS-Arid Agriculture University, Rawalpindi, Punjab, Pakistan

Supriya Bhalerao
Interactive Research School for Health Affairs, Bharati Vidyapeeth Deemed (to be) University, Pune, India

Pushpa Bharati
Dept. of Food Science & Nutrition, College of Community Science, University of Agricultural Sciences, Dharwad, India

Purabi Bose
Researcher and Filmmaker, IUFRO Deputy Coordinator Social Aspects of Forest & Coordinator Gender in Forest Research; IASC Council Member; IUCN CEESP's Deputy Chair for Theme on Governance, Equity and Rights

Palanisamy Bruntha Devi
Department of Food Science and Technology, Pondicherry University, Puducherry, India

Hamid Ezzatpanah
Department of Food Science and Technology, Science and Research Branch, Islamic Azad University, Tehran, Iran

Dilip Ghosh
Nutriconnect, Sydney, NSW, Australia; Food Nutrition Partner, Auckland, New Zealand, New Zealand; NICM, Western Sydney University, Sydney, NSW, Australia; Health Foods and Dietary Supplements Association (HADSA), Mumbai, India; Ambassador-Global Harmonization Initiatives, Vienna, Austria

T.K. Srinivasa Gopal
Centre of Excellence in Food Processing Technology, Kerala University of Fisheries and Ocean Studies, Cochin, India

Sudhakar T. Johnson
Professor of Biotechnology and Center for Innovation, Incubation and Entrepreneurship, currently resides at 2-B2, Second Floor, Swarna Residency, Currency Nagar, Vijayawada - 520008, India

Dambar Bahadur Khadka
Central Campus of Technology, Tribhuvan University, Dharan, Nepal

Uma Koirala
Gender Studies Program, Tribhuvan University, Kathmandu, Nepal

Uma N. Kulkarni
Dept. of Food Science & Nutrition, College of Community Science, University of Agricultural Sciences, Dharwad, India

A. Jyothi Lakshmi
Protein Chemistry and Technology Department, CSIR-Central Food Technological Research Institute, Mysuru, India

Jiwan Prava Lama
Nepal Agribusiness Innovation Centre, Kathmandu, Nepal

Chathudina J. Liyanage
Department of Food Science and Technology, Faculty of Applied Sciences, Sabaragamuwa University of Sri Lanka, Belihuloya, Sri Lanka

Muhammad Nadeem
Department of Environmental Sciences, COMSATS University Islamabad, Vehari Campus, Vehari, Punjab, Pakistan

D.B. Anantha Narayana
Ayurvidye Trust, and, Member, Expert Committee (Nonspecified Foods and Food Ingredients), Food Safety Standards Authority of India (FSSAI), Ministry of Health and Family Welfare, Govt. of India, Bengaluru, India

M. Niamul Naser
Department of Zoology, Faculty of Biological Sciences, University of Dhaka, Dhaka, Bangladesh

Kalpana Platel
CSIR-Central Food Technological Research Institute, Mysuru, India

Jamuna Prakash
Ambassador for India, Global Harmonisation Initiative, Vienna, Austria

V. Prakash
Ramaiah University of Applied Sciences, Bangalore, India; IFRIFANS, Mysore, India

Prathapkumar Halady Shetty
Department of Food Science and Technology, Pondicherry University, Puducherry, India

R.B. Smarta
Interlink Marketing Consultancy Pvt. Ltd., Mumbai, India; Hon. Secretary, Health Foods And Dietary Supplements Association (HADSA), Mumbai, India

Ketki Wagh
Ayurveda Preventive Medicine & Yoga Consultant, RK University, Rajkot, Gujarat, India

Viduranga Y. Waisundara
Australian College of Business & Technology - Kandy Campus, Sri Lanka

About the editors

Jamuna Prakash

Fellow, International Union of Food Science and Technology; Visiting Professor, Zhejiang Gongshang University, P.R. China; Ambassador for India, Global Harmonization Initiative

Dr. Jamuna Prakash is serving as Visiting Professor for International Union of Food Sciences & Technology and Department of Food Science & Biotechnology, Zhegiang Gongshang University, China. A former Professor of Food Science & Nutrition at University of Mysore, India, with vast teaching and research experience, and she is a Fellow of IUFOST and National Academy of Agricultural Sciences, India. She has had an exemplary academic career with many awards and accolades and credited with more than 250 research and review papers, 15 books/book chapters, more than 400 presentations, and successful completion of many research and educational projects. Her research interests are compositional analysis of foods, product formulation, sensory evaluation, nutrient digestibility and bioavailability, nutrition status of population, and food behavior. She is a member of many National and International committees and a life member of many professional organizations, and she serves as Indian Ambassador for Global Harmonization Initiative, Austria.

Viduranga Waisundara

Australian College of Business & Technology—Kandy Campus, Sri Lanka

Dr. Viduranga Waisundara is currently the Deputy Principal of the Australian College of Business & Technology—Kandy Campus, Sri Lanka. She obtained her PhD from the Department of Chemistry, National University of Singapore in Food Science & Technology in 2010. She was a lecturer at Temasek Polytechnic, Singapore from July 2009 to March 2013. Following this, she relocated to her motherland of Sri Lanka and spearheaded the Functional Food Product Development Project at the National Institute of Fundamental Studies from April 2013 to October 2016. Thereafter, she was a Senior Lecturer on a temporary basis at the Department of Food Technology, Faculty of Technology, Rajarata University of Sri Lanka from January 2017 to July 2018. Dr. Waisundara is the present Global Harmonization Initiative Ambassador for Sri Lanka.

Vishweshwaraiah Prakash

Vice President, International Union of Nutritional Sciences; Scientific Chair, International Union of Food Science and Technology; Adjunct Professor, Ramaiah University of Applied Sciences, India; Adjunct Professor, Institute of Chemical

Technology, India; Visiting Professor, Zhejiang Gongshang University, China; Founder Board Member, Global Harmonization Initiative; Distinguished Scientist of Council of Scientific and Industrial Research, India

Dr. Vishweshwaraiah Prakash is currently the Vice President of IUNS (2017–21); President of ISNANN, IFRIFANS, INDIA; Chairman, India Region of European Hygienic Engineering Design Group, Germany; Adjunct Professor at RUAS, Bangalore, India; and Adjunct Professor at ICT, Mumbai, India. He was Former Director of CFTRI, Mysore, and Distinguished Scientist of CSIR, India. He has received more than 65 National and International awards including one of the high Civilian Awards Padmashree, Coveted Bhatnagar Award for Science and Technology and Rajyothsava awards and several Lifetime Achievement Awards from organizations like FICCI, IUFoST, in India and abroad. He is currently serving in the editorial board of many Food Science and Technology and Nutrition Journals and is in the editorial board of numerous books. He is also Chairman, Scientific Council of IUFoST. He has 212 peer reviewed research publications, 55 patents filed, is the author of 12 books, and has 9 more books in pipeline.

Preface

Following the publication of the book *Regulating Safety of Traditional and Ethnic Foods*, published in 2016 (Prakash et al., 2016), the editors were asked why they had not included nutrition and health aspects of such foods. This is because a little is widely known about these aspects, and today scientists and many others, in particular, those who travel to far-away countries, are interested to know about these aspects.

Nutrition is a globally active and far-reaching area of scientific research that begins with local geography, history, culture, resources, and genetics and goes all the way through to the development of food and beverage products and their nutritional benefit to individual consumers and communities. With the world being turned into one big village, interest in traditional and ethnic foods has been rising and so have the claims about their nutritional values and health-promoting effects. Today, traditional foods often are produced in a way that deviates from the ways used in the long past, when unknowingly microbes were exploited to make healthy and nutritious food products. In principle, there is much knowledge about traditional and ethnic foods, but it is scattered around the world and in the mind and sometimes just in the notes of many people. It may have been published in an infinite number of journals, magazines, and books. This knowledge often is hard to retrieve if retrievable at all. Much of it may disappear if not captured in time. The editors had the difficult task to identify the authors capable of doing what was needed, by collecting and summarizing scattered information.

For a long time, food traditions were seen as based on beliefs without evidence about any of the supposed or believed nutritional and health aspects. It was widely recommended to trust only the information that has been carefully checked scientifically by modern methods, preferably in the western world. The vast experience and knowledge of many populations that for often very good reasons adjusted to certain diets have been largely ignored. Only in the past decade, serious research has started to find out about the claims made, and scientists started to investigate the claims and beliefs based on the composition of the foods used and the way they were traditionally prepared. Responding to the requests, it was decided to try to capture information about traditional and ethnic foods from all countries in the world. The intention was to cover, for all countries, information such as the history of eating habits and the reasons for these habits. The information is important to understand, for example, why some foods are only suitable for some people but not for others as is the case with cow's milk. Large populations lack β-galactosidase and hence cannot digest such milk. Other aspects to be covered are common nutrition and health issues; the abundance or scarcity of certain types of food, also depending on the season and including preservation strategies; environmental sustainability issues; regulatory issues and proposals to harmonize regulations; to end with a future outlook.

The initial idea had been to produce a single volume, similar to the book on the safety of the foods, and the publisher expected that approximately 250 pages would be the size of the book. After discussing the coverage and the fact that there would be huge differences between countries and even within countries or regions, the proposed size of the book became 500 pages and then, following more discussions, it was rapidly growing to the idea of a series that would do justice to all cultures in the world. The final plan turned out to a need of 26 volumes of about 300 pages; therefore, instead of a book, it became a series of 26 books of which this is the first volume about Asia, covering the southern part of the continent.

Huub Lelieveld
President, Global Harmonization Initiative

Reference

Prakash, V., Martin-Belloso, O., Keener, L., Astley, S., Braun, S., McMahon, H., Lelieveld, H., 2016. Regulating Safety of Traditional and Ethnic Foods. Academic Press/Elsevier, Waltham; Oxford, ISBN: 978-0-12-800605-4.

PART 1

History of Traditional Foods in South Asia

CHAPTER 1

Eating habits, food cultures, and traditions in South Asia Region

V. Prakash[1,2]
[1]Ramaiah University of Applied Sciences, Bangalore, India
[2]IFRIFANS, Mysore, India

The book series on *Nutritional and Health Aspects of Traditional and Ethnic Foods* covers globally the various regions in different volumes. This particular volume pertaining to South Asia entitled *Nutritional and Health Aspects of Food in South Asian Countries* covers some of the countries in the region such as India, Sri Lanka, Nepal, Bangladesh, Pakistan, and Iran with individual country's different aspects of traditional and ethnic foods. The Global Harmonization Initiative has the focus to address the subject with a holistic angle of culture, tradition, nutrition, health, sustainability, functionality, role of traditional wisdom, health, and wellness, nutraceutical potential, underutilized foods in remote area, and more importantly safety and regulatory requirements for a sustainable scale-up of traditional foods, global and regional challenges, and future outlook of traditional and ethnic foods for South Asia.

The history of traditional and ethnic foods is documented in the culture and civilization of these countries beyond 5000 years covering the various angles of these foods in different seasons with different agricultural practices especially the edible plant parts, the role of functional ingredients and culinary, and the diurnal routines of eating habits to mention a few that has the value of well-established sustainable practices from generation to generation. This also establishes the eating habits and links it to traditional wisdom and benefit on the one hand especially in countries such as India and other Southeast Asian Countries as traditional medicine (*Ayurveda* in India for example). This strategically links through several foods with health. It is necessary for the modern-day population to know the heritage of foods globally and especially in the South Asian regions. Moreover, the total number of medicinal manuscripts worldwide is approximately 100,000 documents. The magnitude of knowledge baffles any person and is not just culinary science but also food engineering in its own environment of technology with appropriate vessels made out of different materials. Therefore in categorizing this knowledge, this particular volume makes a humble attempt to introduce to the reader basically the depth of knowledge that South Asia has in this important area of traditional and ethnic foods, the history, the documentation, the practices,

Nutritional and Health Aspects of Food in South Asian Countries
DOI: https://doi.org/10.1016/B978-0-12-820011-7.00001-0

and the sustainable systems through the various introductory write-ups of several authors in this chapter about the individual country's practices in traditional and ethnic foods such as nutrition, health, wellness, and food safety aspects. This should not be construed as a comprehensive document, but it is important that the reader must ensure extra reading with the references provided to get more insight into the individual countries with a holistic approach.

Introduction of the food cultures and tradition with reference to *Nutritional and Health Aspects of Traditional and Ethnic Foods of South Asia* is reflected in a brief write-up in the chapter by the authors from India, Sri Lanka, Nepal, Bangladesh, Pakistan, and Iran. The authors who have covered these in about two pages are listed below for each country before the beginning of each chapter for each country: India—Jamuna Prakash; Sri Lanka—Viduranga Waisundara; Nepal—Jiwan Lama; Bangladesh—S.M. Nazmul Alam; Pakistan—Anwar Ahmed, and Iran—Hamid Ezzatpanah. Each author has covered this area extensively to give a glimpse of the individual country's diversity in the country chapters of this book. The common regulatory issues and the future outlook are covered separately in Part 8, Common regulatory and safety issue and future outlook for South Asia region, with respect to safety requirements from the point of a global and regional challenge, and reach out of functional and nutritional foods based on traditional wisdom is dealt with separately. These are covered to bring a holistic outlook on the subject of traditional and ethnic foods in this book.

Thus the various chapters from different countries regarding traditional and ethnic foods from the point of view of nutritional, health, and wellness aspect opens a huge opportunity and a large window for the possible reach of traditional and ethnic foods in the health sector especially gut health and immune modulation, prevention of diseases, and health benefits road map interfacing through modern scientific tools. This will help to generate rationale and scientific evidence of the benefits with a clear mandate of global policy issues in the research and development, energy, food engineering and technologies for application, scale-up of traditional and ethnic foods manufacture covering trends in packaging and ultimately food safety issues, quality assurance, and standards including waste disposal and eco-friendly technologies that make it sustainable for wider reach of these traditional and ethnic foods for better nutrition and health in the region of South Asia and the global market complying with the local and global regulations.

PART 2

Food, Nutrition, and Health in India

CHAPTER 1

Introduction

Jamuna Prakash
Ambassador for India, Global Harmonisation Initiative, Vienna, Austria

Culinary traditions define the culture of a nation and are closely linked to the health and well-being of its populace. Traditional diets also reflect the agricultural patterns, seasonal variations, availability, and accessibility to foods as well as the processing techniques followed through centuries. Indian traditional diets have undergone a transition as expected on account of changing sociodemographic profiles, agriculture, advances in food processing, and availability of processed foods, although the basic food combinations remain the same. It is interesting to examine the health and nutritional status of population, nutritional sufficiency of the traditional diets, the traditional food preservation techniques practiced, the food habits of tribal populations, the food-related culture and rituals and their significance, the functional components of traditional diets, the role of *Ayurveda*, in health and diseases (the ancient medical science followed in India), and the contribution of foods from marine sources to nutrition. This chapter presents a bird's eye view of these aspects of Indian traditional diets.

The present health and nutrition situation of the Indian population indicates an overall reduction in the prevalence of severe nutritional deficiencies, although subclinical deficiencies do prevail. There has been an alarming increase in noncommunicable diseases, on account of many factors, specifically, the lifestyle changes, the diet being one of them. The country battles with malnourished children with stunted growth, chronic energy deficiency in adults, micronutrient deficiencies, iron deficiency anemia, and obesity. India is self-sufficient in food production, although poor socioeconomic conditions deprive a section of the population with adequate food, giving rise to nutritional insecurities. A wide variety of food grains (cereals, millets, and pulses), fruits, vegetables, and oilseeds are grown along with a record milk production and resultant abundance of milk products. Livestock is a big industry too with easy availability of eggs, poultry, meat, and fish.

Indian traditional diets usually comprise dishes prepared using cereals, pulses, vegetables, and a serving of curd (yogurt). The diets are diverse in terms of varieties of foods used, a large number of cereals and millets used as staples, a variety of legumes used for making the additional courses, and many vegetables used for making accompanying dishes. In general, it is a healthy blend of many foods. Spices add on to the

Nutritional and Health Aspects of Food in South Asian Countries
DOI: https://doi.org/10.1016/B978-0-12-820011-7.00002-2

unique blend of flavor. Apart from being nutritionally rich, the food combinations also enrich the diet with many inherent bioactive components, the plant pigments, nondigestible constituents, bioactive peptides, essential oils, etc. Notable is the use of unrefined foods in natural form in traditional cuisine, which are rich in nonnutrient bioactives. Statewise differences are observed in the types of foods eaten. Wheat predominates in the Northern part of India, whereas rice is a more common staple in South India. Millets are also used in some states. The dishes prepared are very unique and different in each ethnic group. Nutritionally, diets are good provided foods are chosen from all groups and adequate quantity is eaten.

Food preservation was practiced traditionally and is used even today, the common techniques being, drying, pickling, salting, and fermentation. These ensured proper utilization of food resources, extending the shelf life of surplus agricultural produce as well as providing newer novel foods with enhanced nutrition. India is also known for its pockets of tribes, who still follow the practice of foraging forest foods and depending on food resources entirely from forest regions. Their food habits are quite different from the urban population with a major dependence on naturally grown unique foods collected from the forest. A section on this dealt as a case study will familiarize readers with their unique food culture.

Vegetarian diets have been unique to Indian culture, and are still followed by a large section of populations. Vegetarianism has been practiced on account of religious reasons for many centuries in many ethnic populations. Vegetarian diets can be healthy, provided foods are selected appropriately. Even in so-called meat-eaters, or nonvegetarians, the frequency of eating meat is very low, sometimes restricted to once a week due to economic reasons or religious practices. India is also bestowed with a large sea coast; hence, marine foods are a source of nutrition to the coastal population. Fish is eaten as a staple providing high-quality proteins, essential vitamins, minerals, as well as fish oils rich in ω-3 fatty acids. Usage of fish is customary especially in coastal areas, with an abundance of fish and other marine foods, and it is an economical way of getting required nutrition for the local populace.

In Indian food culture, food and water were given a prominent place. Religious rituals required the offering of the best food to God. Fasting and feasting were common and associated with special days. There were specific rules followed for cooking and eating of food that indicated adherence to certain standards of hygiene and sanitation. Rituals were mandated to ensure food safety in all food handling protocols. Sharing of food was considered sacred and no needy person was turned away hungry from home, thus ensuring food security to all. The food culture followed the principles of Ayurveda, wherein foods were prescribed based on the nature (body type) of an individual and were modified depending on the seasons. The foods were defined in terms of their properties, and the selection of foods was based on these specific properties. Interestingly, Ayurveda describes six types of basic taste quality (*rasa*) of foods, which has been acknowledged much later in modern science. A healthy meal is supposed to be a combination of all tastes and texture.

As in other parts of the world, India is also witnessing dietary and nutrition transitions with direct visible impacts on the health of people. As expected, these changes are on account of globalization of food chain, availability of different foods and cuisines and desire to experiment with new food cultures, advances in food processing and an enormous increase in number of processed foods available, easy access to fast food vendors, increase in disposable income, and consequent expenditure on catered or processed foods. Although the type and number of foods available have increased, the nutritional quality of diet is decreasing at an alarming rate due to the overconsumption of energy-dense foods, salt, sugar, fat, refined foods, and trans fats. At one end of the spectrum, there is malnutrition and, at the other, obesity is increasing due to overeating. The consumer needs to be educated regarding unhealthy processed foods and the nutritional superiority of our traditional diets as well as rich culture.

CHAPTER 2

Diet-related nutrition and health issues in Indian population

A. Jyothi Lakshmi[1] and Jamuna Prakash[2]
[1]Protein Chemistry and Technology Department, CSIR-Central Food Technological Research Institute, Mysuru, India
[2]Ambassador for India, Global Harmonisation Initiative, Vienna, Austria

Contents

2.1 Introduction

Food is the "basic right of every human being," at the same time, "we are what we eat," that is, the food we eat reflects our nutritional status and in turn our health and well-being. Innovation, being the key to research and development, has conquered every field of life for which food and nutrition are not an exception. Economic inequalities, technological intervention and selective outreach, and globalization associated with diminishing health and nutritional awareness have impelled toward the adoption of faulty or imbalanced dietary practices. Lifestyle changes associated with reduced physical activity due to less labor-intensive activities, mechanization, and stress to cope with the changing work cultures in all strata have impacted on compromised nutrition. These uninterrupted changes in lifestyle accompanied by faulty feeding practices are increasing the occurrence of overnutrition and obesity leading to the increasing prevalence of noncommunicable diseases at one end and persisting occurrence of

Nutritional and Health Aspects of Food in South Asian Countries
DOI: https://doi.org/10.1016/B978-0-12-820011-7.00003-4

undernutrition (though with a notable reduction in severe forms) due to inadequate food intake at the other end. This dual burden of malnutrition faced by our country poses the challenges to the health and nutrition professionals as "food and nutrition" is the root cause for it, although it is backed by various other factors. The extent of dietary influences on the magnitude of various health and nutrition issues prevalent in India will be discussed in the subsequent sections.

2.2 Historical overview

The dietary surveys conducted by National Nutrition Monitoring Bureau (NNMB) periodically, that is, from 1975 onwards have shown a decade wise gradual decrease in consumption of energy-based foods, that is, cereals, sugar, and jaggery have slid down, whereas protein and micronutrient-based foods (iron and vitamin A, and some B-complex vitamins) such as pulses, vegetable, and fruits that were below adequacy levels, have remained the same over the four decades. Energy and protein consumption patterns of households declined by 20% with a shift from the adequacy to inadequacy zone (NNMB, 2012). These observations also confirm that the diets were cereal-based and lacked protective nutrients from the past four decades (Table 2.1).

The partial improvement in nutritional status could be attributed to various factors such as attaining self-sufficiency in food production through the green revolution, providing food grains to poor families at subsidized rates through the public distribution system and through the inception of direct national nutrition programs to children, pregnant women, and school children. The major national nutrition intervention programs that were incepted from 1960 onwards are compiled in Table 2.2.

Table 2.1 An overview of nutritional status of preschool children from 1970s to 2012 (NNMB, 2012).

Nutritional indicator		Prevalence from 1975 to 2012
Children	• Severe protein-energy malnutrition	Kwashiorkor and marasmus have become rare
	• Underweight	Reduced from 75.5% to 41%
	• Stunting	Reduced from 82% to 45.7%
	• Wasting	Reduced from 27% to 16.0%
Adults	• Chronic energy deficiency	Reduced by 26% in female and 20% in male
	• Obesity/overweight	Increased by fivefold in adults
Vitamin A deficiency		Bitot's spots have become negligible
Vitamin B-complex deficiency		Angular stomatitis is significantly declined
Prevalence of diabetes, hypertension, and cancer		Has increased and still increasing

Table 2.2 National nutrition programs and the target groups.

National nutrition program	Beneficiaries
Applied nutrition program	Promoting the production and consumption of protective foods for pregnant and lactating mothers and children
Integrated Child Development Services Scheme	Provides supplementary nutrition to preschoolers (500 kcal of energy and 12–15 g protein/day), extra nutrition for severely malnourished children, nonformal education for preschoolers, health checkups, immunization, referral services, and nutrition and health education for both children and pregnant women (600 kcal and 18–20 g protein/day)
Nutrition program for adolescent girls	Girls <35 kg and pregnant women <45 kg will be provided with 6.0 kg take-home ration/month for three consecutive months in a year
National nutritional anemia prophylaxis program	Provision of iron supplements Children, 1–5 years—20 mg elemental iron + 0.1 mg folate/day Children, 6–10 years—30 mg iron + 0.25 mg folate Adolescents, 12–18 years—100 mg iron + 0.5 mg folate/day Pregnant women—60 mg iron + 0.5 mg folate/day for 100 days
Weekly iron and folic acid supplementation program for nonschool going adolescents	Iron folic acid tablets on a weekly basis for 12–18-year girls for 52 weeks Biannual deworming tablets
National prophylaxis program for prevention of vitamin A deficiency	For all children 6–11 months, 100,000 IU; 1–5 years old—200,000 IU of vitamin A on a 6-monthly basis. On diagnosis of vitamin A deficiency—a megadose of 200,000 IU of vitamin A immediately and the next dose 1–4 weeks later
National iodine deficiency disorder control program	Universal salt iodization in the country—30 ppm at the manufacturing level and 15 ppm at the consumption level
Mid-day meal program	Provide one full meal to school children providing one-third of the calorie and half of the protein requirement per day
Nutrition program for adolescent girls (*Kishori shakti yojna*)	Targeted for adolescent girls of 11–18 years, it covers awareness on watch over menarche, half-yearly general health check-up, training on minor ailments, deworming, prophylactic measures against anemia, goiter, vitamin deficiencies, and supplementary nutrition

The national nutritional studies conducted from past 4 to 5 decades at global, national, societal, and individual levels have clearly shown that the qualitative and quantitative dietary adequacy is the major determinant of the health and nutritional status of our populace. Dietary adequacy is dependent on socioeconomic, agroclimatic, environmental, and physiological factors. The lead national health and nutrition surveys—NNMB and National Family Health Survey (NFHS) surveys that report the health and nutritional status from pregnancy have reported that the effect of faulty feeding practices originates "in utero" and percolates through the life cycle in varied forms depending on the prevailing factors.

Consumption of a balanced diet leads to normal health and nutritional status, but the dietary patterns vary widely across the nation due to diversity in domicile, food availability, accessibility, affordability, and other priorities. Lack of nutritional nutritional awareness to judge the veracity of dietary suggestions from social media and peer pressure can result in a wide spectrum of nutritional imbalances ranging from undernutrition to overnutrition and obesity leading to the developmental impairments of organs and finally the onset of chronic degenerative diseases. The effect of dietary imbalances including micronutrient deficiencies in different population groups, namely pregnant women, children, and adults are summarized in the following sections with epidemiological data and associated observations.

2.3 Dietary intake and nutritional and health status of pregnant women

Pregnancy requires additional nutrients for meeting the growth and developmental needs of the fetus, for meeting the mother's own requirements, and to establish good nutrient stores for postpartum requirements of lactation. Dietary surveys have shown that diets of a sizeable proportion of pregnant women meet around 50% of recommended dietary allowances (RDAs) of protein and calories (Fig. 2.1) (NNMB, 2012). Micronutrient inadequacies including iron and folic acid were reported in more than 75% of the mothers. The iron–folic acid supplements provided by the government was consumed completely by only 30% of the mothers. This is well reflected in the prevalence of anemia by 58.7% of pregnant women (NFHS-4, 2015–16).

Specific nutrient deficiencies during pregnancy apart from affecting the growth of the fetus are also known to cause genetic alterations resulting in adverse health impairments in later life (Table 2.3).

Poor maternal nutritional intake during pregnancy negatively impacts fetal genetic trajectory and restricts fetal growth. It affects the vascularity of the placenta that effectively transports nutrients to the offspring and results in low birth weight that has profound adversities in later life (Table 2.4).

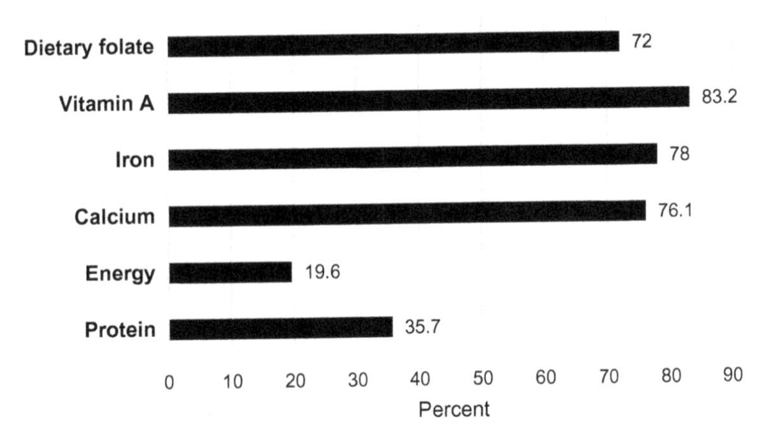

Figure 2.1 Percent of pregnant women obtaining <50% of the recommended dietary allowance of major nutrients through diet (NNMB, 2012).

2.4 Dietary adequacy of under five children and adults

Dietary imbalances have been attributed to be the direct cause for the prevalence of malnutrition in India. These are in common frank inadequacies of the critical nutrients leading to undernutrition and deriving disproportionate calories from the macronutrients leading to overweight and obesity associated with micronutrient deficiencies.

Children below 5 years who have a high growth rate associated with higher calorie requirements per unit body weight were reported to have a dietary inadequacy of energy (23%–41%) and micronutrients (Table 2.5). Calorie inadequacy was reported along with protein inadequacy or in isolation in 40%–50% of the children both in longitudinal and cross-sectional studies (NNMB, 2012; Kulsum et al., 2008). Energy inadequacy was reported among preschoolers even in families where the nutrient adequacy levels were better among adults and older children. Micronutrient inadequacy was reported in a much higher proportion of the children. Inadequate intake of iron, vitamin A, and folic acid was of a higher level among the preschool children. Among adults too, a similar trend of inadequacy was evident, around 30% of them showed different proportions of calorie and protein inadequacy. The quantitative inadequacy of iron ranged from 33% to 45% and vitamin A around 80%. Most diet surveys have clearly shown that cereals and pulses are the major sources of all nutrients, and diets lack in sufficient quantities of protective foods such as fat, milk, vegetables, and fruits. The qualitative inadequacy (amino acid content) and poor digestibility also contribute for compromised nutrition that is reflected in deficiencies and functional impairments (Bamji & Nair, 2016; Lakshmi et al., 2005; Kulsum et al., 2009).

Table 2.3 Impact of specific nutrient deficiencies in mother on infant's later life: few observations.

Implications of macronutrient deficiencies
• Protein inadequacy leads to the deficiency of amino acids and impairment of one-carbon metabolism and DNA methylation • Protein deficiency leads to cardiometabolic disorders in later life of the infant, including higher blood pressure • Maternal undernutrition produces infants with thin lean mass and higher adipose percentage with insulin • Deficiency of protein and micronutrients along with excess fat affected kidney development in infants (Wood-Bradley et al., 2015)
Implications of micronutrient deficiencies
• Iron deficiency anemia is associated with adverse birth outcomes such as preterm delivery, low birth weight, and growth restriction (Allen, 2000). It is associated with the cardiovascular risk of the offspring during pregnancy • Inadequate intake of folic acid during the first trimester of pregnancy was reported to cause neural tube defects (Wasserman et al., 1998). Deficiency of folic acid and vitamin B_{12} is associated with raised homocysteine levels that restrict fetal growth • Higher folate and lower vitamin B_{12} are associated with offspring adiposity and insulin resistance • Raised level of serum homocysteine due to dietary deficiencies of folic acid, vitamins B_{12} and B_6 (perhaps B_2), involved in its metabolism, seems to be an important etiological factor for cardiovascular and other chronic diseases (Raman, 2016) • Imbalance or deficiency of B vitamins is known to have shown increased homocysteine levels that are indicative of cardiovascular disease in adult life (Yajnik et al., 2008; Krishnaveni et al., 2014; Yajnik et al., 2014) • Vitamins A and D influence gene expression by interacting with nuclear receptors, folic acid, and vitamin B_{12} through epigenetic mechanisms. Deficiencies of these nutrients distract both the mechanisms altering the cellular processes in critical times during fetal development and influence the structure and function of organs and systems and contribute to long-term effects on disease susceptibility termed as programing • Synapse formation and myelination during the critical periods of brain development and nutrient deprivation during this period cause irreversible brain dysfunction (Georgieff, 2007) • Zinc deficiency is known to affect the regulation of the autonomic nervous system as well and hippocampal and cerebellar development (Vazir and Boindala, 2016). PEM and zinc deficiency are reported to cause stunting, affecting learning and poor cognitive development (Özaltin et al., 2010)

2.5 Undernutrition

The nutritional status of the population for whom the dietary inadequacies are reported confirms the presence of undernutrition determined based on anthropometric indices that are alarmingly high in children below 5 years and also in adults.

Acute and chronic forms of undernutrition, which originate during early infancy, increase by fivefold by the end of 11 months (Table 2.6) and continue at the same

Table 2.4 Consequences of imbalanced nutrition during pregnancy.

The implications of low birth weight/intrauterine growth retardation
• The secondary factor for 40%–80% neonatal deaths • Risk factor for perinatal morbidities • Increased risks of disorders/disruptions of child growth development—neurologic disorders, learning disabilities, childhood psychiatric disorders, and mental retardation • Increased morbidities in the long run (Goldenberg and Culhane, 2007) • Long-term disability imposes a high economic burden on households depriving them of proper nutrition (Abu-Saad and Fraser, 2010) • Increases the risk of type 2 diabetes during adulthood (Whincup et al., 2008). Low metabolic capacity coupled with high metabolic load posed due to faulty dietary habits is reported to lead to high levels of body fat and glycemic load increases the risk for diabetes (Unnikrishnan et al., 2016) • Subjects showed higher insulin resistance and higher glucose at 4 years of age. A follow-up at 8 years showed that those who had the highest current weight also had higher insulin resistance and worst cardiovascular profile (Bavdekar et al., 1999)
Low birth weight with higher adiposity
• Cord blood contained higher levels of leptin, insulin, and lower adiponectin that strongly suggests a higher risk of diabetes in their adulthood (West et al., 2014; Yajnik et al., 2002)
Implications of maternal overnutrition
• Excess energy intake leads to a birth weight >4 kg in infants due to fetal hyperinsulinemia • Fetal overnutrition due to hyperinsulinemia programs the offspring for type 2 diabetes • The infants are born larger and develop obesity, insulin resistance, impaired glucose tolerance, and diabetes at a younger age
Implications of gestational diabetes
• Infants born with a larger size at birth and with higher subcutaneous adiposity showed higher insulin and glucose levels and had glucose resistance at nine years. • In addition, mothers with vitamin B_{12} deficiency had a higher risk of being diabetic 5 years postpartum in comparison to those without vitamin B_{12} deficiency (Krishnaveni et al., 2010)

Table 2.5 Percent adequacy of dietary intake of nutrients in children (under five) and adults.

Subjects	Protein	Energy	Calcium	Iron	Vitamin A	Dietary folate
Adults	80–100	80–88	55–62	55–77	20–22	53–61
Children <5 years	>100	69–77	33–41	52–55	15–19	60–72

pace up to 5 years old. Children between 6 and 23 months receiving an adequate diet were only 9.6%, which is the period of onset of malnutrition (NFHS-4, 2015–16). With this higher prevalence rate, India contributes to about 40% of stunted and 50% of wasted children in the world (UNICEF, 2013). Around 4.6% of children were

Table 2.6 Prevalence of under nutrition in India in different age groups (%).

Age group	Underweight	Stunted	Wasted	Reference
Infancy (0–11 months)	7–32	6–35.2	25	NNMB (2012)
Children (<5 years)	35.8	38.4	21.1	NFHS-4 (2015–16)
	41.1	45.7	15.5	NNMB (2012)
Undernutrition among adults				
Chronic energy deficiency	**Women**	**Men**	**Reference**	
	35.5	34.2	NFHS-4 (2015–16)	
	33	32	NNMB (2012)	

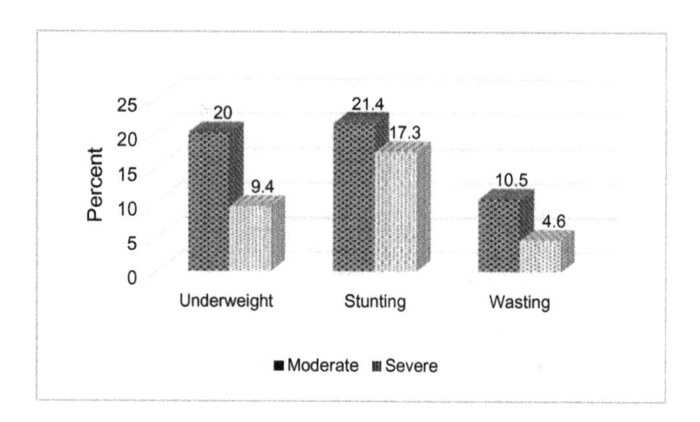

Moderate: < Mean – 2 SD to < Mean- 3 SD; Severe: < Mean – 3 SD

Figure 2.2 Prevalence (%) of undernutrition—0–59 months (RSOC, 2013–14).

reported to be subjected to severe acute malnutrition with very low weight for height (Fig. 2.2). Around one-third of the adult population was found to be chronic energy deficient (CED) as per both the surveys. Overnutrition leading to obesity was also observed in 15.8% of adult population (NFHS-4, 2015–16).

2.6 Micronutrient deficiencies

Different from macronutrient deficiencies, micronutrient deficiencies cannot be visualized unless they are clinically manifested, by then the unfavorable consequences in impaired growth, immunity, learning and cognitive ability, and work performance, in general, would have witnessed the adversities. The economic losses due to micronutrient deficiencies in India indexed as DALYs are estimated to range from 0.8% to 2.5% of GDP. Micronutrient deficiencies are estimated to cost India around $2.5 billion per year (PHFI, 2015). Therefore these deficiencies are termed as "hidden hunger" (Bamji and Nair, 2016). Among the micronutrient deficiencies, iron deficiency anemia, vitamin A deficiency, and zinc deficiencies are the major ones. Ocular manifestations of vitamin A deficiency such as Bitot's spots and night blindness are observed among children at <1% among preschool children and 1%–2% among older children and pregnant women (NNMB, 2012). However, a higher percentage of our population showed low serum retinol levels indicative of a higher degree of vitamin A deficiency going asymptomatic. Iron deficiency anemia based on hemoglobin levels was found to be high with 69.5% among children, 55.3% in women, and 58.5% in pregnant women (PHFI, 2015; NFHS-4, 2015–16). One of the well-proven and researched etiologies for iron deficiency anemia is poor bioavailability from plant-based diets in addition to low intake of iron. Research has shown that the bioavailability of iron from the habitual Indian diets containing different staple cereals ranged between 3% and 8% in different age groups (Nair et al., 2013). Intake of other nutrients such as ascorbic acid, zinc, vitamin A, and folic acid is also inadequate in the dietaries of this population.

Iodine deficiency disorders were among the micronutrient deficiencies prevalent among the local population and are still prevalent in India, with <5% in six states and >0.5% in Maharashtra and West Bengal among the states covered by NNMB surveys. ICMR survey has indicated that no state or union tertiary in India is free from iodine deficiency (Pandav et al., 2013). Human brain development is completed before 3 years old and iodine deficiency during pregnancy or early childhood would lead to irreversible brain damage. The salt iodization program came to existence in 1992, and since then the deficiency has reduced drastically.

2.7 Undernutrition and cognition

Cognitive functions depend on the combined activity of several neurons, several biochemical pathways, and enzymes that require proper nourishment. Improving the nutritional status of stunted infants before 2 years of life could improve the cognitive function of children (Crookston et al., 2013) although correcting the nutritional status at later stages of life was not found to be beneficial (Carba et al., 2009). Multiple micronutrient supplementation during pregnancy showed a better impact on child nutrition than individual nutrient supplementation. Trials with fish oil supplementation showed that α-linoleic acid, docosahexaenoic acid, and eicosapentaenoic acid were important components of myelination and synaptogenesis (Vazir and Boindala, 2016).

2.8 Overnutrition and allied health ailments

Owing to the improvement in the economic status over the last four decades, there has been a reduction in CED by 20%–27% with an associated fivefold increase in overweight and obesity (Vijayaraghavan, 2016). The shift observed in the type of malnutrition has led to a different spectrum of health issues. The economic liberalization of India has brought in false-positive lifestyle changes such as increased ownership of vehicles, sedentary occupation cultures for long hours, less exposure to sunlight, and absence of proper compensated recreational physical activity (Anjana et al., 2014). An increase in the availability of processed foods in both organized and unorganized sectors was reflected in the compound annual growth rate of 8.4% from 2005–06 to 2009–10 (Rais et al., 2013). Increased marketing of food has increased the availability of packaged and processed foods containing more salt, sugar, and preservatives. The transitional dietary changes have led to increase in the occurrence of chronic degenerative diseases. The prevalence of diabetes and obesity is on a rise and is becoming an epidemic in human history, and India is considered to be the third-largest country in this context (Zimmet, 2017).

2.9 Influence of diet and nutrition on the increasing occurrence of disease

Increased food availability and accessibility in India lead to an unhealthy nutrition transition that is reported to accelerate the noncommunicable diseases. Data from major dietary surveys have revealed the components of transition diets and the impact is depicted in Table 2.7.

Obesity is characterized by excess adipose tissue accumulation resulting from an imbalance in energy intake and expenditure. High body mass index (BMI) is an important risk factor contributing to diabetes in India and has doubled from 1990 to 2016, during which diabetes has increased almost in every state. Improvement in food security and increased disposable income has led to dietary transitions of the population from traditional millet and coarse cereal-based foodstuffs to highly refined cereal-based foods that are energy-intense, nutrient-poor, and high-carbohydrate diets leading to increased BMI among our population (ICMR, 2018; Popkin, 2001; Mohan et al., 2011). Nearly 20% of the local population are obese as per the latest survey (Table 2.8).

2.9.1 Diabetes mellitus

The burden of diabetes has steadily increased over the last decades at the global and national levels for which India has contributed a major part. Diabetes is identified as one of the four priority noncommunicable diseases targeted for action due to its growing disease burden (ADA, 2015). It has become one of the major threats in the industrialized world not only among adults but also among adolescents and children (Rao et al., 2014). Surveys including that conducted by ICMR have revealed the prevalence of 5.5%–7.7% between 1990 and 2016, whereas the NFHS survey has shown still

Table 2.7 Transition in the dietary pattern and health consequences.

Observation	Imbalance of dietary nutrients	Consequences	Reference
Increased consumption of refined grains—polished rice and refined wheat flour replacing whole grains	Increased refined carbohydrates, reduced dietary fiber and micronutrients	Increased glucose and insulin concentrations Increased digestibility of carbohydrates, increased risk for diabetes	NSSO (2010); NNMB (2012); Kapil and Sachdev (2012)
Reduced consumption of protective foods such as pulses, milk, vegetables, and fruits	Low amounts of proteins, fiber, and micronutrients	Contributes to increased GI	NNMB (2012)
Increased consumption of visible fats and oils Processed, baked, and fried foods have increased	FAO data suggest that energy from fat has increased from 14% to 19% and vegetable oils from 6% to 10% Trans fat consumption above the safety level of 1.1% of energy	Contributes to obesity, altered lipid profile, and cardiovascular diseases	FAO (2004) Misra et al. (2009)
Sugar-sweetened beverages and energy drinks have increased Consumption of processed foods has increased	Per capita sugar consumption from sweets and beverages has increased to 25 kg/capita/annum. This increases the consumption of sugar, salt, and preservatives.	Increases risk of obesity and other chronic diseases	Gulati and Misra (2014)
Changed lifestyle with reduced exposure to sunlight	Increase in vitamin D deficiency	Negative impact on the glycemic index	Adams and Hewison (2010)

higher prevalence. Prediabetes and diabetes in India are as high as 13% in some Indian regions (Anjana et al., 2017). Diabetes contributes to 3.1% of all deaths in India. Asian Indians were found to have the peak prevalence of diabetes 10 years earlier compared to their other Asian counterparts, and the take-off point for the increased prevalence of diabetes among Asian Indian individuals was 25–34 years as per the ICMR study (ICMR, 2018). There is sufficient evidence of an "Asian phenotype" in diabetes, and the progression from prediabetes to diabetes appears to occur faster in this population. The clinical and biochemical features that dispose Asians to a higher risk are higher

Table 2.8 Prevalence of overweight and obesity (%).

Age group	Obesity (BMI >25)	Diabetes (Blood glucose 140 to >160)	Hypertension	Reference
Women	20.6	8.6	8.8	NFHS-4 (2015–16)
Men	18.9	11.9	13.6	
Adults	–	69.2 million	–	IDF (2015)
All	–	–	One-fifth of Indian population	Bhansali et al. (2015)

waist circumference, higher waist-to-hip ratio, more subcutaneous and visceral fat, and higher insulin resistance than individuals of US origin (Bajaj et al., 2014). Almost an equal or higher proportion of the population is also subjected to hypertension in the same population.

Diet has shown a strong correlation on the onset, progression, severity, and secondary complications of diabetes. There is vast literature on the association of dietary constituents and the occurrence of diabetes with traditional and current transitional diets. The association between single dietary ingredients and/or constituents and diabetes has been extensively studied, and a few studies are cited in Table 2.9.

The main features observed in the transition dietaries in urban areas have shown a higher proportion of refined cereals and junk foods and sweetened beverages. The predictive risk of developing metabolic syndrome was found to be 7.9% with elevated fasting blood glucose levels accelerating diabetes (Radhika et al., 2009; Unnikrishnan et al., 2016).

2.9.2 Cardiovascular disease

Cardiovascular diseases have become the leading cause of disease burden and deaths globally for which India is not an exception. These diseases contributed to 28.1% of the total deaths and 14.1% of the disability-adjusted life years (DALYs) in India (India State-Level Disease Burden Initiative CVD Collaborators, 2018). Increased consumption of saturated fatty acids such as palmitic and myristic acids, lauric acid, trans fatty acids, high sodium intake, and unfiltered boiled coffee have all shown to increase the risk of cardiovascular disease (Ding et al., 2014). High intake of fruits and vegetables conferred 48% protection against cardiovascular disease and 30% of risk reduction from myocardial infarction. Consumption of green leafy vegetables was associated with a lower risk of ischemic disease. Replacing saturated fatty acids with carbohydrates is known to reduce the risk of cardiovascular disease (Siri-Tarino et al., 2010).

Meta analyses to assess the comparative effect of different types of dietssuch as Dietary Approaches to Stop Hypertension (DASH) diet, Mediterranean diet, Low sodium and Vegetarian diet were assessed. All diets were effective in reducing blood

Table 2.9 Association of major dietary constituents and the onset of diabetes.

Dietary constituent	Biochemical change
The quality and quantity of carbohydrates	Higher glycemic index and glycemic load diets along with low dietary fiber content are known to increase insulin demand and further lead to pancreatic β-cell exhaustion (Radhika et al., 2009) One to two servings of sugar-sweetened beverages per day is known to cause insulin resistance, impair β cell function, increase inflammation, and increase the risk of diabetes by 26% (Malik et al., 2010) Substituting brown rice over white rice significantly lowered blood glucose and insulin levels (Mohan et al., 2011)
Quality and type of fats	Fatty acids influence glucose metabolism by altering cell membrane function, enzyme activity, insulin signaling, and gene expression Replacing saturated fats and trans fatty acids with unsaturated fats has beneficial effects on insulin sensitivity and is likely to reduce the risk of type 2 diabetes Linoleic acid from the n-6 series improves insulin sensitivity, while saturated fats are known to impair insulin activity. The effect of the ratio of ω-6 and ω-3 fatty acids on the insulin sensitivity and metabolic abnormalities are controversial (Bradley, 2018)
Protein quality and quantity	Proteins are believed to induce insulin secretion both by the direct stimulation of pancreatic β-cells by amino acids and via incretin hormones expressed in response to meal composition • Coingestion of a protein and amino acid mixture with carbohydrates in type 2 diabetes subjects can increase the plasma insulin response 2–3-fold (Loon et al., 2003) • The ratio of animal and plant protein in a meal can affect insulin secretions • Among amino acids, branched-chain amino acids (BCAA) and phenylalanine are known to affect insulin secretion, and the effect was higher with BCAA alone • The glucose-lowering and insulinotropic effect of amino acids were more effective when ingested with glucose. BCAAs, arginine, and glutamic acid, when ingested with glucose, were found to function as secretagogues • Among dietary proteins, legumes, soya, and whey proteins were more effective in regulating glucose levels • Whey protein was found to be superior in the regulation of glucose homeostasis by—increasing satiety, preventing postprandial glucose spikes, and increased postprandial insulin response. Whey proteins lead to the subsequent synthesis and secretion of the incretin hormones, glucose-dependent insulinotropic polypeptide (GIP), and glucagon-like peptide-1 (GLP-1) in healthy subjects. (Pal et al., 2014; Gunnerud et al., 2013; Ricci-Cabello et al., 2014)

pressure and lipid levels at varying levels. DASH diet have shown more promising evidences in reducing hypertension, LDL and total cholesterol but no effect was seen in triglycerides (Eckel, Jakicic, Ard, de Jesus, Miller, & Hubbard, et al., 2014).

DASH diet comprises of whole grains, higher fresh fruits and vegetables, low fat dairy products and lesser quantity of sodium, fat and meat products.

Mediterranean diet comprises of higher proportion of whole grains, legumes, fresh fruits and vegetables, moderate quantity of fish, olive oil, low fat dairy products, small quantities of red wine, while red meats are avoided (Shai et al., 2008). In this type of dietary intervention, recurrent cardiovascular diseases (CVD) was reduced by 70%. Indian migration study carried out in four cities of India to assess the impact of vegetarian diets showed lower levels of total cholesterol, blood glucose, and blood pressure (Shridhar et al., 2014).

2.9.3 Diet and hypertension

Excess dietary salt intake account for 17%–30% risk for hypertension, which in turn is associated with stroke, direct vascular damage, obesity, stomach cancer, osteoporosis, kidney stones, and thirst (WHO, 2013). According to a nationwide India diabetes study, one-fifth of the Indian population is hypertensive and consumes dietary salt higher than the recommended 6 g/person/day (Bhansali et al., 2015). Radhika et al. (2009) observed that salt intake significantly correlates with the prevalence of hypertension in the Chennai urban population. NNMB report (2012) indicate that 20% of hypertensives in rural area consume more than 5 g of salt/person/day. Adults with type 2 diabetes or at least 3 CVD risk factors on Mediterranean diets showed a reduction of blood pressure by 6–7/2–3 mm Hg (Eckel et al., 2014). DASH diet is used as an effective dietary measure to manage hypertension (Sacks and Campos, 2010).

2.9.4 Diet and cancer

Around 0.55 million deaths occur annually in India, the most commonly prevalent fatal forms of cancer in India are oral, pharynx and lung in men, and cervix, breast, and stomach cancer in women (Dikshit et al., 2012). Overweight and obesity as an outcome of imbalanced nutrition are reported to be one of the contributing factors for cancer. Association of dietary factors and the occurrence of cancer from cross-sectional epidemiological studies are indicated in Table 2.10.

Consequences of noncommunicable diseases such as diabetes, cardiovascular disease, cancer, and mental health between 2012 and 2030 in India is estimated to be US $4.58 trillion (Bloom et al., 2011). The losses are a sum of reduced savings, medical expenses at both household and national level, loss of productivity due to sick workers, increase in DALYs in younger age groups and, on the whole, the cost of the

Table 2.10 Association of dietary imbalances and the occurrence of different types of cancer.

Type of cancer	Dietary associations
Reduced risk for oral, esophageal, breast, endometrial, and cervical cancers in Indian migrants in Singapore	High intake of vegetables, fruits, fish, eggs, and diets high in carotenoids and nutrients such as vitamins C and E (Sinha et al., 2003)
Increased prevalence of upper aerodigestive cancer	Reduced intake of vegetables/fruits, pulses, fish, and low intakes of vitamin A, C, and B complex and selenium (Krishnaswamy et al., 2016)
Increased risk of breast cancer and ovarian cancer	• Increased energy, saturated fat, and reduced physical activity and vice versa • Protective association of green tea and reduction of risk of ovarian cancer • Dried fish, high temperature foods, chilies, and spicy foods • (Crane et al., 2015)

diseases is known to cause 5%–10% loss of GDP. A reduction of 0.5% loss of economy is known to increase mortality by 10% (Patel et al., 2011).

2.10 Future outlook

Diet is the sole source of all nutrients that further determines the nutritional status and health status of the individual from "in utero" to elderly both in health and sickness and this fact is proven through epidemiological, clinical, long-term, cross-sectional, and community-based studies. Well-controlled nutrition intervention studies have further confirmed that certain impairments due to specific nutrient deficiencies can be reversed through the replenishment of the nutrients through dietary interventions that have better compliance and sustainability. Clinical trials have also shown better management of disease conditions with dietary modifications. The social network is playing a prominent role in creating health and nutrition awareness, although there is no regulation to validate the claims. There is no scarcity of knowledge or the professionals; however, appropriate outreach of research outcomes to the beneficiaries is a limiting factor. To overcome the persistent ill effects of malnutrition in our country, the integration between the nutritionists, medical professionals, food scientists, policymakers, and food manufacturers has to be strengthened. The beneficiaries who are the stakeholders need to be sensitized about ill-effects of malnutrition percolating through generations and modification of genetic substance through the widely reachable and acceptable social media.

References

Abu-Saad, K., Fraser, D., 2010. Maternal nutrition and birth outcomes. Epidemiol. Rev. 32, 5–25.

ADA (American Diabetes Association), 2015. Classification and diagnosis of diabetes. Diabetes Care 38, S8–S16.

Adams, J.S., Hewison, M., 2010. Update in vitamin D. J. Clin. Endocrinol. Metab. 95, 471–478.

Allen, L.H., 2000. Anemia and iron deficiency: effects on pregnancy outcome. Am. J. Clin. Nutr. 71 (5 Suppl.), 1280S–1284S.

Anjana, R.M., Pradeepa, R., Das, A.K., Deepa, M., Bhansali, A., Joshi, S.R., et al., 2014. Physical activity and inactivity patterns in India – results from the ICMR INDIAB study (Phase-1) [ICMR-INDIAB-5]. Int. J. Behav. Nutr. Phys. Act. 11, 26–32.

Anjana, R.M., Deepa, M., Pradeepa, R., Mahanta, J., Narain, K., Das, H.K., et al., 2017. Prevalence of diabetes and prediabetes in 15 states of India: results from the ICMR-INDIAB population-based cross-sectional study. Lancet Diabetes Endocrinol. 5, 585–596.

Bajaj, H.S., Pereira, M.A., Anjana, R.M., Deepa, R., Mohan, V., Mueller, et al., 2014. Comparison of relative waist circumference between Asian Indian and US adults. J. Obes. 2014, 1–10. Available from: https://doi.org/10.1155/2014/461956. Article ID461956.

Bamji, M.S., Nair, M., 2016. Food-based approach to combat micronutrient deficiencies. Proc. Indian Natl. Sci. Acad. 82, 1529–1540.

Bavdekar, A., Yajnik, C.S., Fall, C.H., Bapat, S., Pandit, A.N., Deshpande, V., et al., 1999. Insulin resistance syndrome in 8-year-old Indian children: small at birth, big at 8 years, or both? Diabetes 48, 2422–2429.

Bhansali, A., Dhandania, V.K., Deepa, M., Anjana, R.M., Joshi, S.R., Joshi, P.P., et al., 2015. Prevalence of and risk factors for hypertension in urban and rural India: the ICMR–INDIAB study. J. Hum. Hypertens. 29, 204–209.

Bloom, D.E., Cafiero, E., Llopis, E.J., Gessel, S.A., Bloom, L.R., Fathima, S., et al., 2011. The Global Economic Burden of Non-Communicable Diseases. World Economic Forum and Harvard School of Public Health, Geneva.

Bradley, B.H.R., 2018. Dietary fat and risk for type 2 diabetes: a review of recent research. Current Nutr. Rep. 7, 214–226.

Carba, D.B., Tan, V.L., Adair, L.S., 2009. Early childhood length-for-age is associated with the work status of Filipino young adults. Econ. Hum. Biol. 7, 7–17.

Crane, T.E., Khulpateea, B.R., Alberts, D.D., Basen-Engquist, K., Thompson, C.A., 2015. Dietary intake and ovarian cancer risk: a systematic review. Cancer Epidemiol. Biomark. Prev. 23, 255–273.

Crookston, B.T., Schott, W., Cueto, S., Dearden, K.A., Engle, P., Georgiadis, A., et al., 2013. Post-infancy growth, schooling, and cognitive achievement: young lives. Am. J. Clin. Nutr. 98, 1555–1563.

Dikshit, R., Gupta, P.C., Ramasundarahettige, C., Gajalakshmi, V., Aleksandrowicz, L., Badwe, R., 2012. Cancer mortality in India: a nationally representative survey. Lancet 379, 1807–1816.

Ding, M., Bhupathiraju, S.N., Satija, A., van Dam, Hu, F.B., 2014. Long-term coffee consumption and risk of cardiovascular disease: a systematic review and a dose-response meta-analysis of prospective cohort studies. Circulation 129, 643–659.

Eckel, R.H., Jakicic, J.M., Ard, J.D., de Jesus, J.M., Miller, H.N., Hubbard, V.S., et al., 2014. 2013 AHA/ACC guideline on lifestyle management to reduce cardiovascular risk: a report of the American College of Cardiology/American Heart Association Task Force on Practice Guidelines. J. Am. Coll. Cardiol. 63 (25-PA), 2960–2984.

FAO (Food and Agriculture Organization), 2004. The State of Agricultural Commodity Markets. Source: www.fao.org/3/a-y5419e.

Georgieff, M.K., 2007. Nutrition and the developing brain: nutrient priorities and measurement. Am. J. Clin. Nutr. 85, 614S–620S.

Goldenberg, R.L., Culhane, J.F., 2007. Low birth weight in the United States. Am. J. Clin. Nutr. 85 (2), 584S–590S.

Gulati, S., Misra, A., 2014. Sugar intake, obesity, and diabetes in India. Nutrients 6, 5955–5974.

Gunnerud, U.J., Ostman, E.M., Bjorck, I.M.E., 2013. Effects of whey proteins on glycaemia and insulinaemia to an oral glucose load in healthy adults; a dose–response study. Eur. J. Clin. Nutr. 67, 749–753.

ICMR (Indian Council of Medical Research), 2018. Public Health Foundation of India, Institute for Health Metrics and Evaluation. GBD India Compare Data Visualization. <http://vizhub.healthdata.org/gbd-compare/india> (accessed 18.03.18.).

IDF (International Diabetes Federation), 2015. Diabetes Atlas, seventh ed. Belgium.

India State-Level Disease Burden Initiative CVD Collaborators, 2018. The changing patterns of cardiovascular diseases and their risk factors in the states of India: the Global Burden of Disease Study 1990–2016. Lancet Glob. Health 6, e1339–e1351.

Kapil, U., Sachdev, H.P.S., 2012. Urgent need to orient public health response to rapid nutrition transition. Indian J. Commun. Med. 37, 207–212.

Krishnaswamy, K., Vaidya, R., Rajgopal, G., Vasudevan, S., 2016. Diet and nutrition in the prevention of non-communicable diseases. Proc. Indian Natl. Sci. Acad. 82, 1477–1494.

Krishnaveni, G.V., Veena, S.R., Hill, J.C., Kehoe, S., Karat, S.C., Fall, C.H., 2010. Intra-uterine exposure to maternal diabetes is associated with higher adiposity and insulin resistance and clustering of cardiovascular risk in Indian children. Diabetes Care 33, 402–404.

Krishnaveni, G.V., Veena, S.R., Karat, S.C., Yajnik, C.S., Fall, C.H., 2014. Association between maternal folate concentrations during pregnancy and insulin resistance in Indian children. Diabetologia 57, 110–121.

Kulsum, A., Lakshmi, J.A., Prakash, J., 2008. Food intake and energy protein adequacy of children from an urban slum in Mysore, India – a qualitative analysis. Malays. J. Nutr. 14, 163–172.

Kulsum, A., Lakshmi, J.A., Prakash, J., 2009. Dietary adequacy of Indian children residing in an urban slum – analysis of proximal and distal determinants. Ecol. Food Nutr. 48 (3), 161–177.

Lakshmi, J.A., Begum, K., Saraswathi, G., Prakash, J., 2005. Dietary adequacy of Indian rural pre-school children: influencing factors. J. Trop. Pediatr. 51, 39–44.

Loon, L.J., Kruijshoop, M., Menheere, P.P., Wagenmakers, A.J., Saris, W.H., Keizer, et al., 2003. Amino acid ingestion strongly enhances insulin secretion in patients with long-term type 2 diabetes. Diabetes Care 26, 625–630.

Malik, V.S., Popkin, B.M., Bray, G.A., Després, J.P., Willett, W.C., Hu, F.B., 2010. Sugar-sweetened beverages and risk of metabolic syndrome and type 2 diabetes: a meta-analysis. Diabetes Care 33, 2477–2483.

Misra, A., Chowbey, P., Makkar, B.M., Vikram, N.K., Wasir, J.S., Chadha, D., et al., 2009. Consensus statement for diagnosis of obesity, abdominal obesity and the metabolic syndrome for Asian Indians and recommendations for physical activity, medical and surgical management. J. Assoc. Physicians India 57, 163–170.

Mohan, V., Joshi, S.R., Seshiah, V., Sahay, B.K., Banerjee, S., Wangoo, S.K., et al., 2011. Current status of management, control, complications and psychosocial aspects of patients with diabetes in India: results from the DiabCare India 2011 Study. Indian J. Endocrinol. Med. 18, 370–378.

Nair, K.M., Brahmam, G.N.V., Radhika, M.S., Dripta, R.C., Ravinder, P., Balakrishna, N., et al., 2013. Inclusion of guava enhances non-heme iron bioavailability but not fractional zinc absorption from a rice-based meal in adolescents. J. Nutr. 143, 852–858.

NFHS-4 (National Family Health Survey), 2015–16. [Internet]. Mumbai: International Institute for Population Sciences (IIPS) and Macro International; 2009. Available from: <http://www.rchiips.org/nfhs/nfhs4.shtml>.

NNMB (National Nutrition Monitoring Bureau), 2012. Diet and Nutritional Status of Rural Population, Prevalence of Hypertension and Diabetes Among Adults and Infant and Young Child Feeding Practices – Third Repeat Survey, NNMB Technical No. 26, National Institute of Nutrition.

NSSO (National Sample Survey Organization), 2010: Migration in India, Report No. 533, Ministry of Statistics and Program Implementation, Government of India, New Delhi.

Özaltin, E., Hill, K., Subramanian, V., 2010. Association of maternal stature with offspring mortality, underweight, and stunting in low- to middle-income countries. J. Am. Med. Assoc. 303, 1507–1516.

Pal, S., Radavelli-Bagatini, S., Hagger, M., Ellis, V., 2014. Comparative effects of whey and casein proteins on satiety in overweight and obese individuals: a randomized controlled trial. Eur. J Clin. Nutr. 68, 980–986.

Pandav, C.S., Yadav, K., Srivastava, R., Pandav, R., Karmarkar, M.G., 2013. Iodine deficiency disorders (IDD) control in India. Indian J. Med. Res. 138, 418–433.

Patel, V.S., Chatterji, D., Chisholm, S., Ebrahim, G., Gopalakrishna, C., Mathers, V., et al., 2011. Chronic diseases and injuries in India. Lancet 377, 413–428.

PHFI, 2015. India Health Report-Nutrition, 2015. Public Health Foundation of India, New Delhi.

Popkin, B.M., 2001. The nutrition transition and obesity in the developing world. J. Nutr. 13, 871S–873SS.

Radhika, G., Van Dam, R.M., Sudha, V., Ganesan, A., Mohan, V., 2009. Refined grain consumption and the metabolic syndrome in urban Asian Indians (Chennai Urban Rural Epidemiology Study 57). Metabolism 58, 675–681.

Rais, M., Acharya, S., Sharma, N., 2013. Food processing industry in India: S&T capability, skills and employment opportunities. J. Food Process. Technol. 4, 260. Available from: https://doi.org/10.4172/2157-7110.100026.

Raman, R., 2016. Nutritional modulation of gene function in disease susceptibility: homocysteine-folate metabolism pathway. Proc. Indian Natl. Sci. Acad. 82, 1413–1424.

Rao, K.R., Lal, N., Giridharan, N.V., 2014. Genetic & epigenetic approach to human obesity. Indian J. Med. Res. 140, 589–603.

Ricci - Cabello, I., Ruiz-Pérez, I., Rojas-García, A., Pastor, G., Rodríguez-Barranco, M., Goncalves, C., 2014. Characteristics and effectiveness of diabetes self-management educational programs targeted to racial/ethnic minority groups: a systematic review, meta-analysis and meta-regression. BMC Endocr. Disord. 14, 60–65.

RSOC, 2013–14. Government of India (2015). Rapid Survey on Children 2013–2014 – India Fact sheet, Ministry of Ministry of Human Development. <http://wcd.nic.in/issnip/National_Factsheet_RSOC_02-07-2015.pdf>.

Sacks, F.M., Campos, H., 2010. Diet therapy in hypertension. N. Engl. J. Med. 362, 2102–2112.

Sinha, R., Anderson, D.E., McDonald, S.S., Greenwald, P., 2003. Cancer risk and diet in India. J. Post Grad. Med. 49, 229–235.

Siri-Tarino, P.W., Sun, Q., Hu, F.B., Krauss, R.M., 2010. Saturated fat, carbohydrate, and cardiovascular disease. Am. J. Clin. Nutr. 91, 502–509.

Shai, I.R.D., Schwarzfuchs, D., Henkin, Y., Shahar, D.R., Witkow, S., Greenberg, I., et al., 2008. Loss with a low-carbohydrate, Mediterranean, or low-fat diet. N. Engl. J. Med. 359, 229–241.

Shridhar, K., Dhillon, P.K., Bowen, L., Kinra, S., Bharathi, A.V., Prabhakaran, D., et al., 2014. The association between a vegetarian diet and cardiovascular disease (CVD) risk factors in India: The Indian Migration Study. PLoS ONE 9, 1–8.

UNICEF, 2013. Improving Child Nutrition, The Achievable Imperative for Global Progress UNICEF. New York.

Unnikrishnan, R., Anjana, R.M., Mohan, V., 2016. Diabetes mellitus and its complications in India. Natl. Rev. Endocrinol. 12, 357–370.

Vazir, S., Boindala, S., 2016. Nutrition, brain development and cognition in infants, young children and elderly. Proc. Indian Natl. Sci. Acad. 82, 1495–1506.

Vijayaraghavan, K., 2016. The persistent problem of malnutrition. Proc. Indian Natl. Sci. Acad. 82, 1341–1350.

Wasserman, C.R., Shaw, G.M., Selvin, S., Gould, J.B., Syme, S.L., 1998. Socioeconomic status, neighbourhood social conditions, and neural tube defects. Am. J. Public Health 88, 1674–1680.

West, J., Wright, J., Fairley, L., Sattar, N., Whincup, P., Lawlor, D.A., 2014. Do ethnic differences in cord blood leptin levels differ by birthweight category? Findings from the born in Bradford cohort study. Int. J. Epidemiol. 43, 249–254.

Whincup, P.H., Kaye, S.J., Owen, C.G., Huxley, R., Cook, D.G., Anazawa, S., et al., 2008. Birthweight and risk of type 2 diabetes: a quantitative systematic review of published evidence. J. Am. Med. Assoc. 300, 2885–2897.

WHO, 2013. Global Action Plan for the Prevention and Control of Noncommunicable Diseases: 2013–2020. 2013. <http://apps.who.int/iris/bitstream/10665/94384/1/9789241506236_eng.pdf> (accessed 08.03.18.).

Wood-Bradley, R., Barrand, S., Giot, A., Armitage, J., 2015. Understanding the role of maternal diet on kidney development; an opportunity to improve cardiovascular and renal health for future generations. Nutrients 7, 1881–1905.

Yajnik, C.S., Lubree, H.G., Rege, S.S., Naik, S.S., Deshpande, J.A., Deshpande, S.S., et al., 2002. Adiposity and hyperinsulinemia in Indians are present at birth. J. Clin. Endocrinol. Metabol. 87, 5575–5580.

Yajnik, C.S., Deshpande, S.S., Jackson, A.A., Refsum, H., Rao, S., Fisher, D.J., et al., 2008. Vitamin B_{12} and folate concentrations during pregnancy and insulin resistance in the offspring: The Pune Maternal Nutrition Study. Diabetologia 51, 29–38.

Yajnik, C.S., Chandak, G.R., Joglekar, C., Katre, P., Bhat, D.S., Singh, S.N., et al., 2014. Maternal homocysteine in pregnancy and offspring birthweight: epidemiological associations and Mendelian randomization analysis. Int. J. Epidemiol. 5, 1487–1497.

Zimmet, P.Z., 2017. Diabetes and its drivers: the largest epidemic in human history? Clin. Diabetes Endocrinol. 3, 1–8.

CHAPTER 3

Nutritional sufficiency of traditional meal patterns

Pushpa Bharati and Uma N. Kulkarni
Dept. of Food Science & Nutrition, College of Community Science, University of Agricultural Sciences, Dharwad, India

Contents

3.1 Introduction

3.1.1 Definition and importance

Traditional foods include an array of food preparations or raw food commodities, the use of which is deep-rooted in once personal traditional practices and habits. These foods are best described as foods that have been consumed for ages and are a blend of culture, traditions, and customs. Such foods are generally based on local staples with more manual and less minimal industrial processing. The local climatic, agricultural, and economic conditions determine the production and processing of staples into traditional food products that represent culture and lifestyle (Anonymous, 2008). The resulting traditional product depicts heritage and represents a specific region where it is

Nutritional and Health Aspects of Food in South Asian Countries
DOI: https://doi.org/10.1016/B978-0-12-820011-7.00004-6

transmitted by their ancestors. The European Food Information Resource Network project defines traditional foods as those with specific features that distinguish them clearly from other similar products of the same category in terms of use of traditional raw material/primary products/traditional composition/traditional production and/or processing methods. Traditional food products are distinguished for their composition, production, and processing methods resulting in culinary depiction. They have evolved through trial and error over many centuries of cultural, social, economic, and sensory experiences (Achaya, 1994).

India has a rich treasure of traditional foods woven intricately into the fabric of culture over generations. Indian traditional foods vary with a broad base of food groups covering cereals, pulses, fruits, vegetables, dairy, and meat as well as their products, the majority of which are influenced by culture, region, and season exhibiting diversities (Achaya, 1994). The functional properties of Indian traditional foods emerged from the oldest medicinal system Ayurveda (Sarkar et al., 2015) and were specific to each food. Functional foods are foods that have a potentially positive effect on health beyond basic nutrition to provide optimal health and reduce the risk of diseases. Traditional foods are not just foods that nurture physical health and offer preventive nutrition but also take care of mental health (Prakash, 2015).

3.1.2 Regional variations in Indian traditional meal pattern

Traditional food choices usually depend on regional preferences that are governed by staples. About 30% of Indians are vegetarian. Even though the proportion of nonvegetarians is increasing, the quantity consumed is meager and is insufficient to contribute to nutritional benefits.

The geographic division of India into North, South, East, and West indicates the variations in the staple foods and their preparation methods. Food patterns in north India were strongly influenced by Central Asian and Mughlai cuisines. In Kashmir, the main course is rice with a delicious semisolid side dish prepared with a green leafy vegetable. States such as Punjab, Haryana, and Uttar Pradesh consume unleavened flatbread (chapati) prepared with a variety of flours such as wheat, rice, refined wheat flour, and Bengal gram flour. Besides chapati, varieties of wheat-based unleavened bread that vary in the method of preparation are also popular.

Western India has its unique taste with varieties of desserts. Rajasthan and Gujarat cuisines, though lack in fresh vegetables, are favored with an immense variety of cooked split lentils and pickles/preserves. Maharashtra combines both north as well as south cuisine, that is, rice and wheat or millet. Mumbai cuisine is marked with a variety of fishes available along the coastal line. The delicacies include Bombay Prawn and Pomfret. Goa is influenced by Portuguese cooking style with sweet and sour Vindaloo, duck baffad, sorpotel, egg molie, etc.

The Eastern India with Bengali and Assamese styles of cooking has rice and fish as staple food. A special delicacy known as "Hilsa" is prepared by wrapping staple in the pumpkin leaf and cooking. Bamboo shoot is commonly consumed. Milk-based sweets include those prepared with agglutinated milk and sweetener.

Southern states of India use spices, fishes, and coconuts as most of them have access to coastal lines. Tamil Nadu uses tamarind to impart tangy taste to the dishes. Andhra Pradesh and Telangana use rice as a staple with generous use of chilies for pungency. Kerala delicacies include lamb stew and "*Appams*" (pancake prepared with fermented rice batter and coconut milk), Malabar fried prawns as well as sweetened coconut milk. Another common dish is "*Puttu*," which is a glutinous rice powder steamed like a pudding in a bamboo shoot (Michel & Kumar, 2013).

However certain common aspects of Indian dietaries are the following:

- Chicken and goat meat are popular all over India, depending on affordability. Beef is consumed only by Christians and Muslims and pork by Christians only. Meat is usually not eaten on all days of the week, but occasionally. Fish is popular in coastal areas consumed nearly 7 days a week.
- Fruits are usually consumed fresh. Traditionally, the processing of ripened fruits is rare.
- Desserts made from milk, sugar, rice, or split legumes, using clarified butter (*ghee*), nuts, and spices such as cardamom, nutmeg, and mace are common on special occasions.
- Clarified butter may be served with rice as a flavor enhancer and to augment palatability. Sesame, peanut, mustard, coconut, and other vegetable oils are generally used for cooking. Pickles and crispy wafers (*papad*) are often used as accompaniments.
- Water is served with meals. "Milky" coffee and tea with sugar are consumed as popular beverages.
- Spices used include coriander seeds, asafetida, cumin seeds, mustard seeds, fenugreek seeds, cinnamon, clove, ginger, pepper, chili, garlic, turmeric, saffron, and cardamom. Religion and religious festivals in all groups in India play a major role in food avoidances or inclusions.

3.2 Historical overview

3.2.1 Old consumption pattern

The traditional food of India has been widely appreciated for its fabulous use of herbs and spices. Indian cuisine is known for its large assortment of dishes. The cooking style varies from region to region and is largely divided into South Indian and North Indian cuisine.

The traditional meal pattern included breakfast, main meal, beverages, and light dinner. Indian bread—unleavened flats prepared with either wheat or sorghum, fermented rice-based traditional dishes, flattened rice, and puffed rice suitably seasoned or cooked constitute breakfast items. Rice or dry pan-roasted unleavened flatbread with boiled and seasoned split lentils, chicken, or fish was the main course of meals in most of the days. Vegetables included okra, a variety of gourds, eggplant, snake beans, various leaves, potato, and tapioca/cassava. Fruits included mangoes, tamarind, plantain, papaya, and those available seasonally (https://metrosouth.health.qld.gov.au/sites/default/files/content/heau-cultural-profile-indian.pdf). Indians loved fried snacks prepared with gram flour or split legumes employing various spices consumed with a hot beverage. More of peanuts, fewer cashews, and rarely other nuts in different forms are a delicacy. The beverages—water, coffee, tea, and juice—were part and parcel of Indian cuisine. However, deep-fried snacks were always restricted for special occasions such as festivals, thereby restricting the calorie intake.

Cultural differences existed between people belonging to different regions, religions and social groups, as well as between individuals within any culture. Takeaways were uncommon and also families eating out were rarely observed. Baked goods were rare so also a number of bakeries. The celebration of foods and religious food practices varied. For example, cakes and sweets were not eaten regularly. Practices varied according to region and occasion. Rice cooked with meat or vegetables and spices called Biryani is a popular festive food but was avoided during Hindu festivals. Meat and fish are also avoided on certain days of the week as part of religious observances. Religious traditions laid importance on fasting. In the Hindu tradition, people choose to fast for various purposes. Fasting or abstaining from food, itself has a significant place in Indian culture irrespective of religion.

3.2.2 The changing Indian diet with the progression of age

Major shifts in dietary patterns are occurring throughout the world from basic staples toward more diversified diets resulting in health consequences. Populations in those countries undergoing rapid transition are experiencing nutritional transition. The diverse nature of this transition may be the result of differences in sociodemographic factors and other consumer characteristics. Among other factors including urbanization and food industry marketing, the policies of trade liberalization over the past two decades have implications for health by virtue of being a factor in facilitating the "nutrition transition" that is associated with rising rates of obesity and chronic diseases such as diabetes, cardiovascular disease, and cancer (Kearney, 2010).

Over the past 50 years, India has changed remarkably with double the population (Roser, 2019) and so has its economy. This has impacted the food patterns of people. As a matter of course, diets vary and evolve over time. Factors such as income, food prices, individual preferences and beliefs, and cultural traditions as well as geographical, environmental, social, and economic factors have all influenced changes in diet, both on an individual and on a national level. A very brief glance into some of the major changes in India's recent history can offer some insight into the factors affecting dietary changes in the past 50 years.

Not too long before the official start point for these figures, in 1961, India had faced one of the world's worst recorded food disasters, the Bengal Famine in 1943 (Alaeddini and Olia, 2004). Shortly after, by the end of World War II, poverty and hunger were in abundance and this resulted in various malnutrition-related epidemic disorders. Poverty drove people to walk long distances and eat a simple diet. The food imports therefore concentrated largely on cereal grains. This no doubt had a lasting impact on the eating habits of those affected. The upsurge of the Green revolution in the 1960s with a better package of practices in field crops resulted in enormous production of food grains thereby increased per capita availability of food grains adding to energy increment. A decade later in the 1970s, the "White Revolution" by the National Dairy Development Board made milk and other dairy products more easily and widely accessible. The usage of butter, cheese, and ghee enhanced the diet especially of the urban Indians, thus pushing up the averages for the national daily intake of dairy and animal products.

Many processed and convenience foods such as pickles and crispy wafers (*papad*) are now easily available as well as Western foods such as pizzas, burgers, and fries (Plummer, 2017). All such factors are playing their part in bumping up the national average of fat and sugar intake (Anonymous, 2017).

3.3 Geography and natural agricultural landscape of India

4.3.1. Cropping system and food grain production
4.3.2. Shift in food consumption patterns

3.3.1 Cropping system and food grain production

Indian soil types, rainfall, temperature, and climatic conditions determine the cropping pattern. Crop cultivation is decided by its suitability to agroclimatic conditions. In India, there are three distinct crop seasons namely *Kharif*, *Rabi*, and *Zaid*. This multiplies the availability of arable land and is the uniqueness of Indian agriculture. The *Kharif* season starts with Southwest Monsoon under which tropical crops are cultivated. The *Rabi* season starts with the onset of winter in October–November and ends in March–April. *Zaid* is a short duration summer cropping season beginning after harvesting of *Rabi* crops.

Types of cropping systems in India: There are two types of crop cultivation practices followed in India (Anwar, 2019).

- *Monocropping or Monoculture*: It involves the cultivation of the single crop on farm every year.
- *Multiple cropping*: It is the cultivation of two or more crops on farmland in one calendar year with scientific methods of management. It includes intercropping, mixed cropping, and sequence cropping.

The diversified agroclimatic zone is unfortunately not giving sufficient production in spite of intensive planning in Indian agricultural practices. Implementation of modern cropping patterns and cropping system can increase production and productivity. Farmers' inclination toward commercial crops can have better economic returns. The production of individual crops will noticeably increase, thereby attaining food and nutritional security.

In India, the agroecosystem is classified into different zones. Major crops cultivated in different zones include millets and oilseeds in Arid zone; rice, peanuts, and coconut with fish as major component in coastal zone; rice, wheat, cotton, and sugarcane in irrigated zone; rice, wheat, coarse cereals, oilseeds, and cotton in rainfed zone; rice, maize, wheat, fruits, and other horticulture crops in Hilly and mountainous region.

In India, the different zones of agroecosystem are classified as follows (Sinha, 2014).

- The Arid zone—Gujarat and Rajasthan grow millets and oilseeds;
- Coastal zone—Andhra Pradesh, Tamil Nadu, Orissa, Karnataka, Kerala, Goa, and Maharashtra grow rice, groundnuts, and coconut with fish as a major component;
- Irrigated zone—Bihar, Haryana, Punjab, Uttar Pradesh, West Bengal, Karnataka, Andhra Pradesh, Telangana, and Maharashtra grow rice, wheat, cotton, and sugarcane;
- Rainfed zone—Assam, Bihar, Madhya Pradesh, Maharashtra, Orissa, West Bengal, Karnataka, Andhra Pradesh, Gujarat, Rajasthan, Tamil Nadu, Uttar Pradesh, and Gujarat grow rice, wheat, coarse cereals, oilseeds, and cotton.
- The Hill and mountainous region—North-Eastern states, Assam and West Bengal, Uttarakhand, Uttar Pradesh, Himachal Pradesh, and Jammu and Kashmir grow rice, maize, wheat, fruits, and other horticulture crops.

The food grain production including cereal and pulses increased from 52.56 to 301.93 million tons from 1950–51 to 2016–17 (Table 3.1). Looking into the country's projected population by 2050; the additional requirement will be to the tune of 430 million mouths to feed. Crop production has to be increased to meet the growing needs at an annual average of 2%, which is close to the current growth trend.

Agricultural crop production has been increasing every year, and India is among the top producers of wheat, rice, pulses, sugarcane, and cotton. It ranks first in milk production because of operation flood, and it is also the second leading producer of fruits and vegetables. About 25% of the world's pulses production was contributed by India in 2013. Apart from these, it also added to the world's 22% of rice production

Table 3.1 Production* of major agricultural crops in India (million tons) (Anonymous, 2017a).

Crops	1950–51	1960–61	1970–71	1980–81	1990–91	2000–01	2010–11	2011–12	2012–13	2013–14	2014–15	2015–16	2016–17
Cereals	44.15	73.4	104.09	125.92	171.09	197.78	247.98	263.95	261.04	270.05	259.04	257.79	278.98
Pulses	8.41	12.7	11.82	10.63	14.26	11.08	18.24	17.09	18.34	19.25	17.15	16.35	22.95
Oilseeds	5.16	6.98	9.63	9.37	18.61	18.44	32.48	29.8	30.94	32.75	27.51	25.25	32.1
Cotton#	3.04	5.6	4.76	7.01	9.84	9.52	33	35.2	34.22	35.9	34.8	30.01	33.09
Jute and Mesta $	3.31	5.26	6.19	8.16	9.23	10.56	10.62	11.4	10.93	11.68	11.13	10.52	10.6
Sugarcane	57.05	110	126.37	154.25	241.05	295.96	342.38	361.04	341.2	352.14	362.33	348.45	306.7
Tobacco	0.26	0.31	0.36	0.48	0.56	0.34	0.8	0.75	0.66	0.74	0.84	0.8	--

*Fourth advance estimates #—million bales of 170 kg each; $—million bales of 180 kg each.

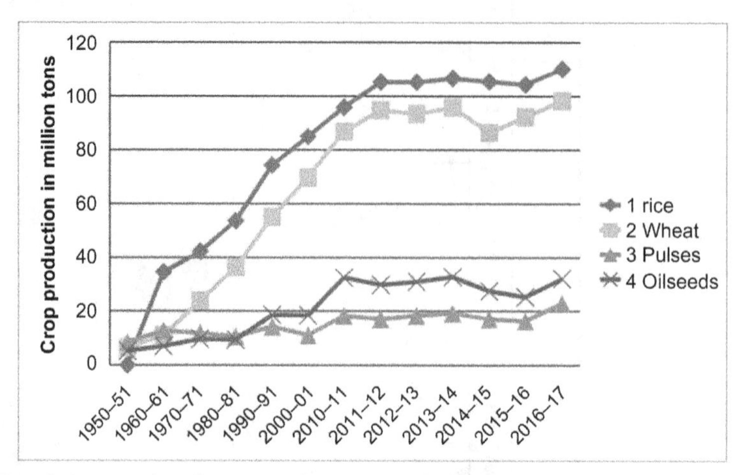

Figure 3.1 Trends in agricultural crop production in India (million tons) (Anonymous, 2017a).

and 13% of wheat production. The green revolution in the 1960s and 2015–16 enhanced production of wheat and rice that accounted for 78% of the food grain production in the country (Fig. 3.1). However, productivity is less compared to China, Brazil, and the United States. The multiple cropping system and cropping in different seasons increase the economic returns for the sustainability of farmers.

3.3.2 Shift in food consumption patterns

Several changes have undergone over the past 50 years in the eating habits of the average Indian. The life expectancy has increased as indicated by statistics produced by FAOSTAT. The consumption pattern of countries across the world is analyzed over a period of the past five decades (1961–2011) by the Food and Agriculture Organization of the United Nations (Anonymous, 2019).

An average Indian consumed a total of 2010 kcal in 1961 (Fig. 3.2). The diet covered 378 g of grains (43%), 199 g of vegetables, fruits, and starchy roots (23%), 108 g of dairy and eggs (12%), 108 g of sugar and fat (12%), 17 g of meat (2%), and 68 g as other foods (8%). With the progression of decades, the average Indian consumption of energy increased to 2458 kcal. The diet consisted of 416 g of grains (32%), 450 g of vegetables, fruits, starchy roots (34%), 235 g of eggs and dairy (18%), 129 g of sugar and fat (10%), 29 g of meat (2%), and 58 g as other foodstuffs (4%).

The per capita consumption of protein in the past 25 years has increased from 55 g per person to 59 g per person (from 1990 to 2015) with increasing protein from an animal source (9 g/day to 12 g/day). The contribution of dietary energy from cereals and roots has decreased from 66 g per day to 59 g per day. The average Indian is consuming more calories than it was observed 50 years ago. The intake of eggs, dairy, and plant produce has increased more than twice during this period. Although the Indian

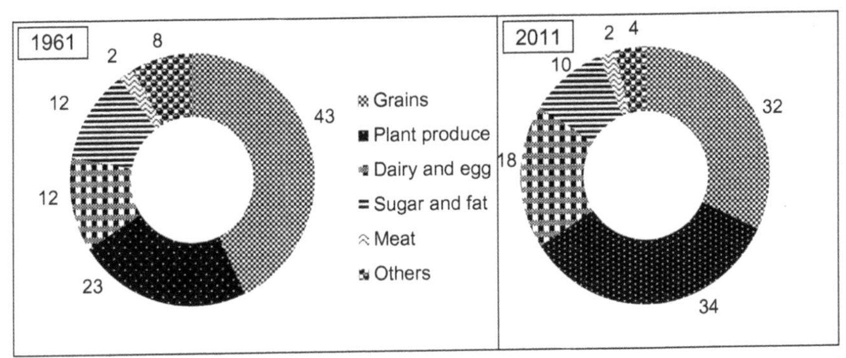

Figure 3.2 Average daily food consumption of Indians in 1961 and 2011 (Anonymous, 2017b).

diet is vegetarian-based, the consumption of meat and animal-based products has increased. The consumption of grains has decreased. The per capita consumption of sugar and fat has increased. Still, India remains one of the countries with most vegetarian people in the world. The nation's life expectancy was only 42 years in 1960 compared to 68 years in 2015 indicating improvement in the quality of diets over the years (Roser, 2019).

About 8.7% of the world's diabetics (or 69.2 million people) live in India as reported by the World Health Organization (Anonymous, 2016). This implies that the quality of life has decreased with an increase in morbidity patterns and lifestyle disorders. Indian food is authentically proven to be healthy. It is rich in nutraceuticals, antioxidants, and bioactive compounds that Western countries aspire for. However, not all traditional Indian foods are the healthy and judicious selection is necessary. With an innovative marketing database, Indian consumers are updated with the latest research information about food when compared to 50 years ago with more choices. However, more choice does not imply better choice (Plummer, 2017).

In most of the communities, food is bound to cultural and religious practices. To build once own cultural competence, understanding the food and food practices of different cultures is a must. Nomadic people migrate quite often, which impose to change their food habits. The reductions in physical activity add to impaired health in the future. The common health problems, morbidity pattern, and nutrition-related chronic diseases such as type 2 diabetes and heart disease are showing an increasing trend (Guha, 2006).

The economic growth of India has envisaged an enormous increase during the past decades. India's average per capita calorie consumption has increased (Fig. 3.3), but protein intake has been fluctuating between 53 and 58 g (Fig. 3.4) with modest changes. However, the per capita fat consumption has registered a higher growth varying from 39 to 49 g. The diversifying diets with more fruit/vegetable and animal-based food share the increased calorie and protein source in the Indian diet with the decline of cereal and pulse consumption (Thakur, 2017).

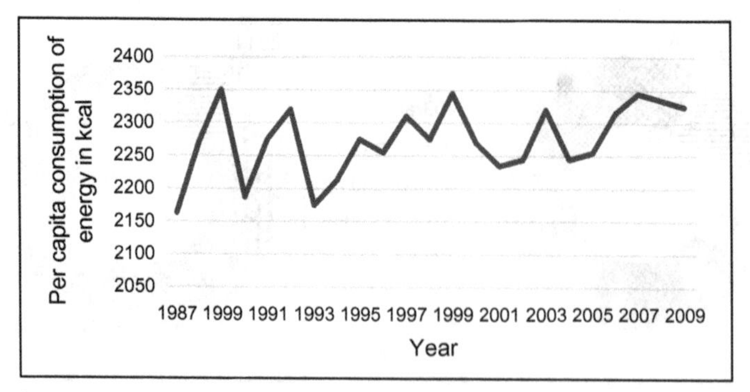

Figure 3.3 Trends in per capita consumption of energy (kcal) in Indians (Anonymous, 2017).

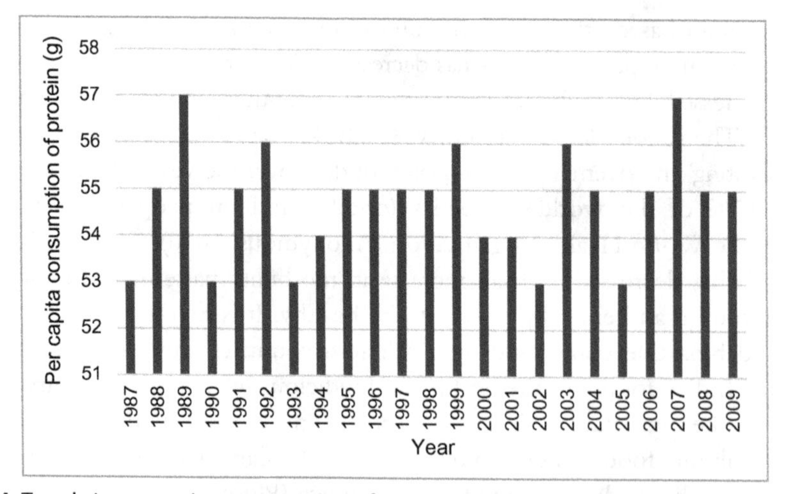

Figure 3.4 Trends in per capita consumption of protein (g) in Indians (Anonymous, 2017).

3.4 Cultural depiction of food consumption

With a rich heritage, Indian dining etiquette has the foundation of traditions handed from generation to generation without proper documentation. Behind every tradition are centuries of invasions, conquests, religious beliefs, political changes, and social customs. People from the Indus valley cooked wild grains with herbs and plants, most of them are staples today. The Mughals saw food as an art and introduced the fragrance of rose water, the texture of yogurt and clarified butter, and the use of spices. Further, Mughals showed that eating is meant to be pleasurable (David, 2009).

Indian food is different from the rest of the world not only in taste but also in cooking methods. It is a perfect blend of various cultures and ages. Just like Indian culture, food in India has also been influenced by various civilizations, which have contributed their share in its overall development and the present form. Foods of India are better known for their spiciness. Throughout India, be it North or South, spices are used generously in cooking. Every single spice used in Indian dishes carries one or the other nutritional as well as nutraceutical properties.

Ayurveda endorses the habit of eating food with hands. It is a sensory experience and eating with hands evokes emotion and passion. Vedic knowledge denotes hands as the most precious organ. The thumb indicates space, the forefinger–air, the middle finger–fire, the ring finger–water, and the little finger–earth. Eating with fingers stimulates these five elements and helps in bringing forth digestive juices in the stomach. The nerve endings on the fingertips are known to stimulate digestion. Feeling the food becomes a way of signaling the stomach that the food is reaching the stomach. Besides India, eating with hands is a common practice in some parts of Africa and the Middle East.

An authentic Southern meal is mostly served on a plantain leaf, especially in Kerala. Eating food on a plantain leaf is considered healthy. Placing hot food on the leaves emanates several nutraceuticals that enrich the food. Plantain leaves contain large amounts of polyphenols: a natural antioxidant found in many plant-based foods. It also adds to the aroma of food and enhances the taste. Traditionally, water is sprinkled on the plantain leaves before use as an act of purification. The use of plantain leaves dates back to a time before metal became a mainstay. People found it more hygienic to use fresh leaves that were disposable instead of wooden utensils. They could easily carry dishes such as curries or chutneys. Moreover, sitting on the floor and eating was recommended, as the repeated bending of the spine was known to improve blood circulation.

The Bohri Muslim community follows a tradition of eating from one huge platter/plate. The meal begins by sitting around the platter and passing the salt. Every dish sits in the center of the plate and the members pull out their share.

The Royal Feast—"*Wazwan*" is royal cuisine and culture of Kashmir. In the Kashmiri language, "*waz*" means a highly skilled cook and "*wan*" refers to shop. Traditionally, it consists of 36 courses and each of them is unique. The complexity and variety of food are not to be matched elsewhere. The meal ends on a sweet note with "*Phirni*"—a dish of milk and rice cooked to a pudding consistency and flavored with nuts and dry fruits, along with "*Kahwa*"—a green tea flavored with spices.

3.5 Traditional foods and their composition

3.5.1 Food groups under Indian traditional meal pattern

Indian traditional foods are based on cereal, pulse, oilseeds, fruits, vegetables, herbs, spices, and dairy products. These foods serve energy-yielding, bodybuilding, and protective functions. Whole grain cereals and millets are the most important sources of macronutrients, viz. carbohydrate, protein, and fats. These are traditionally used for preparing varieties of food products consumed during all meals of the day. Pulses and legumes have been an integral part of the traditional Indian food system. They serve as sources of protein besides energy and micronutrients (vitamins and minerals). Oilseeds apart from fat-soluble vitamins A, D, E, K, also provide protein, B-vitamins, and essential minerals. The products exclusively derived from cow or buffalo milk are essential traditional foods in India. Milk is an important source of nutrition for infants and children and is equally ubiquitously consumed by adults. It is used as such or as curds (Indian yogurt) and as an ingredient in a variety of beverages such as tea/coffee, sweet porridge, and many regional sweet preparations such as *Rasgolla*, *Sandesh*, and *Pedha* prepared with coagulated or condensed milk. Vegetables and fruits provide vitamins B, C, and K, β-carotene, and minerals such as calcium, phosphorus, potassium, iron, and zinc as well as fiber. Many fruits such as plantain, apple, pineapple, papaya, citrus fruits, and guava form part of traditional Indian food and are never subjected to cooking, thereby enhancing nutrient availability. Animal foods are rich in protein with essential amino acids that aid in bodybuilding and maintenance. In addition, many spices and their blends that enhance the aroma of food are used.

3.5.2 Traditional foods and their composition

Traditionally foods are consumed not only to meet physiological requirements but also as a means for pleasure and to provide emotional and social satisfaction wherein the family members sit together for sharing a meal. India is the country where multiple recipes form one meal (served on a plate called "*thali*"), and one course comprises several side dishes. The *thali* is a wholesome meal that is found in many regions such as Rajasthan, Gujarat, or down South, complete with light and delicious curries, local greens, cooked split legumes, rice, and Indian bread. Accompaniments such as homemade chutneys, pickles, and crisp wafers are a must. It defines the system of Indian meals prepared and eaten in most households across the country. The beauty of the *thali* is that while it is a significant part of our culture, it offers a scientific approach to nutrition. A view at any plate meal represents the food pyramid of today with carbohydrates from grains, fiber from fruits and vegetables, and nutrients from dairy products such as curds. It is a balanced diet where variety is at its best (Vasudeva, 2017).

Plate meal or "*thali*" with assorted delicious regional dishes is a common consumption pattern for lunch/dinner. One dish for a meal is rarely found in Indian cuisine in any part of the country. The *thali* signifies cultural significance besides being a complete meal in itself. Local delicacies are prepared and served traditionally across the geographical borders. Typical *thali* comprises a main dish (generally a staple cereal/millet), which basically is a source of major nutrients, while several side dishes including snacks, sweets, and dessert serve as the treasure of micronutrients and nutraceutical components, thus providing nutritional benefit to the consumer. Indian plate meals are seasonal and traditional local delights that concentrate on the typical method of preparation, which generally is elaborate. Each Indian *thali* is unique in terms of ingredients used, method of preparation, combination of dishes served, and style of consumption (Sarkar, 2018).

West Bengal, Sikkim, Assam, Arunachal Pradesh, Meghalaya, Manipur, Nagaland, Mizoram, Tripura, and Orissa are the states of East India. The typical character of this region is that these are surrounded by beaches and mountains; thus seafoods constitute a major component. Rice is the major crop grown due to the heavy rainfall received. People are both vegetarians and nonvegetarians with a strong influence on Chinese and Mongolian cuisine. Several green leafy vegetables and fruits are included in their meals, thereby balancing the nutritional requirements. Method of preparation being simple, foods are generally boiled or steamed. Fish followed by pork finds a place in the East Indian *thali*. Sweet dishes are a part of every meal. Rice, vegetables, fruits, mustard seeds, and oil are common ingredients while cumin seeds, onion seeds, mustard seeds, fennel seeds, and fenugreek seeds are the most preferred spices. Chilies grown here are less pungent, and both green and red varieties are used. Sweet dishes are based on milk, coconut, and gram flour. *Momos* (steamed, meat-, or vegetable-filled wontons) and *Thukpa* (a clear soup) are popular dishes. Tomato pickle, fish curry, and puffed rice spicy snack are also commonly seen on menus. *Sandesh* (made of coagulated milk and sugar) and *Rasgolla* (coagulated milk dumplings in syrup), as well as creamy rice pudding—*Kheer* are common sweets and desserts.

The states included in the western region are Rajasthan, Gujarat, Maharashtra, and Goa. Rajasthan and Gujarat have hot, dry climates, while Goa and Maharashtra are coastal and partly arid. Coastal regions of Goa have a lush green coastline with abundant availability of fresh fish and seafood. Coconut is the major oil crop. Vindaloo—a fiery, spicy dish and Xacuti—a curry prepared with complex spicing including white poppy seeds, coconut, and red chilis are local dishes that testify the fact that it was a Portuguese colony until the 1960s. All states of Western India have a diverse style of food preparation and consumption. In Maharashtra, coastal areas cuisine includes fresh coconut-based hot and sour curries with fish and seafood. Part of Maharashtra uses a lot of dry coconuts. Goan food is rich, piquant, and strongly flavored by coconut, red chilies, and vinegar. Gujarati food being sweetish and vegetarian, Rajasthani food is hot and spicy with non-vegetarian dishes based on red meat. Gujarati *thali* (a large plate) consists of many different vegetable dishes, rice, unleavened flat Indian bread, sweets, and a fried crispy snack based on Bengal gram flour known as Farsan. In Gujarat and Rajasthan, corn, lentils, and gram flour, dry red chilies, fermented milk, yogurt, sugar, and nuts constitute staple ingredients; in Maharashtra, fish, rice, coconut, and peanuts; in Goa, fish, pork, and rice. Sunflower, canola, peanut oil, and ghee are commonly used cooking oils. Dry red chilies, sugar, sesame seeds, coconut, nuts, and vinegar are the common spices used.

South Indian states, namely, Andhra Pradesh, Tamil Nadu, Kerala, and Karnataka are bordered by the coastal belt. The rainfall is abundant and areas have a hot, humid climate. The specialty of South Indian meals is the serving of meals on a plantain leaf. The states witness a huge supply of rice, fish, fresh fruits, and vegetables. The cuisine of Andhra Pradesh is known for its spiciness, while Tamil Nadu has largely vegetarian "*Chettinad*" cuisine. Malabari cooking is from Kerala, Regal Nizami food is from Hyderabad. Hyderabadi food is full of nuts, dried fruits, and exotic, expensive spices like saffron. Rice is combined with spicy red gram soup with vegetables (*Sambaar*) or hot sour soup (*Rasam*) or yogurt. The meal is accompanied with fryums—deep-fried crispy lentil pancakes. Either boiled rice or "*Idlis*" (steamed cakes made from rice batter), "*Dosas*" or "*Uttapams*" (pancakes made from a batter of rice and black gram flour), and dumplings of millets are used as the main part of a meal. Dhals (decorticated lentils) are also a part of most meals. Vegetable oils such as coconut, sunflower, or groundnut are cooking oils. The use of pure clarified butter on the table is a common practice thus augmenting energy intake. Curry leaves, mustard, coriander, cumin seeds, Asafetida, pepper and peppercorns, tamarind, chilies, and fenugreek seeds are frequently used spices.

North Indian region includes Jammu and Kashmir, Himachal Pradesh, Punjab, Uttaranchal, Uttar Pradesh, Haryana, Bihar, Jharkhand, Chattisgarh, and Madhya Pradesh. Temperature variations could be extreme in some areas with too hot summer and too cold winters. There is an abundance of fresh fruits and vegetables. Mughlai and Kashmiri's styles of cooking are popular and prevalent. North Indian curries are generally thick, moderately spicy and creamy gravies with generous use of nuts and other thickeners. Dairy products such as milk, cream, cottage cheese, ghee (clarified butter), and yogurt play an important role in the cooking of both savory and sweet dishes. Wheat-based products are generally preferred over rice-based items for the reason that the climate is suitable for production of wheat and not rice. Hence, North India is famous for "*tandoori roti*" and "*naans*" (bread made in a clay tandoor oven), stuffed "*paratha's*" (flaky Indian bread with different kinds of vegetarian and nonvegetarian fillings), and "*kulchas*" (bread made from the fermented dough). Rice is also made into elaborate *biryanis* and *pulaos* (pilafs). Vegetable oils such as sunflower and canola are common cooking oils. Mustard oil is rarely used and only in some states of the region. Ghee is normally reserved for cooking on special occasions. Coriander seeds, cumin, dry red chilies, turmeric, cardamom, cinnamon, cloves, and aniseed/fennel constitute important spices. "*Mutter Paneer*" (a curry made with cottage cheese and peas), "*Samosas*" (spicy deep-fried snack with different kinds of fillings), and "*chaat*" (hot-sweet-sour snack made with potato, chickpeas, and tangy chutneys) are common dishes.

3.5.3 Sufficiency of traditional foods in terms of nutrients

A wide variety of traditional food combinations exists across the northern, southern, eastern, and western states of India. A typical day starts with a beverage (tea/coffee or milk), followed by a traditional breakfast, lunch, evening tea with snacks, and dinner. The traditional meal pattern is always associated with a variety of accompaniments and is nutritious. Depending on the single-serving size, the traditional food combinations yield 60–604 kcal of energy. The carbohydrate, protein, fat, calcium, and iron contents are in the range of 20.5–85.0 g, 1.4–21.6 g, 1.4–28.1 g, 2.4–235.9 mg, and 0.44–22.8 mg, respectively.

On average, traditional East Indian thali provides 1100 kcal of energy, 27 g protein, 25 g fat, 50 mg calcium, and 14 mg of iron. The Western Indian thali provides 1100 kcal, 34 g protein, 50 g fat, 110 calcium, and 10 mg of iron. The South Indian thali provides 1400 kcal of energy, 25 g protein, 55 g fat, 180 mg calcium, and 8 mg iron. On an average, North Indian thali provides 1345 kcal of energy, 45 g protein, 60 g fat, 280 mg calcium, and 25 mg iron Thus irrespective of region, Indian traditional thalis provide 1100–1400 kcal of energy, 25–45 g of protein 25–60 g of fat, 50–280 mg of calcium, and 8–25 mg of iron.

3.5.4 Benefits of traditional foods for health, social, and economic aspects

The food groups categorized under Indian traditional meal patterns exert a wide range of health benefits. Today, there is growing recognition that food plays more roles than just being a source of macro- and micronutrients. The Functional Food Centre (Anonymous, 1998) defines functional food as "natural or processed foods that contain known or unknown biologically active compounds"; these foods, in defined, effective and nontoxic amounts, provide a clinically proven and documented health benefit for the prevention, management, or treatment of chronic diseases. Apart from providing functional as well as nutraceutical benefits, traditional foods help to mitigate the hidden hunger of micronutrients.

A significant determinant of the health effects of whole grains is their nondigestible carbohydrate component. The nondigestible carbohydrates of food act as dietary fibers especially, β-glucan and resistant starch, are perhaps the most important functional components that modulate the glycemic index of food (Tappy et al., 1996). The functional components of cereals, viz. rice bran with γ-oryzanol and wheat bran with insoluble fiber helps in the management of lifestyle disorders. Pulses and legumes aid in combating protein-energy malnutrition. Pulses alone or in a combination of cereals reduce the glycemic index of food that is beneficial for diabetics. The isoflavones and dietary fiber present in pulses serve as functional components. Oilseed and their oil do contain functional components. Flaxseed is rich in ω-3 fatty acids, and rice bran oil contains γ-oryzanol as a functional component.

Probiotics are commonly consumed as a part of fermented food products such as yogurt, fermented milk, and curds and form functional components. Curd (Indian yogurt), a popular fermented product prepared from milk using lactic acid bacteria, is rich in B complex vitamins, folic acid, and riboflavin and confers a wide range of health benefits due to the presence of probiotic bacteria (Sarkar et al., 2015). The so-called "healthy bacteria" have been classified as probiotics and are defined as live microbial food ingredients that are beneficial to health. Many fruits form part of traditional Indian food and are rich sources of flavonoids, minerals, vitamins, carotenoids, electrolytes, and other bioactive compounds that have an impact on human health. Among fruits and vegetables—carrot with dietary fiber, carotenoids, cruciferous vegetables with dithiolthiones, green leafy vegetables with β-carotene and lutein, tomato with lycopene, grapes with resveratrol, alliums with sulfur compounds, and a wide range of polyphenols and glucosinolates designate as functional foods. The components present in fruits and vegetables are essential for digestion, bone development, hematopoiesis, immunity development, etc. Among animal foods, fishes such as tuna, salmon, and mackerel are rich in ω-3 fatty acids and thus aid in reducing low-density lipoprotein levels, increase high-density cholesterol levels, and thereby reduce the problems of cardiovascular diseases.

Spices and herbs used in Indian traditional cuisine bring to food a large number of bioactives that render foods functional, besides improving the palatability. These include turmeric—curcuminoids, pepper—piperine, clove, and cinnamon—eugenol, ginger—gingerol and shogol, fenugreek—disogenin, 4-hydroxy isoleucine, and galactomannan, garlic—flavonoids, diallyl sulfate, alliin, ajoene, and allicin, and cinnamon—cinnamtannin B1. The sulfur compounds confer a wide array of therapeutic effects including antimicrobial, anticancer, antidiabetic, antiinflammatory, and antioxidant activities as well as the ability to improve cardiovascular health (Rivlin, 2006; Milner, 2010; Bayan et al., 2014). They also exert beneficial effects against nauseating discomforts, platelet aggregation and cardiovascular diseases, dyslipidemia, inflammation, oxidative stress, and hypertension (Singletary, 2010). In addition, reports indicate antimutagenic property in vivo (Nirmala et al., 2007) and in vitro (Panpatil et al., 2013). Spices are known to possess gastroprotectant, hepatoprotectant, and antidiabetic effects in addition to hypocholesterolemic activity (Singletary, 2010; Meghwal and Goswami, 2012) and reduced risk of cardiovascular diseases (Canene-Adams et al., 2005) and hypertension (Ranasinghe and Galappaththy, 2016). They are used as a general tonic or stimulant, food preservative, cosmetic agent, carminative, diuretic, blood purifier, antiphlegm, and remedy for cough, cold, sinusitis, pain, and intestinal and liver disorders (Krishnaswamy, 2006).

Apart from serving as functional foods, the traditional foods of India seem to be exerting nutraceutical effects. Nutraceuticals are natural phytochemicals that render foods functional. These include ω-3 fatty acids that are neuroprotective and anticardiac; curcumin in turmeric has anticancer, antioxidant, antidiabetic, and antiinflammatory activities and neuroprotective properties; resveratrol, a stilbenoid type of plant polyphenol found in a variety of berries, particularly in the skin and seed of grapes, is known for antioxidant potential (Ungvari et al., 2009); quercetin is a naturally occurring polyphenol found in onions, apples, black and green tea, beans, grapes, berries, vegetables, and fruits and affords protection against certain types of cancer, inflammatory conditions, cardiovascular diseases, diabetes, and aging as well as aiding in bone formation (Boots et al., 2008; Brackman et al., 2010); piperine, an alkaloid found in black pepper, provides inhibitory potential against detoxification enzymes and inhibition of intestinal p-glycoproteins responsible for efflux of drugs (Patil et al., 2011); eugenol, a phenolic compound found in medicinal plants, exhibits antimutagenic, anticancer, antifungal, antiviral, antibacterial, antiparasitic, antiinflammatory (Raja et al., 2015), and antidiabetic effects (Srinivasan et al., 2014). The immense health benefits, nutraceutical contents, and bioactives in Indian traditional foods reduce the medical expenses of communicable as well as noncommunicable diseases, morbidity, and mortality rate that adds to the family income. The economic benefits reflect savings for a better future. Apart from this, reverting back to traditional meal patterns can create opportunities for entrepreneurship, eating outlets or eateries leading to the growth of the economy.

Traditional meal patterns served social functions too. These foods have always been the central part of our community, social, cultural, and religious life. It has been an expression of love, friendship, happiness at religious, social, and family get together.

3.6 Future for traditional foods

Indian traditional foods vary in processing methods, ingredients, and combinations. Traditionally, the ingredients used in Indian diets are manually processed including grinding, milling, and retained more natural ingredients. The increasing population, urbanization, industrialization, and women working outside homes have a created high demand for convenience foods and ready-to-eat foods. The foods ingredients are now being mechanically processed; they induce heat or alterations in nutrients with structural modification and thereby can reduce the nutrient bioavailability. For example, oils obtained from cold-pressed cakes have better fatty acid content compared to those obtained from hot press cakes. Modification of the structure of the nutrients during processing is another example. The structure of starch and protein get modified due to the generation of heat that affects the nutritional profile. Traditional foods are also now available in the market. However, they may not provide the same nutritional profile that was endorsed in ancient times. These market available traditional foods are prepared with ingredients that are not organic, unlike olden days. The organic agriculture has been modernized into inorganic cultivation, to get more yields with less land, the resources including land, water, and fertility are burdened with the application of heavy pesticides and insecticides. The residual effect of these chemicals is evidenced by various research studies. Moreover, to attract consumers, food products are adulterated and promoted with changes in color, size, taste, etc. The Indian culture is more inclined toward a sit-down eating pattern with family or friends, different from the counterparts from the developed world who are likely to grab their foods on-the-go or adopted to sit around the table and eat. Particularly, in metropolitan cities among the younger generation, the sit-down eating pattern is slowly vanishing. Many processed and convenience foods such as pickles and crisp wafers that were prepared at home without additives are now easily available in markets loaded with food additives crossing the permissible limits. The popularization of junk foods such as pizzas, burgers, and fries that are entering into a go-grab pattern is gaining momentum over traditional patterns. All such factors are playing their part in accelerating fat and sugar consumption at the national level. This is reducing the health benefits and nutraceutical content of traditional foods. However, reverting back to traditional foods may not fetch the same nutritional benefits, as the processing of food ingredients in traditional methods causes drudgery on the part of processors. Hence, it is high time to revisit the originality of traditional foods, which are better than the novel foods with respect to health.

References

Achaya, K.T., 1994. Indian Food: A Historical Companion. Oxford University Press, New Delhi, India.

Alaeddini, M.A., Olia, M., 2004. Green revolution in India; an experience. Proc of the Fourth Intern Iran & Russia Conf on Agriculture and Natural Resources. Shahrekord University, Shahrekord, Iran, pp. 1118–1122.

Anonymous, 1998. Functional Foods. Functional Food Center, USA, <https://in.linkedin.com/company/functional-food-center-functional-food-institute>.

Anonymous, 2008. Promotion of traditional regional agricultural and food products: a further step towards sustainable rural development. In: Proc Twenty-Sixth FAO Regional Conf Europe: 2008, June 26–27: 2008, Innsbruck, Austria: 2008. pp. 8–17.

Anonymous, 2016. World Health Day-2016. <http://www.searo.who.int/india/mediacentre/events/2016/en>.

Anonymous, 2017. FAOSTAT. <http://www.fao.org/faostat/en/#data/FBS/report>.

Anonymous, 2017a. Pocket book of Agricultural Statistics-Directorate of Economics and Statistics. Ministry of Agriculture and Farmers Welfare, GOI, New Delhi, p. 27.

Anonymous, 2017b. What the World Eats? <https://www.nationalgeographic.com/what-the-world-eats/>.

Anonymous, 2019. FAOSTAT. <http://www.fao.org/faostat/en/#home>.

Anwar, S., 2019. Cropping Patterns and Cropping Systems in India. <https://www.jagranjosh.com/general-knowledge/cropping-patterns-and-cropping-systems-in-india-1517395777-1>.

Bayan, L., Kouliv, P.H., Gorji, A., 2014. Garlic: a review of potential therapeutic effect. Avicenna J. Phytomedicn. 4, 1–4.

Boots, A.W., Haenen, G.R.M.M., Bast, A., 2008. Health effects of quercetin: from antioxidant to nutraceutical. Eur. J. Pharmacol. 585, 325–337.

Canene-Adams, K., Campbell, J.K., Zaripheh, S., Jeffery, E.H., Erdman, J.W., 2005. The tomato as a functional food. J. Nutr. 135, 1226–1230.

David, M., 2009. Eating for Pleasure. <https://experiencelife.com/article/eating-for-pleasure/>.

Guha, A., 2006. Ayurvedic Concept of Food and Nutrition. <https://opencommons.uconn.edu/som_articles/25/>.

Kearney, J., 2010. Food consumption trends and drivers. Philos. Trans. Royal Soc. B. 365 (1554), 2793–07.

Krishnaswamy, K., 2006. Turmeric: The Salt of the Orient is the Spice of Life, vol. 1. Allied Publishers Pvt. Ltd, New Delhi, India, pp. 1–238.

Meghwal, M., Goswami, T.K., 2012. A review on the functional properties, nutritional content, medicinal utilization and potential application of fenugreek. J. Food Process. Technol. 3, 181.

Michel, M., Kumar, P., 2013. Trends and Pattern of Consumption of Value Added Foods in India, 2013 June. Available from: <http://www.nhcgroup.com/indian-food-culture>.

Milner, J.A., 2010. Garlic. In: Paul, M.C., Joseph, M.B., Marc, R.B., Gordon, M.C., Mark, L., Joel, M., et al.,Encyclopedia of Dietary Supplements, second ed. Marcel D, New York, pp. 314–325.

Nirmala, K., Krishna, T.P., Polasa, K., 2007. In vivo antimutagenic potential of ginger on formation and excretion of urinary mutagens in rats. Int. J. Cancer Res. 3, 134–142.

Panpatil, V.V., Tattari, S., Kota, N., Nimgulkar, C., Polasa, K., 2013. In vitro evaluation on antioxidant and antimicrobial activity of spice extracts of ginger, turmeric and garlic. J. Pharmacogn. Phytochem. 2, 143–148.

Patil, U., Singh, A., Chakraborty, A., 2011. Role of piperine as a bioavailability enhancer. Intern. J. Recent Adv. Pharm. Res. 4, 16–23.

Plummer, L., 2017. 50 Years of Food in India: Changing Eating Habits of a Rapidly Changing Nation (of Foodies). <https://www.thebetterindia.com/98604/india-eating-habits-food-50-years-culture/>.

Prakash, V., 2015. Role of functional foods and beverages in health and wellness. Paper presented at International Symposium Diet, Lifestyle & Health: 2015, November 20–21, Colombo, Sri Lanka.

Raja, M.R.C., Srinivasan, V., Selvaraj, S., Mahapatra, S.K., 2015. Versatile and synergistic potential of eugenol: a review. Pharm. Anal Actap. 6 (5), 1–6.

Ranasinghe, P., Galappaththy, P., 2016. Health benefits of Ceylon cinnamon (*Cinnamomum zeylanicum*): a summary of the current evidence. Ceylon Med. J. 61, 1–5.

Rivlin, R.S., 2006. Is garlic alternative medicine? J. Nutr. 136, 713S–715S.

Roser, M., 2019. Future Population Growth (Cited 2019). Published Online at Our World In Data.org. Retrieved from: <https://ourworldindata.org/future-population-growth>.

Sarkar, P., Kumar, L.D.H., Dhumal, C., Panigrahi, S.S., Choudhary, R., 2015. Traditional and ayurvedic foods of Indian Origin. J. Ethnic Foods 2, 97–109.

Sarkar, P.V.,2018. What is the Thali Way of Eating Indian Food? <https://www.thespruceeats.com/put-together-a-thali-3976523>.

Singletary, K., 2010. Ginger—an overview of health benefits. Nutr. Today 45, 171–183. <https://www.researchgate.net/publication/232129720_Ginger_An_Overview_of_Health_Benefits>.

Sinha, 2014. Agro-Ecological Regions of India – Meaning and Determining <http://www.yourarticlelibrary.com/agriculture/agro-ecological-regions-of-india-meaning-and-determining/42300>.

Srinivasan, S., Sathish, G., Jayanthi, M., Muthukumaran, J., Muruganathan, U., Ramachandran, V., 2014. Ameliorating effect of eugenol on hyperglycemia by attenuating the key enzymes of glucose metabolism in streptozotocin-induced diabetic rats. Mol. Cell. Biochem. 385, 159–168.

Tappy, L., Gügolz, E., Würsch, P., 1996. Effects of breakfast cereals containing various amounts of â-glucanfibers on plasma glucose and insulin responses in NIDDM subjects. Diabetes. Care 98, 31–34.

Thakur, M., 2017. An Analysis of Changing Food Consumption Pattern in India: Pre and Post Reforms Period. <https://www.academia.edu/.../>. An Analysis of Changing Food Consumption Pattern in India.

Ungvari, Z., Labinskyy, N., Mukhopadhyay, P., Pinto, J.T., Bagi, Z., Ballabh, P., et al., 2009. Resveratrol attenuates mitochondrial oxidative stress in coronary arterial endothelial cells. Am. J. Physiol. Heart Circ. Physiol. 297 H 1876–1881.

Vasudeva, S., 2017. Eating With Your Hands and Other Indian Food Traditions NDTV. <https://food.ndtv.com/food-drinks/a-bite-at-a-time-foods-traditions-from-ancient-india-1206447>.

Further reading

Anonymous, 2015. Food and Cultural Practices of the Indian Community in Australia – A Community Resource. <https://metrosouth.health.qld.gov.au/sites/default/files/content/heau-cultural-profile-indian>.

Coates, P.M., Brackman, F.G., Edgar, A., 2010. Pygeum. In: Paul, M.C., Joseph, M.B., Marc, R.B., Gordon, M.C., Mark, L., Joel, M., Jeffrey, D.W. (Eds.), Encyclopedia of Dietary Supplements, second ed. Marcel D, New York, pp. 650–655.

CHAPTER 4

Forest foods for tribals in selected regions of India and their sustainability

Purabi Bose
Researcher and Filmmaker, IUFRO Deputy Coordinator Social Aspects of Forest & Coordinator Gender in Forest Research; IASC Council Member; IUCN CEESP's Deputy Chair for Theme on Governance, Equity and Rights

Contents

4.1 Introduction

Almost 250 million people, a majority from indigenous and tribal regions rely on forest resources (FAO, 2015). Different from the urban or rural population, forest-dependent indigenous people forage forests to collect edible foods. In many hunting and gathering tribal communities, foraging wild forest food has been a traditional practice. This is true for tribal communities currently living in various countries, particularly in the global south. For the urban population, the foods for consumption are products that are purchased from the supermarkets. In contrast, tribal communities buy only a few food products and cultivate some of the food, while most of the food is obtained from foraging forests and natural resources (Bose, 2019).

Nutritional and Health Aspects of Food in South Asian Countries
DOI: https://doi.org/10.1016/B978-0-12-820011-7.00005-8

Many studies have highlighted the significance of a wide variety of wild foods from forest and other natural resources and its importance in the diets of local communities (Paumgarten and Shackleton, 2011; Anglesen et al., 2014; IFPRI, 2014). The challenge, however, is that little has been done to protect the rapidly changing food and nutritional security that is affected due to market demand, deforestation, land-use change, or lack of tenure, access, and control over forest food resources (Sayer et al., 2013; Vira et al., 2015). This chapter poses two questions: (1) How forest "wild" food demand in urban areas is affecting traditional food and nutrition security of tribals? (2) How is diet quality influenced by cultural mainstreaming and sustainability aspects? One of the main arguments is that with the increase in market demand for traditional forest wild food, the nutritional quality of diets for local forest-dwelling tribal communities is reduced.

The precise meaning of "forest food" is open to different interpretations. For the purpose of this chapter, the term wild refers to untamed objects that exist autonomously from the human impact that is derived mainly from wilderness areas. In other words, forest foods are not domesticated by humans but derived from wild species that occur in self-maintaining populations in natural or seminatural ecosystems. Censkowsky et al. (2007) refer to wild forest products to the practice as gathering a noncultivated native or naturalized resource from its natural habitat. The distinction is challenging given that some products that are collected from nature might have been subject to manipulation, or wild products in one country might be cultivated in another (Censkowsky, 2007; Wiersum, 2017). Pimentel et al. (1997) estimate that about US$ 90 billion in nontimber forest products (NTFPs) are harvested each year.

Lack of forest tenure and governance represents a risk to forest dwellers, and it is thus necessary to identify its impact on indigenous people with different food cultural acceptability and nutrition security (Bose, 2019). This chapter looks into the food and nutrition security aspect of traditional foods in tribal India. The chapter starts with a description of the study population and provides empirical evidence and then moves step by step toward a sustainable future of traditional food and nutrition.

4.2 Study population and methodology

The study specifically highlights the plights of a lesser-known indigenous hunting-gathering tribe, particularly vulnerable tribal groups (PVTGs). During the early 1970s, the Government of India created a separate category of so-called less developed tribal groups as primitive tribal groups and it was renamed to PVTGs due to debate about the word "primitive." Each of the 75 PVTGs is heterogenous, a few similar characteristics include physical isolation often living in remote forest areas, the absence of written language, and minimalistic lifestyle.

The four PVTGs case studies that have been identified for the study area represent a diversity of population and landscapes, each from Central, East, West, and South India. Detailed qualitative interviews were conducted during 2016 and 2017 by the author, who was accompanied by a translator and a camera person. The investigators spent a minimum of 2 weeks with each tribe, including walking with them in their forest areas. Two complementary methods were used—semistructured interviews and maintenance of diaries for each community. This collection diary gave a rough estimate of the diversity of wild plants and animals including birds and aquatic habitats.

Participant observations helped in understanding the pattern of food consumption, type of food, and method of consumption (raw, preserved, cooked, other techniques). The narration about traditional food is recorded from men, women, the elderly, and youths of the tribal villages in their local languages. A qualitative manual data analysis was used, given that data collection was largely qualitative in content.

4.3 Findings

All the four tribal groups are traditional hunter-gatherers and have continued the tradition of foraging forest foods despite several restrictions from the Forest Department of Government of India. The findings are presented in a briefcase study format.

4.3.1 Baigas from Chhattisgarh, Central India

The Baigas live inside the Tiger Reserve project in the Achanakmar Wildlife Sanctuary of Chhattisgarh in Central India. One of the important plants commonly accessed by Baigas is drumstick (*Moringa oleifera*). Due to lack of electricity and minimum kitchen equipment, the leaves, flowers, and fresh pods are sun dried and stored and customarily used for cooking. Drought resistant, hardy, and nutritious traditional coarse millets such as wild rice, finger millet (*Eleusine coracana*), and "*Kodo*" millet (*Paspalum scrobiculatum*) form the customary staple diet. They boil it with wild tubers and fruits and consume it. Due to an increase in demand for *kodo*, pearl (*Pennisatum glaucum*), and finger millet as superfoods in the market, Baigas are now trading organic coarse millets for cash or barter them for polished rice.

NTFPs such as *bholim* are used as medicine while weaver ants (*Oecophylla smaragdina*) are enjoyed as a snack food. During the monsoon, Baiga men collect a special type of mushroom, known as "*Pihiri*" (variety of *Phallus rubicundus*) from the forest, which is now recognized as a superfood. An NGO staff explained, "Baigas are selling these days rare and exotic wild food, *Pihiri*, to barter for soap and cooking oil, or even *enouwa* (alcohol). Outsiders are recognizing the forest food's value while Baigas lack the information that they are sacrificing their best nutritional diet for nothing." Moreover, Baigas are in the brink of facing displacement from the Tiger Reserve wherein they would not only lose their traditional land rights but access to traditional food and nutrition from the commons.

4.3.2 Kurumbas from Nilgiris, Tamil Nadu, South India

Traditionally hunting and gathering communities, the Kurumbas of this study are a resettled community after relocation from reserved to nonreserved forest areas. Two households interviewed practice cash crops, including coffee, pepper, turmeric, and ginger. All the study households living in the forest area have claimed the individual tenure rights from the Forest Department. The respondents mentioned that they are dependent on the forest. Wild honey was one of the key NTFPs for livelihood. Women respondents observed that they are increasingly shifting toward rice as compared to their traditional staple diet of finger millet. The women explained, "This is different from our traditional activities of collecting forest foods. We are learning from the other non-*adivasis* (non-tribal) to prosper and eat properly cooked food. This adaptation is good to be recognized as one of the mainstream population."

The key issue in the focus group discussion was the change in lifestyle from hunting and gathering (a cash-free system) to a small farm with a focus on cash and land as property. Despite restrictions imposed by government officials, the Kurumbas occasionally hunt birds and other small wild animals from the forests for food. Often, they share wild foods among kinfolk, thereby distributing the responsibility collectively.

4.3.3 Paudi Bhuyan from Odisha, East India

An elderly Paudi Bhuyan woman, explained: "We do not have a fixed meal consumption concept such as breakfast, lunch, and dinner. Rather the clans ate collectively as and when foods were available. Nowadays, after we've been settled, we began learning the concept of individual households, mid-day meals for children and a slow transition towards a mainstream diet due to exposure as wage labourers." Many customary foods disappear, according to a youth, due to changes in work and lifestyle, and lack of access to forest resources.

According to Paudi Bhuyan men, wild meat and vegetables such as yam when prepared by simple techniques of steaming, boiling, fermenting, or roasting on open wood fires provide sufficient nutrition for people to remain healthy and satisfied with the taste. The respondents attributed health issues to lack of access to their customary diet of diverse seasonal wild foods, particularly medicinal herbs that previously were accessible from the forest. In a focus group discussion, they voiced: "Our young generation feels stigmatized because of our foraging culture, mainly for wild small animals such as rabbits and pigs. We no longer feel proud of our customary food habits, even though that suited our health much better than the urban-based carbohydrate-rich rice and wheat food we eat now."

4.3.4 Katkaris, dry deciduous forests of Maharashtra, West India

A majority of Katkaris depend on seasonal forest food, which according to them is not only delicious but also healthy due to medicinal properties (see Table 4.1). "We wake up in the morning and have millet porridge with some dried wild meat. It keeps us going for all day long." They have been traditionally drying the Moringa leaves and

Table 4.1 Nontimber forest produce used by Indian tribal population and associated challenges.

PVTGs	Forest food—sustainably collected by the tribals	Superfood demand	Risks related to superfood
Baigas	Wild rice, finger and kodo millet, honey, mahua (*Madhuca longiflora*), fowl, weaver ants, custard apple, *bholim*, and wild mushroom	Finger and kodo millet. *Bholim* and weaver ants are of rare medicinal value making it one of the most expensive forest foods	Baigas barter nutritious organic finger and kodo millet rich in mineral and vitamins for rice and maize
Paudi Bhuyans	Bamboo shoots, Chenhek (*Garcinia cowa*), wild pigs, insects, rabbit, dog, fish, crab, highland rice, fowl, lemons, wild edible leafy vegetables such as ai-du (*Amomum dealbatum*)	Bamboo shoots—are regarded as high in phytonutrients and help to get phenolic acids into the human body. It is good for weight loss due to high fiber and low energy content	Taking away of bamboo shoots by urban trades, thereby causing environmental degradation and depriving Paudi Bhuyans of their much-needed forest produce
Katkaris	Pearl millet, moringa, guava, cow pea, fowl, and other forest foods include *vilayati imli* (*Pithecellobium dulce*), and jamun fruit (*Syzygium cumini*)	Moringa and jamun are regarded as high medicinal value for diabetes, antifungal, antiviral, antidepressant, and antiinflammatory properties	Commercial exploitation of moringa leaves and jamun fruits. Katkaris are left without these nutritious leaves and fruits
Kurumbas	Honey, birds and small wild animals, banana flowers, jackfruit dried seeds	Honey—pure organic wild forest honey with medicinal value	Kurumbas are pushed to barter for nonnutritious food

use it as an herb in our food every day. With the increase in awareness among the urban population, the demand for Moringa leaves has increased in recent years making it a "marketable" product. Katkaris, when in need of money, sell the moringa flowers, drumstick, and leaves in the market.

Jamun fruits are collected by Katkaris, and they have various techniques for preserving using natural methods due to lack of electricity or piped gas for cooking. "Our children used to drink jamun juice that we have made it traditionally including raw mango juice, but these days aerated cold drinks are influencing our children's food habits," says a Katkari mother of two adolescent children.

4.4 Discussion

4.4.1 Traditional food and nutrition of particularly vulnerable tribal groups

The PVTGs for generations have developed techniques that preserve food and nutrition from forests. Forest "wild" food discussed in this chapter from the perspective of PVTGs shows that their so-called "primitive" food is becoming a modern culture (Bose, 2016).

4.4.1.1 *Farming techniques and land use*

All the PVTGs mentioned in this chapter are 80% dependent only on forest food different from rural communities. A few of them use subsidized food grains and cultivate small family farms less than half hectares of forestland. They use a traditional manual technique of throwing the seeds on the cleared field rather than sowing and without using any chemicals. Diversity of crops in farming helps them to cope with climate variability impact but also helps them to have diversity on their plates. Swidden cultivation or "*jhum*" as it is known locally is a way to manage the biodiversity, wherein they cut and burn a small patch of forest and farm for 5–7 years before leaving the land to regenerate. The vegetables and fruits grown in such farms demand no or fewer pesticides and fertilizers. Therefore the food safety and nutrition component due to organic products remain uncompromised. Edible insects, such as spiders and grasshoppers among others, are carefully roasted in the sand and/or dried in sun using rock salt to ensure the nutritive value is retained. Often, children are encouraged to eat these edible insects as snacks.

4.4.1.2 *Eating habits*

Different from modern-day western notions, many tribal communities in South Asia and elsewhere in the world have strong community sharing and cooking traditions. For all the PVTGs, the sense of food habits is closely interlinked to sharing foods with their neighbors and kinships. Studies have shown that many traditional diets were rich sources of micronutrients such as calcium, iron, vitamin A (as β-carotene), and folate (Ghosh-Jerath et al., 2015). Moreover, the PVTGs being gatherers consumed only when they were hungry, and community eating of hunting food, such as wild pig, for example, helped them to use the resources of cooking wise in addition to sharing the burden and risk of food insecurity. Different from rural settings of India, tribal men and women eat and drink equally without any gender-biased or taboo associated with eating habits.

4.4.1.3 *Cooking techniques*

Paudi Bhuyan tribe, for example, among other PVTGs commonly use fermentation technique. They believe that bamboo shoots, which are collected from the forest, when fermented produce a sour bitter taste making it rich in probiotic properties good for the human body (Jeyaram et al., 2010). Similarly, Kurumbas ferment millets and wild rice to prepare various steamed items without any use of fat or oil. The use of traditional stone to grind and store the fermented millets produces a rich bacterial population beneficial for digestion and maintenance of body temperature. Given that most tribal communities lack basic kitchen utensils and depend on wood fuel for cooking, the utility of resources is maximized. Baiga tribe uses smoking to cook a particular type of wild small animal that is hunted once a year and shared as a community meal with high protein content.

4.4.1.4 Preservation techniques

Food preservation techniques in the PVTGs though may differ based on the cultural and ethnic diversity of the tribe, but more or less they all use traditional techniques such as drying, fermenting, water-covering, cooling, freezing, and salting. Sweet is rarely or never used except those who have access to honey or other forms of the traditional wild sweetening agent. Mahua flowers are brewed to make alcohol using a fermenting traditional herb while the seeds are processed manually to extract oil for cooking purposes. The traditional knowledge of preservation techniques has dual emphasis, as this study finds out, one that of food safety to ensure food is hygienic and secondly to maintain the nutritional components without compromising on taste.

4.4.1.5 Game meat and fish

The rest of India has a different food culture compared to the traditional food culture of the PVTGs. It is well known that fish plays a big role in providing ω-3 fatty acids that help in improving human health, particularly because of high protein and fat content. The PVTGs with free access to natural resources and those who have not yet been displaced (different from Baiga PVTGs mentioned in this chapter) also have better access to eat game meat. This food culture makes them different from the rest of India. The food security provisions of subsidized grains (Reji, 2013) fail to understand that a higher protein intake diet of PVTGs is not suitable for only grain, often genetically modified, imported food provided by the government under the provisions of the Right to Food Act (Bose and van der Meulen, 2014).

4.4.2 Modern transition in food and culture

A modern diet such as rice, wheat, lentils, and sugar that are provided as subsidized food reduces forest food diversity. This transition has not only the direct impact on indigenous food system knowledge but also on the health of the next generation that mainly lives on carbohydrate-rich supplies from government shops. For PVTGs, unlike mainland India, forest and food have been an integral part of their livelihood and food security. The risk of modern transition in food and culture relates to pesticides, chemicals, and salt and sugar, and it leads to a high risk of diabetes, which these communities have never been exposed earlier.

4.4.3 Future of traditional food for tribal communities

There is a need that the traditional food system is documented to understand the rapid decline in biodiversity and nutrient-based diet. Gathering, storing, preserving, and cooking food without losing its nutrients are part and parcel of indigenous food systems. The future is in understanding that eating a healthy diet can be done sustainably without compromising on local ecosystems as shown by this study's indigenous hunting-gathering communities. One of the important aspects that we see in the PVTGs is the wisdom of eating high protein and mineral and micronutrient-rich forest food such as millets to reduce cholesterol.

4.5 Conclusion

This empirical research on rarely studied PVTGs highlighted three categories that impact forest food, particularly women and children: (1) commercialization of forest foods as "superfood" due to its high nutrition value, (2) cultural acceptability wherein tribal people lose out their traditional food due to mainstreaming; and (3) challenges sustainability due to loss of the forest resources. The author argues that food security studies in vulnerable areas with marginal populations demanding a shift in outlook from a primary preoccupation with staple food grains such as rice and wheat (Pingali, 2015; Bose, 2019) toward more food and nutrition value-based traditional food rich in micronutrients and vitamins are needed in tribal India.

The institutions and policies impacting forest food systems in India, such as forest, land, agriculture, food security, social policies, and market among others, have developed rather in an ad hoc way over the past 70 years. As a result, institutional pluralism and proliferation of policies have multiplied in inefficient ways, creating contradictions, gaps, and inconsistencies within and between them. To better understand how local indigenous and tribal communities manage their forest landscapes for sustaining their traditional healthy diet, the author recommends more in-depth research on "traditional food of indigenous peoples and its nutritional benefits."

References

Anglesen, A., Jagger, P., Babigumira, R., Belcher, B., Hogarth, N.J., Bauch, S., et al., 2014. Environmental income and rural livelihoods: a global-comparative analysis. World Dev. 64, S12–S28.

Bose, P., 2016. Hipster Hunger for Superfoods is Starving India's Adivasis. Scroll (December 9). <https://scroll.in/magazine/821786/hipsters-hunger-for-superfoods-is-starving-indias-adivasis>.

Bose, P., 2019. India's Right to Food Act: human rights for tribal communities' forest food. In: Urazbaeva, A., et al., (Eds.), The Functional Field of Food Law. European Institute Food Law Series, vol. 11. Wageningen Academic Publishers, pp. 55–72. , <https://www.wageningenacademic.com/doi/10.3920/978-90-8686-885-8_3>.

Bose, P., van der Meulen, B., 2014. The law to end hunger now: food sovereignty and genetically modified crops in tribal India – a socio-legal analysis. Penn State Law Rev. 118 (4), 893–918.

Censkowsky, U., Helberg, U., Nowack, A., Steidle, M., 2007. Overview of World Production and Marketing of Organic Wild Collected Products. International Trade Center UNCTAD/WTO and International Federation of Organic Agriculture Movements (IFOAM), Geneva, Switzerland.

FAO, 2015. The State of Food Insecurity in the World. Meeting the 2015 International Hunger Targets: Taking Stock of Uneven Progress. FAO, Rome.

Ghosh-Jerath, S., Singh, A., Kamboj, P., Goldberg, G., Magsumbol, S.M., 2015. Traditional knowledge and nutritive value of indigenous foods in the Oraon tribal community of Jharkhand: an exploratory cross-sectional study. Ecol. Food Nutr. 54 (5), 548–568.

IFPRI, 2014. Towards Sustainable, Healthy and Profitable Food Systems: Nutrition and the Sustainable Management of Natural Resources. UNSCN, Technical Note No. 4. Global Nutrition Report: Actions and Accountability to Accelerate the World's Progress on Nutrition. International Food Policy Research Institute, Washington, DC.

Jeyaram, K., Romi, W., Singh, T.A., Devi, A.R., Devi, S.S., 2010. Bacterial species associated with traditional starter cultures used in fermented bamboo shoot production in Manipur state of India. Int. J. Food Microbiol. 143, 1–8.

Paumgarten, F., Shackleton, C.M., 2011. The role of non-timber forest products in household coping strategies in South Africa: the influence of household wealth and gender. Popul. Environ. 33 (1), 108–131.

Pimentel, D., McNair, M., Buck, L., Pimentel, M., Kamil, J., 1997. The value of forests to world food security. Hum. Ecol. 25 (1), 91–120.

Pingali, P., 2015. Agricultural policy and nutrition outcomes – getting beyond the preoccupation with staple grains. Food Secur. 7 (3), 583–591.

Reji, E.M., 2013. Community grain banks and food security of the tribal poor in India. Dev. Pract. 23 (7), 920–933.

Sayer, J., Sunderland, T., Ghazoul, J., Pfund, J., Sheil, D., Meijaar, E., et al., 2013. Ten principles for a landscape approach to reconciling agriculture, conservation, and other competing land uses. Proc. Natl. Acad. Sci. USA. 110 (21), 8349–8356.

Vira, B., Wilburger, C., Mansourian, S., 2015. Forests and Food: Addressing Hunger and Nutrition Across Sustainable Landscapes. Open Books Publisher and IUFRO, Cambridge, UK.

Wiersum, K.F., 2017. New interest in wild forest products in Europe as an expression of biocultural dynamics. Hum. Ecol. Interdiscip. J. 45 (6), 787–794.

CHAPTER 5

Traditional preserved and fermented foods and their nutritional aspects

Palanisamy Bruntha Devi and Prathapkumar Halady Shetty
Department of Food Science and Technology, Pondicherry University, Puducherry, India

Contents

5.1 Introduction

India is rich in natural resources and has been known for its diverse culture and traditions since historical times. India is also known for its amazingly diverse food culture and culinary practices. Ethnic foods can be of three major types. Foods that are cooked using variety of cooking practices and consumed fresh, traditionally preserved foods for better flavors, aroma and long shelf life, ethnic fermented foods that give diversity as well as nutritional superiority to the product. Indian traditional foods, both fermented and unfermented, constitute the main component of daily diet giving diversity as well as ensuring the nutritional requirements of the individual. Food preservation has been in practice for many centuries spanning to early civilization (Tamang and Samuel, 2010). Preservation gives an opportunity to extend the shelf life of perishable as well as seasonal raw materials and also gives an opportunity to make a regional product to be transported to far-flung areas. Ancient food preservation methods are still practiced in India at the household as well as at the local level. These are practiced by using the traditional knowledge passed through generations. Traditionally, drying, pickling, dry salting, smoking, and fermentation are carried out to preserve all types of plant and animal resources such as fruits, vegetables, cereals, pulses, milk, fish, and meat. Fermentation is one of the oldest food-processing methods used since ancient time initiated either by the spontaneous and back-slop process. Asia in general and India, in particular, is home to a wide variety of traditional

Nutritional and Health Aspects of Food in South Asian Countries
DOI: https://doi.org/10.1016/B978-0-12-820011-7.00006-X

fermented foods. Fermented foods are known to give diversity, improve nutritional value, reduce antinutritional substances, and, more importantly, are known to be the sources of crucial probiotics (Tamang, 2010). Food preservation practices vary from region to region with the same substrate or with smaller variations in the raw materials used. This chapter focuses on traditional food preservation methods with respect to historical background, culture and traditions, and diversity as well as nutritional and health benefits.

5.2 Historical overview

Indian agriculture has been traditionally nonintensive and organic. Indian traditional and religious texts gave the highest importance to culinary aspects of food and also have linked the food and health, evidenced by documents such as *Nala's Pakashastra* and Indian system of medicines such as *Siddha*, where food is used as a principle for treating diseases (Sarkar et al., 2015).

Different preservation methods are employed during the ancient time to preserve perishable and seasonal foods by using simple methods. Postharvest processing and preservation have been minimal, limiting to drying, storage and manual milling of cereals and millets, manual processing of pulses, cold processing of oilseeds, and drying and pickling of vegetables and fruits. Indigenous structures such as *Bakhara* (made of wood), *Kanaja* (made of bamboo), *Kothi* (made of clay, wheat straw, and cow dung), *Sanduka* (wooden box storage structure), earthen pots, and *Gummi* (bamboo and mud-based structure) are used traditionally for storing and preserving the food grains since ancient period. These structures are made using locally available materials such as mud, bricks, cow dung, paddy and wheat straw, reeds, wooden logs, and bamboo sticks. Storage structures are constructed in various sizes and shape according to their region, climatic conditions, and function (Mann et al., 2016). Hand pounding is used for cereals and millets, which are known to preserve most of the essential nutrients. Since ancient times, parboiling of rice has been carried out in Southern India by steeping the paddy in hot water, steaming, drying until suitable moisture and milled. Traditionally, *Ghanis* (crude oil extracting equipment) is used for extracting the oil from oilseeds, and the *Kachighani* oils (crude oil extracted using *Ghani*) are considered to be rich in functional elements such as fatty acids and vitamins (Achaya, 1994). Interestingly, most of the traditional methods are coming back owing to their retention of nutrients and flavors.

Fermentation is one of the widely used traditional strategies for processing and preservation and also to bring diversity to the food products. Since ancient times, earthen pots are used for the fermentation process, as it imparts a unique flavor and texture to the fermented food (Samanta et al., 2011). During 6000–4000 BC period onwards, the usage of *Dahi* (homemade yogurt), fermented milk, which is recorded in Hindu's sacred books such as *Rig Veda* and *Upanishad* (Aiyar, 1953), is in practice. In 3000 BC, wide usage of buttermilk and butter are recorded in *Bhagavad-Gita* and

Vaishanavik literature. *Idli*, a popular fermented rice-black gram-based food of South India is cited by the poet Chavundaraya (during 1025 AD) (Iyengar, 1950). Another similar cereal–pulse-based food, *Dhokla*, the popular fermented breakfast food of Northern India prepared with rice and Bengal gram dhal is stated as early as 1066 AD (Prajapati and Nair, 2003). In Tamil Sangam literature from India during the sixth century, *Dosa*, a cofermented product of rice and dhal, is mentioned (Srinivasa, 1930). These citations take back the histological origin of some of the traditional fermented foods.

5.3 Culture and traditions

History of Indian civilization and religious texts such as the *Bhagavad-Gita, Ramayana*, and *Manusmriti* provide information that food culture forms an integral part of cultural heritage. India has one of the most divergent historic civilization rich in diversities of cultures and traditions. Variations are documented in customs, languages, cultural practices, ethnic wear, festive celebrations, food, and cuisine from region to region throughout the country. The beauty of India also lies in diversity in ethnicity and rich food culture (Asrani et al., 2019). It is well known for wide diversity for food culture including ethnic foods, traditionally preserved foods, ethnic fermented foods, and beverages (Rao et al., 2005; Sekar and Mariappan, 2007). Consumption of traditional foods is also in practice for many thousands of years even though the method of preparation varies from region to region. Religious ethnic foods play an important part in Indian food culture through a close link between traditional foods and religious festivals. Each ethnic group, as well as the religious subset, follows unique traditional food habits closely linked to the religious customs. Various environmental factors, availability of raw materials, geographical location, and preference to the food make the Indian ethnic food unique (Kwong and Tamang, 2015). There are specific traditional foods for different seasons, different health conditions, and age groups.

5.4 Traditional food preservation methods in India

In India, in spite of modernization, traditional practices are still being used in the villages. Drying, fermentation, pickling, dry salting, and smoking are some of the most common methods followed for preserving foods traditionally both in household and small- and medium-scale food industries, as these methods are easier, less expensive, and do not need modern infrastructure facilities (Fig. 5.1) (Tamang et al., 2016).

Drying is the processing of dehydrating foods by removing the moisture content to an extent that prevents microbial activity. Mostly, traditional drying is done under direct sunlight, and sometimes temperature control equipment is used. Fruits, vegetables, spices, legumes, nuts, meat, and seafood are traditionally preserved by sun drying (Sekar and Mariappan, 2007). Throughout India, dried fish products are famous and

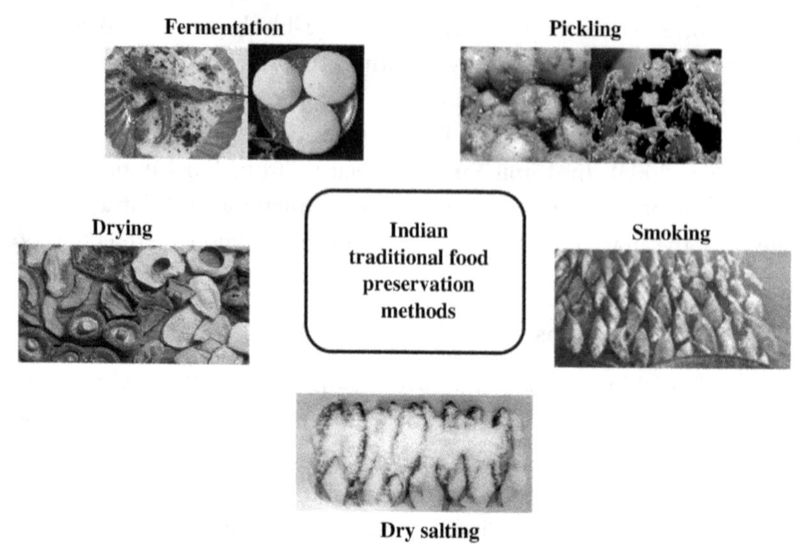

Figure 5.1 Traditional food preservation methods in India.

practiced since the ancient period by drying fishes under direct sun and wind for several days. The shelf life of this product varies from several months to a year, and it depends on the species used and is mostly done by fisherman families since the ancient period. The dried fish name varies from region to region, for example, *Sukho Bangdo* in Konkan region, *Karuvadu* in Tamil, *Suka masa* in Marathi. *Sidra* and *Sukuti* are sun-dried fish products in the North-Eastern part of India (Thapa, 2016). *Vadam*, the dried ground rice, and *Vathal*, the dried vegetable products, are common in South India. *Mormilagai*, a sun-dried chili, is prepared by soaking in buttermilk overnight and drying in sun for few days. This can be stored for many months in air-tight containers, and this type of preservation is also used for a few other vegetables such as bitter gourd and turkey berries. *Aampapad*, a dried mango pulp preserve, is prepared by spreading pulp on the sheet as thin film and rolled into shapes after drying.

The fermentation process is one of the most commonly used preservation technologies traditionally from ancient times. This process is carried out to improve the shelf life of the product, which also augments the digestibility, nutritive value, texture, taste, and aroma of the food (Tamang, 2015). Fermentation is done by either spontaneous or backslopping method, and mainly lactic acid bacteria, yeast, and some fungi are involved. In the backslopping method, traditionally people are using starters to prepare ethnic fermented foods in the Northeastern region of India, especially Sikkim and Meghalaya. *Marcha* and *Thiat* are some of the amylolytic starters that are used to prepare various ethnic fermented beverages and often sold in the market as starters. The technique of preparing these starters is a traditional practice that is still existing in these states and is a vital part of their sociocultural heritage; otherwise, it would disappear with time (Sha et al., 2017). Due to this cultural practice, now we are able to explore the microbial diversity scientifically of these starters that existed ethnically from many hundred years ago. Fermented foods are categorized widely based on the substrates used, viz. cereal- and/or pulse-based, fruits and vegetables, dairy, fish- and meat-based products. However, regionwise products differ in the preparation process and usage of substrates. Common traditional foods preserved by fermentation are discussed in subsequent "Typical food and food products" section. *Idli, Dosa, Dhokla, Bhatura, Misti, Dahi, Kadhi, Papad, Jalebis, Kinema, Khaman, Lassi, Vada, Grundruk,* and *Sinki* are widely consumed fermented foods in India (Rao et al., 2005; Savitri and Bhalla, 2007). *Ngari, Hentak, Tungtap,* and *Shidal* are fermented fish products of North Eastern India (Thapa, 2016).

Pickling is a process of preservation by anaerobic fermentation in brine, oil, or vinegar. Mostly vegetables and few fruits are preserved by this method. Mango, citrus fruits, and cucumbers are extensively preserved by pickling. Pickles also occupy a very important part in Indian meal as spicy condiments and appetizers. Different type of jars and clays are used for preparing pickles (Joshi and Bhat, 2000).

Dry salting, fermentation, or pickling techniques are used traditionally in India, as these do not involve any complicated process or expensive instruments. The lower salt concentration of 2%–5% encourages the fermentation process, while the higher salt concentration of around 20%–30% prevents the microbial activity, thereby preserving the food with its original freshness. Predominately, fishes are preserved by the dry salting method traditionally. Smoking is a process of preservation by exposing the food to wood smoke, thereby increasing the flavor, appearance, and shelf-life extension. Smoked fish and meat are ethnic foods of the north-eastern states of India done at the household level. *Karati, Bordia,* and *Lashim* are sun-dried and salted fish products, whereas *Suka ko maacha* and *Gnuchi* are ethnic smoked and dried fish products of the north-eastern states of India (Thapa, 2016).

5.5 Typical foods and food products

India is the center of diverse food culture showing variations within the same product in different locations and regions. Ethnic foods gain a significant role in diverse food culture involving both fermented and nonfermented foods and beverages. Ethnic fermented foods are unique foods of a particular ethnic group prepared by using the native knowledge transferred from generation to generation through their ancestors. Locally available materials are used for the fermentation by either natural or by the usage of starters containing functional microbiota (Tamang, 2010). Exhilarating feature of the Indian fermented food is known to possess functional traits leading to many health benefits apart from providing basic nutrition. Biological functions include the preservation of delicate nutrients, enhancement of nutritional values, bioavailability of minerals, and production of bioactive components such as antioxidants, enzymes,

Table 5.1 Traditional fermented foods of India.

Fermented foods	Substrate	Ethnic region	Nutritional/bioactive component/health benefits	Health benefits	References
Idli	Rice, black gram dal	Southern India	Rich in all essential amino acids Good source of soluble vitamins such as folate, vitamin A, B_1, B_2, and B_{12}, acetoin and volatile fatty acids	Acts as an antiobesity component and consumed for losing weight Dietary supplement for children with malnutrition and kwashiorkor Reduction toward the risk of high blood pressure, cardiovascular diseases, and stroke Micronutrients such as calcium, folate, iron, and zinc help in the prevention of anemia and enable the oxygenation of the blood thereby nourishing the bone and muscle. Dietary fiber along with carbohydrates supports good digestion and formation of bulky stools Substantial increase in the bioavailability of zinc (50%–71%) and iron (127%–277%) and protein content, and production of bioactive compounds such as thiamine, methionine, choline, and riboflavin	Blandino et al. (2003), Ghosh and Chattopadhyay (2011), Hemalatha et al. (2007), Joshi et al. (1989), Purushothaman et al. (1993), and Ray et al. (2016)
Kinema	Soybean	North Eastern India	48% protein per 100 g dry matter; 8 mg thiamine, 12 mg riboflavin, and 45 mg niacin per kg dry matter; rich in phenolic acids, linoleic acid, essential fatty acid and phytosterol, rich in polyglutamic acid.	Cholesterol reducing property	Sarkar et al. (1996, 1998), and Tamang (1992, 2015)

Tungrymbai	Soybean	North Eastern India	45.9% protein per 100 g dry matter; carotene (212.7 μg/100 g) and folic acid (200 μg/100 g)	–	Agrahar-Murugkar and Subbulakshmi (2006) and Tamang (1992)
Hawaijar	Soybean	North Eastern India	26%–27% soluble proteins	Possess medicinal properties such as antiosteoporosis, anticancer, and hypocholesterolemic effects	Somishon and Thahira Banu (2013), and Thingom and Chhetry (2011)
Gundruk	Mustard leaf	North Eastern India	Rich in free amino acids such as glutamic acid, alanine, leucine, lysine, and threonine; rich in organic acids such as lactic, acetic, citric, and malic acids. It also possesses a fine quantity of ascorbic acid, carotene and palmitic, oleic, linoleic, and linolenic acids	Good appetizer, Higher levels of carotene with anticancer properties Induces milk production in mothers	Tamang et al. (2005), Tamang and Tamang, (2010)
Soibum	Bamboo shoot	North Eastern India	Abundant essential amino acids, vitamins, minerals, and fatty acids	Higher phenolic compounds and tannins, and possess antioxidants, anticancer, and antiaging properties	Giri and Janmejay (2000), Jeyaram et al. (2010), Tamang and Tamang, (2009), and Thakur et al. (2016)
Dahi	Milk	All over India	Potential source of vitamin B complex, folic acid, riboflavin, and bioactive compounds such as diacetyl, hydrogen peroxide, and reuterin, bioactive peptide (ACE-I peptide)	Substantially hinders the fall of glucose intolerance, thereby signifying the reduction in risk of diabetes; suppress the growth of undesirable flora such as *E. coli, Bacillus subtilis*, and *Staphylococcus aureus*	Ashar and Chand (2004), Sarkar and Misra (2001), Sharma and Lal (1997), and Yadav et al. (2007)

(*Continued*)

Table 5.1 (Continued)

Fermented foods	Substrate	Ethnic region	Nutritional/bioactive component/health benefits	Health benefits	References
Yogurt	Milk	Northern India	Minerals such as calcium, phosphorus, magnesium, potassium, and proteins function together to build up strong healthy bones	–	Chandan and Kilara (2013)
Lassi	Milk	North India	Possess 8 antioxidant peptides and 14 bioactive peptides	–	Padghan et al. (2017)
Sour rice	Rice	South India	Rich source of vitamin B complex, vitamin K, and minerals such as sodium, potassium, and calcium	Energy rehydrating food; prevents constipation by controlling the bowel movement; maintains the beneficial intestinal microflora Prevents gastrointestinal ailments such as celiac disease, duodenal ulcers, Crohn's disease, candida infection, irritable bowel syndrome, infectious ulcerative colitis	Choi et al. (2014) and Ray et al. (2016)
Dhokla	Rice and Bengal gram dhal	Western and Northern India	50% increase in thiamine and riboflavin content; a rich source of acetoin and volatile fatty acids	Lower glycemic index suitable for diabetic individuals; help in managing age-related diseases and oxidative stress-induced degenerative diseases	Joshi et al. (1989), Ray et al. (2016), and Roy et al. (2009)
Porridge	Pearl millet	South India	Enrichment of ferulic acid		Palaniswamy and Govindaswamy (2016)

Dosa	Rice and dehusked black gram	South India	Substantial increase in the levels of total acids, free amino acids, enzymes, vitamins, folic acid, antimicrobial and antioxidant ingredients	Improves the bioavailability of zinc and iron Helps in managing pre- and postdiabetic conditions due to its lower glycemic load and glycemic index levels Believed to help in increasing fertility, fetus weight, and breast milk. Provides sufficient energy for extended physical stamina and helps in the treatment of rheumatism and neural disorders Cofermentation of finger millet and horse gram and/or pearl millet in *dosa* batter significantly enriches the dietary fiber, calcium, and iron content and also enhances flavor, aroma, and appealing qualities	Blandino et al. (2003), Chelliah et al. (2017), Gupta and Tiwari (2014), and Palanisamy et al. (2012)
Ambali	Finger millet	South India	–	Highly suitable for infants due to its easy digestibility, rich protein, low resistant starch, and high calcium content Increased levels of vitamins and tryptophan, reduced leucine to lysine conversion, and bioavailability of minerals	Mangala et al. (1999), Mbithi-Mwikya et al. (2000), and Kumar et al. (2013)
Hentakis	Fermented fish	Manipur	–	Good for women during the late pregnancy stages or persons retrieving from illness or wounds	Sarojnalini and Vishwanath (1988)
Chyang	Finger millet	Himalayan region	–	Recommended for postpartum to boost their internal strength	Thapa and Tamang (2004)
Ngari	Fermented fish	Manipur	Protein (34.1%), fat (13.2%), carbohydrate (31.6%), Ca (41.7 mg/100 g), Fe (0.9 mg/100 g), Mg (0.8 mg/100 g), Mn (0.6 mg/100 g), and Zn (1.7 mg/100 g)	–	Thapa et al. (2007)

bioactive peptides, and nutraceuticals. Long-term consumption of these foods is reported to impart health benefits such as lowered cholesterol levels, antiatherosclerotic, anticarcinogenic, antidiabetic, antidiarrheal, antiallergic, and immunomodulatory properties (Hotz and Gibson, 2007; Tamang et al., 2012; Sarkar et al., 2015). Fermentation microflora in ethnic foods is also known to have probiotic and prebiotic properties. Another interesting feature of fermented foods is that it aids in the management of beneficial microorganisms in the gut leading to better defense against pathogens and positively modulating the gut–brain axis of the host (Tamang, 2015; Ray et al., 2016). A list of important fermented foods and their nutritional composition and health benefits are detailed in Table 5.1.

5.6 Future outlook

Traditional foods have a strong place in the Indian food plate. Many of these traditionally processed and fermented food products have been consumed for centuries in spite of influences of modern lifestyle and onslaught of westernization. With the passing time, more and more health benefits of traditional foods are being documented and their benefits with respect to the management of metabolic disorders are becoming apparent. Traditional foods are now getting more relevant in the modern food plate and rapidly being identified as health foods. India with diverse traditional foods and recipes can be harvested commercially as health foods for satisfying the rapidly developing market of health and functional foods in the world. There is an urgent need for the documentation of traditional foods that are consumed regionally by small ethnic groups and in-depth studies into the nutritional and health beneficial properties of these products.

References

Achaya, K.T., 1994. *Ghani*: a traditional method of oil processing in India. Food Nutr. Agric. 4, 23.

Agrahar-Murugkar, D., Subbulakshmi, G., 2006. Preparation techniques and nutritive value of fermented foods from the *Khasi* tribes of Meghalaya. Ecol. Food Nutr. 45, 27–38. Available from: https://doi.org/10.1080/03670240500408336.

Aiyar, A.K.Y.N., 1953. Dairying in ancient India. Indian Dairyman 5, 77–83.

Ashar, M.N., Chand, R., 2004. Antihypertensive peptides purified from milks fermented with *Lactobacillus delbrueckii spp. bulgaricus*. Milchwissenschaft 59, 14–17.

Asrani, P., Patial, V., Asrani, R.K., 2019. Production of fermented beverages: shedding light on Indian culture and traditions. Production and Management of Beverages. Woodhead Publishing, pp. 409–437.

Blandino, A., Al-Aseeri, M.E., Pandiella, S.S., Cantero, D., Webb, C., 2003. Cereal-based fermented foods and beverages. Food Res. Int. 36, 527–543. Available from: https://doi.org/10.1016/S0963-9969(03)00009-7.

Chandan, R.C., Kilara, A. (Eds.), 2013. Manufacturing Yogurt and Fermented Milks. second ed. John Wiley & Sons, Chichester, West Sussex, UK.

Chelliah, R., Ramakrishnan, S.R., Premkumar, D., Antony, U., 2017. Accelerated fermentation of *Idli* batter using *Eleusine coracana* and *Pennisetum glaucum*. J. Food Sci. Technol. 54, 2626–2637. Available from: https://doi.org/10.1007/s13197-017-2621-9.

Choi, J.S., Kim, J.W., Cho, H.R., Kim, K.Y., Lee, J.K., Ku, S.K., et al., 2014. Laxative effects of fermented rice extract (FRe) in normal rats. Toxicol. Environ. Health Sci. 6, 155–163. Available from: https://doi.org/10.1007/s13530-014-0200-2.

Ghosh, D., Chattopadhyay, P., 2011. Preparation of *Idli* batter, its properties and nutritional improvement during fermentation. J. Food Sci. Technol. 48, 610–615. Available from: https://doi.org/10.1007/s13197-010-0148-4.

Giri, S.S., Janmejay, L.S., 2000. Effect of bamboo shoot fermentation and aging on nutritional and sensory qualities of *Soibum*. J. Food Sci. Technol. 37, 423–426.

Gupta, A., Tiwari, S.K., 2014. Probiotic potential of *Lactobacillus plantarum* LD1 isolated from batter of *Dosa*, a south Indian fermented food. Probiotics Antimicrob. Proteins 6, 73–81. Available from: https://doi.org/10.1007/s12602-014-9158-2.

Hemalatha, S., Platel, K., Srinivasan, K., 2007. Influence of germination and fermentation on bioaccessibility of zinc and iron from food grains. Eur. J. Clin. Nutr. 61, 342. Available from: https://doi.org/10.1038/sj.ejcn.1602524.

Hotz, C., Gibson, R.S., 2007. Traditional food-processing and preparation practices to enhance the bioavailability of micronutrients in plant-based diets. J. Nutr. 137, 1097–1100. Available from: https://doi.org/10.1093/jn/137.4.1097.

Iyengar, S.H., 1950. Lokopakara of Chavundarava. Oriental Manuscripts Library, Madras, India, pp. 120–134.

Jeyaram, K., Romi, W., Singh, T.A., Devi, A.R., Devi, S.S., 2010. Bacterial species associated with traditional starter cultures used for fermented bamboo shoot production in Manipur state of India. Int. J. Food Microbiol. 143, 1–8. Available from: https://doi.org/10.1016/j.ijfoodmicro.2010.07.008.

Joshi, V.K., Bhat, A., 2000. Pickles: technology of its preparation. In: Verma, L.R., Joshi, V.K. (Eds.), Postharvest Technology of Fruits and Vegetables, vol. 2. The Indus Publ., New Delhi, pp. 777–820.

Joshi, N., Godbole, S.H., Kanekar, P., 1989. Microbial and biochemical changes during *dhokla* fermentation with special reference to flavour compounds. J. Food Sci. Technol. 26, 113–115.

Kumar, R.S., Kanmani, P., Yuvaraj, N., Paari, K.A., Pattukumar, V., Arul, V., 2013. Traditional Indian fermented foods: a rich source of lactic acid bacteria. Int. J. Food. Sci. Nutr. 64, 415–428. Available from: https://doi.org/10.3109/09637486.2012.746288.

Kwon, D.Y., Tamang, J.P., 2015. Religious ethnic foods. J. Ethnic Foods 2, 45–46. Available from: https://doi.org/10.1016/j.jef.2015.05.001.

Mangala, S.L., Malleshi, N.G., Tharanathan, R.N., 1999. Resistant starch from differently processed rice and ragi (finger millet). Eur. Food Res. Technol. 209, 32–37. Available from: https://doi.org/10.1007/s002170050452.

Mann, S., Dixit, A.K., Tushir, S., Bashir, A.A., 2016. Traditional grain storage practices in India: SWOT analysis. In: Navarro, S., Jayas, D.S., Alagusundaram, K. (Eds.), Proceedings of the 10th International Conference on Controlled Atmosphere and Fumigation in Stored Products (CAF2016). CAF Permanent Committee Secretariat, Winnipeg, Canada, pp. 500–503.

Mbithi-Mwikya, S., Ooghe, W., Van Camp, J., Ngundi, D., Huyghebaert, A., 2000. Amino acid profiles after sprouting, autoclaving, and lactic acid fermentation of finger millet (*Eleusine coracana*) and kidney beans (*Phaseolus vulgaris* L.). J. Agric. Food. Chem. 48, 3081–3085. Available from: https://doi.org/10.1021/jf0002140.

Padghan, P.V., Mann, B., Sharma, R., Bajaj, R., Saini, P., 2017. Production of angiotensin-I-converting-enzyme-inhibitory peptides in fermented milks (*Lassi*) fermented by *Lactobacillus acidophillus* with consideration of incubation period and simmering treatment. Int. J. Pept. Res. Ther. 23, 69–79. Available from: https://doi.org/10.1007/s10989-016-9540-x.

Palanisamy, B.D., Rajendran, V., Sathyaseelan, S., Bhat, R., Venkatesan, B.P., 2012. Enhancement of nutritional value of finger millet-based food (Indian *dosa*) by co-fermentation with horse gram flour. Int. J. Food. Sci. Nutr. 63, 5–15. Available from: https://doi.org/10.3109/09637486.2011.591367.

Palaniswamy, S.K., Govindaswamy, V., 2016. *In-vitro* probiotic characteristics assessment of feruloyl esterase and glutamate decarboxylase producing *Lactobacillus* spp. isolated from traditional fermented millet porridge (*kambu koozh*). LWT-Food Sci. Technol. 68, 208–216. Available from: https://doi.org/10.1016/j.lwt.2015.12.024.

Prajapati, J.B., Nair, B.M., 2003. The history of fermented foods. In: Farnworth, R. (Ed.), Handbook of Fermented Functional Foods. CRC Press, New York, pp. 1–25.

Purushothaman, D., Dhanapal, N., Rangaswami, G., 1993. Indian *idli, dosa, dhokla, khaman* and related fermentations. Handbook of Indigenous Fermented Foods. Marcel Dekker, New York, pp. 149–165.

Rao, R.E., Vijayendra, S.V.N., Varadaraj, M.C., 2005. Fermentation biotechnology of traditional foods of the Indian subcontinent. In: Shetty, K., Paliyath, G., Pometto, A., Levin, R.E. (Eds.), Food Biotechnology, second ed. CRC Press Taylor and Francis, Boca Raton, FL, pp. 1759–1794.

Ray, M., Ghosh, K., Singh, S., Mondal, K.C., 2016. Folk to functional: An explorative overview of rice-based fermented foods and beverages in India. J. Ethnic Foods 3, 5–18. Available from: https://doi.org/10.1016/j.jef.2016.02.002.

Roy, A., Moktan, B., Sarkar, P.K., 2009. Survival and growth of foodborne bacterial pathogens in fermenting batter of *dhokla*. J. Food Sci. Technol. 46, 132–135.

Samanta, A.K., Kolte, A.P., Senani, S., Sridhar, M., Jayapal, N., 2011. Prebiotics in ancient Indian diets. Curr. Sci. 101, 43–46.

Sarkar, S., Misra, A.K., 2001. Bio-preservation of milk and milk products. Indian Food Ind. 20, 74–77.

Sarkar, P.K., Jones, L.J., Gore, W., Craven, G.S., 1996. Changes in soya bean lipid profiles during kinema production. J. Sci. Food Agric. 71, 321–328. Available from: https://doi.org/10.1002/(SICI)1097-0010(199607)71. 3<321::AID-JSFA587>3.0.CO;2-J.

Sarkar, P.K., Morrison, E., Tingii, U., Somerset, S.M., Craven, G.S., 1998. B-group vitamin and mineral contents of soybeans during *kinema* production. J. Sci. Food Agric. 78, 498–502. Available from: https://doi.org/10.1002/(SICI)1097-0010(199812)78. 4<498::AID-JSFA145>3.0.CO;2-C.

Sarkar, P., Lokith Kumar, D.H., Dhumal, C., Panigrahi, S.S., Choudhary, R., 2015. Traditional and ayurvedic foods of Indian origin. J. Ethnic Foods 2, 97–109. Available from: https://doi.org/10.1016/j.jef.2015.08.003.

Sarojnalini, C., Vishwanath, W., 1988. Composition and digestibility of fermented fish foods of Manipur. J. Food Sci. Technol. 25, 349–351.

Savitri, Bhalla, T.C., 2007. Traditional foods and beverages of Himachal Pradesh. Indian J. Tradit. Knowl. 6, 17–24. <http://nopr.niscair.res.in/handle/123456789/815>.

Sekar, S., Mariappan, S., 2007. Usage of traditional fermented products by Indian rural folks and IPR. Indian J. Tradit. Knowl. 6, 111–120. <http://nopr.niscair.res.in/handle/123456789/840>.

Sha, S.P., Jani, K., Sharma, A., Anupma, A., Pradhan, P., Shouche, Y., et al., 2017. Analysis of bacterial and fungal communities in *Marcha* and *Thiat*, traditionally prepared amylolytic starters of India. Sci. Rep. 7, 10967. Available from: https://doi.org/10.1038/s41598-017-11609-y.

Sharma, R., Lal, D., 1997. Effect of *dahi* preparation on some water-soluble vitamins. Indian J. Dairy Sci. 50, 318–320.

Somishon, K., Thahira Banu, A., 2013. *Hawaijar* – a fermented Soya of Manipur, India: review. IOSR J. Environ. Sci. Toxicol. Food Technol. 4, 29–33.

Srinivasa, P.T.I., 1930. Pre-Aryan Tamil Culture. University of Madras, Madras, India, pp. 57–70.

Tamang, J.P., 1992. Studies on the Microflora of Some Traditional Fermented Foods of Darjeeling Hills and Sikkim. North Bengal University, Darjeeling (Doctoral dissertation, Ph.D. Thesis.

Tamang, J.P., 2010. Diversity of fermented foods. In: Tamang, J.P., Kailasapathy, K. (Eds.), Fermented Foods and Beverages of the World. CRC Press/Taylor & Francis Group, New York, pp. 41–84.

Tamang, J.P. (Ed.), 2015. Health Benefits of Fermented Foods and Beverages. CRC Press, New York.

Tamang, B., Tamang, J.P., 2009. Traditional knowledge of biopreservation of perishable vegetable and bamboo shoots in Northeast India as food resources. Indian J. Tradit. Knowl. 8, 89–95. <http://nopr.niscair.res.in/handle/123456789/2978>.

Tamang, B., Tamang, J.P., 2010. In situ fermentation dynamics during production of *gundruk* and *khalpi*, ethnic fermented vegetable products of the Himalayas. Indian J. Microbiol. 50, 93–98. Available from: https://doi.org/10.1007/s12088-010-0058-1.

Tamang, J.P., Samuel, D., 2010. Dietary culture and antiquity of fermented foods and beverages. In: Tamang, J.P., Kailasapathy, K. (Eds.), Fermented Foods and Beverages of the World. CRC Press/ Taylor & Francis Group, New York, pp. 1–40.

Tamang, J.P., Tamang, B., Schillinger, U., Franz, C.M., Gores, M., Holzapfel, W.H., 2005. Identification of predominant lactic acid bacteria isolated from traditionally fermented vegetable products of the Eastern Himalayas. Int. J. Food Microbiol. 105, 347–356. Available from: https://doi.org/10.1016/j.ijfoodmicro.2005.04.024.

Tamang, J.P., Tamang, N., Thapa, S., Devan, S., Tamang, B., Yonzan, H., et al., 2012. Microorganisms and nutritional value of ethnic fermented foods and alcoholic beverages of north east India. Indian J. Tradit. Knowl. 11, 7–25. <http://nopr.niscair.res.in/handle/123456789/13415>.

Tamang, J.P., Thapa, N., Bhalla, T.C., Savitri, 2016. Ethnic fermented foods and beverages of India. In: Tamang, J.P. (Ed.), Ethnic Fermented Foods and Alcoholic Beverages of Asia. Springer, New Delhi, India, pp. 17–72.

Thakur, K., Rajani, C.S., Tomar, S.K., Panmei, A., 2016. Fermented bamboo shoots: a riche niche for beneficial microbes. J. Bacteriol. Mycol. 2, 87–93. Available from: https://doi.org/10.15406/jbmoa.2016.02.00030.

Thapa, N., 2016. Ethnic fermented and preserved fish products of India and Nepal. J. Ethnic Foods 3, 69–77. Available from: https://doi.org/10.1016/j.jef.2016.02.003.

Thapa, S., Tamang, J.P., 2004. Product characterization of *kodo ko jaanr*: fermented finger millet beverage of the Himalayas. Food Microbiol. 21, 617–622. Available from: https://doi.org/10.1016/j.fm.2004.01.004.

Thapa, N., Pal, J., Tamang, J.P., 2007. Microbiological profile of dried fish products of Assam. Indian J. Fish. 54, 121–125.

Thingom, P., Chhetry, G., 2011. Nutritional analysis of fermented soybean (*Hawaijar*). Assam Univ. J. Sci. Technol. 7, 96–100.

Yadav, H., Jain, S., Sinha, P.R., 2007. Antidiabetic effect of probiotic dahi containing *Lactobacillus acidophilus* and *Lactobacillus casei* in high fructose fed rats. Nutrition 23, 62–68. Available from: https://doi.org/10.1016/j.nut.2006.09.002.

CHAPTER 6

The dietary practices and food-related rituals in Indian tradition and their role in health and nutrition

Jamuna Prakash
Ambassador for India, Global Harmonisation Initiative, Vienna, Austria

Contents

6.1 Introduction

Indian civilization is one of the oldest civilizations found on earth and can be traced back to nearly 10,000 years with documentary evidence in support of its vibrant tradition and culture. Among the various South Asian cultures, India stands different due to a diverse dietary pattern and existence of vegetarianism. The present-day Indian food patterns evolved over thousands of years following the paleolithic ages of using stone tools for killing animals, use of fire for cooking, agriculture, domesticating animals, and fabricating metal weapons and artifacts for various purposes as in other parts of the world. Documentary evidence in the form of ancient scriptures, cave paintings, and excavated artifacts give us information regarding the various types of foods available, trading, cooking methods, distribution among people, foods to be offered to

Nutritional and Health Aspects of Food in South Asian Countries
DOI: https://doi.org/10.1016/B978-0-12-820011-7.00007-1

Gods, etc. (Achaya, 1994; Narasinga Rao, 2005). Dietary practices and food culture were intricately woven into the fabric of religion to ensure compliance. Food was given prominence in every celebration and was an integral part of many rituals and customs. Offering water and food to God and guests was a rich tradition that continued even today. Vegetarianism has been very unique to Indian culture as well as many beliefs of food avoidances and recommendations for special conditions such as infancy, pregnancy, lactation, and sickness signifying that these were recognized as vulnerable periods requiring extra care. Dietary diversification advocated by modern scientists to make the diet nutritionally richer was being practiced fervently and still continues. The very ritual of eating had many do's and don'ts designed to follow optimum hygiene during food preparation and serving. This chapter discusses some of these aspects of Indian traditional dietary practices in the light of health and nutrition.

6.2 Dietary practices

6.2.1 Vegetarianism

The concept of vegetarianism seems to have originated from India with strong followers in different communities. From earlier evidence, it is clear that during the Harappan civilization and Vedic period meat-eating was practiced and it is only later that meat-eating was looked down upon. In earlier documents, at least 50 different animals have been referred to which were used for sacrifice and there is also a mention of domestic rearing of cattle. There are specific instructions for the slaughtering of animals, distribution of meat, and cooking of meat (Auboyer, 1965, Raychaudhari, 1964, Iyengar, 1912, Kosambi, 1975, Ghurye, 1979). In fact, as stated in the "Ramayana" (an old religious epic), rice cooked with deer meat and spices was the favorite food of Sita (wife of Lord Rama, the legendary King of Ayodhya) (Ghosh, 1976). There may have been two reasons for the emergence of vegetarianism. The early Aryan started questioning the "taking of life" or "killing" for humanitarian reasons. With the spread of Buddhism and Jainism, which advocated nonviolence in any form, these beliefs became stronger and were adopted by the royalties (Horner, 1945). Another reason could have been an abundance of food grains due to planned agriculture and settled civilizations making meat a nonessential item of the meal. Both Harappan and Indus valley civilizations provide adequate evidence for the storage of grains that nearly eliminated the essentiality of meat for everyday diets as recorded by Achaya in his beautiful treatise on the history of Indian foods (Achaya, 1994).

At present, a significant Indian population follows vegetarianism, though the consumption of animal foods is gradually increasing. Vegetarians can either be lacto-vegetarians (consuming dairy products and plant foods) or lacto-ovo-vegetarians (consuming dairy products, eggs, and plant foods). Nearly 29% of the population is lacto-vegetarian, while the rest consume animal foods, though with restrictions (SRS, 2014). In a very strict sense, even among nonvegetarians, the amount eaten may be small or infrequent due to prohibitive cost and self-imposed restrictions on account of religious beliefs. On certain days of the week or certain calendar days, meat foods are not allowed. Plant foods are by far much cheaper and affordable.

Vegetarianism can be associated with two distinct positive influences, one on health and the other, on the environment. The potential health benefits of vegetarian diets and a reduction of risk for many chronic degenerative diseases and total mortality have been documented in many studies during the last three decades (ADA, 2009). A systemic review by McEvoy et al. (2012) brings out the pros and cons of vegetarian diets concluding that vegetarians by far have lower rates of obesity, cardiovascular diseases, and lower lipid levels. A well-balanced diet should take care of possible vitamin deficiencies. Vegetarians have a much larger variety of foods to choose from and diets are varied. Generally, Indian traditional diets are a combination of cereals, pulses, vegetables, dairy foods, and nuts.

The food system is responsible for more than a quarter of all greenhouse gas emissions, while unhealthy diets and high body weight are among the greatest contributors to premature mortality. Industrialized agriculture and mass animal production is associated with various negative influences on the environment and health. Vegetarian diets protect the environment, reduce pollution, and minimize global climate changes (Leitzman, 2003). Springmann et al. (2016) in their analysis of health and climate change cobenefits of global dietary changes for major regions of the world report that as the fraction of animal-sourced foods in our diets is lowered, higher benefits are gained. Transitioning toward more plant-based diets that are in line with standard dietary guidelines could reduce global mortality by 6%–10% and food-related greenhouse gas emissions by 29%–70% by 2050 amounting to an estimated economic benefit of 1–31 trillion US dollars. The water footprints of producing animal meat are also very high and can become a major concern in the future. For example, the water needed to grow 1 kg of food in liters is around 3400 for rice, 1600 for maize, 1300 for bread (wheat) in comparison to beef requiring 15,500, chicken 3900, and pork 4800 L. Vegetables need much lesser: tomato, 180, potato, 250, and cabbage, 200 L per kg. Coarse grains (which were being used traditionally in India) require only one-fourth of water required by rice and wheat for production. Hence, overall, vegetarian diets impose less water stress on the environment (Chapagain and Hoekstra, 2004; Hoestra, 2008).

6.2.2 Recognizing food for their health-promoting properties

Indian culture also offers certain beliefs regarding food, which were handed down from generation to generation. Foods were associated with many medicinal properties, and at times used for curing a disease. For example, foods are classified as having digestive properties, for immune functions, to support growth and development, for energy, for cognitive performances, etc. A detailed description of dietary advice for different disease conditions is also available (Ksemasarma, 2009). Another notable belief was regarding "hot" and "cold" foods. This seems to have been developed during Indo-Aryans and was integrated with the theory of ill-health through a humoral imbalance. This belief seems to have made its way around the world in the course of time. It was deeply entrenched in patterns of seasons, temperature, and geographical locations. Thus a "hot" food of one region may be considered as "cold" of another. Although scientific evidence of such beliefs is lacking, these had a basis of observational concept and a systematic investigation could tell us of their veracity. Another food belief revolves around the foods avoided during vulnerable conditions such as pregnancy, lactation, and sickness. In rural Karnataka, a state in Southern India, the foods avoided during pregnancy are papaya, drumstick leaves, and egg. During lactation, there are a number of foods that are prohibited such as cowpea, potato, brinjal, pumpkin, cold fruits (banana, guava), jackfruit, and papaya. These are linked to the health of newborns. Although there is no scientific basis at present for the avoidance of these foods, the beliefs could have stemmed from certain food allergies or body adaptation to new food in individual cases.

A document written during the 17th century compiling all the available knowledge on therapeutic properties of various foods, as well as the method of preparing dishes from different sources, is a valuable source of knowledge and beliefs pervading at that time and also serves as an authentic source of information (Raghunathsuri, 2012). For example, general therapeutic properties of milk are described as conducive, tasty, unctuous, alleviates "vata" and "pitta" (humoral imbalances as described in Ayurveda, the ancient medical science of India; good for complexion, intellect, growth and nourishment; can be used as an aphrodisiac; is heavy to digest, confers strength, cures tiredness, giddiness, cough, dyspnea and hunger. This is followed by a description of the properties of milk obtained from different animals such as sheep, goat, elephant, camel, and donkey. Further, it also elaborates on how the properties of cow's milk would differ depending on the color of the cow, time of consumption, mode of consumption, time of parturition, etc. Modern science is yet to understand these; however, the compositional differences in milk based on the time of parturition is well known. Recent research also shows that depending upon species of cow, the properties of milk differ as is the case with so-called A1 and A2 milk originating from different species of a cow with different protein structures and the consequent effect on health (Boro et al., 2016).

6.2.3 Dietary diversification

Dietary diversification is considered as a food-based approach to treat malnutrition (Frison et al., 2006). This was being practiced by incorporating a variety of food in the diet. The traditional diet pattern depended on the availability of food, following the cycles of seasons and limited to geographical locations. Man was forced to eat whatever was available, so diets were diversified. The dietary diversity in India is symbolized by significant regional differences in diet patterns. Although the basic structure of diet may remain similar, comprising cereals, pulses, vegetables, milk products, and animal foods, the type of cereals or legume used, the methods of cooking, and the spice combinations vary greatly among regions. However, all diets contribute to a healthy proportion of carbohydrates, proteins, and fats. In the coastal region, we observe a dominance of seafood. India is blessed with nearly 8000 km of the sea coast, where the staple foods are mostly rice and fish, fish being an important source of protein. Legumes or beans are used in lesser quantities. Coastal areas of Kerala, Karnataka, and Tamil Nadu use coconut in cooking abundantly. As we move inland, there are mixtures of cereals and millets used with varieties of legumes. Among cereals, rice, finger millet, and sorghum predominate in Southern states while wheat is the staple in Northern states. Pearl millet is used as a staple in Western India. Vegetables are used depending upon the type grown in local areas. The type of oil used traditionally also differed considerably. The state of Kerala predominantly used coconut oil (which is still common), while Tamil Nadu used gingelly oil. Groundnut oil was used more in Karnataka, Andhra Pradesh, and Gujarat, while Eastern states used mustard oil. The traditionally used oils are now being replaced with other new arrivals such as sunflower, palm, and rice bran oil.

From the nutritional point of view, the diversity of foods has been a significant feature of traditional dietary patterns. For instance, in rural Karnataka, the practice of eating locally available mixed green leafy vegetables that grow naturally in fields with other crops is very common. They are the best examples of dietary diversification not only because of their nutritive value but also because of many health-promoting properties, which have been documented in the literature (Wealth of India, 1992). Nutritional analysis of these green leafy vegetables revealed that, in general, they were rich sources of many nutrients, some being exceptionally rich in iron (*Celosia argentea*, *Centella asiatica*, *Amaranthus tricolor*, and *Digera arvensis*), calcium (*D. arvensis*, *Boerhaavia diffusa*, *Cucurbita maxima*, and *A. tricolor*), magnesium and zinc (*C. asiatica*), and copper (*Delonix elata*, *C. asiatica*, *B. diffusa*, and *Cocculus hirsutus*). These were also very rich sources of total and β-carotene as other conventional greens (Gupta et al., 2005; 2006).

6.2.4 Foods in natural form

With advances in food technology, the amount of processed foods available has increased tremendously. Within an Indian context, this brought about a major change in the type of food eaten during the last 50 years. Although processing has its advantages, it also offers food in a refined form. For example, rice was primarily used in the unpolished form (hand-pounded every day for domestic consumption because of low keeping quality) until about a century ago before the introduction of mechanized paddy hullers. This way, the inherent nutrition of rice grain, was being utilized in totality. Modern technology gave us white polished rice, which is easy to cook, but devoid of many essential nutrients (Gopalan et al., 1996). The separated rice bran is used for extraction of oil, the nutritional virtues of which are well documented (Orthoefer, 2005, Prasad et al., 2011). Refined oils are odorless, colorless with a long shelf life but are also devoid of many natural constituents extracted in crude oil. Roller milling of wheat is a technical marvel but removes the bran and germ, which are most nutritious parts of the grain (Oghbaei and Prakash, 2013, 2016). Processed foods are best when presented in natural form, that is, without removing any edible part of the food. The traditional meal patterns were healthier because of the inclusion of unrefined foods.

6.3 Food consumption patterns

6.3.1 Dietary patterns

Discovery of nutrients, their physiological functions, requirements, and deficiencies were the foundations of modern nutrition science. These were the basis of determining nutrient intakes and subsequently, for foods to be included in daily diets to obtain all the required nutrients. For Indians, the recommended dietary allowances (ICMR, 2010) and food composition database are also available (Gopalan et al., 1996; Longvah et al., 2017). On comparing the present-day recommendations of food intake and what is prescribed in the ancient text, it is evident that the amounts and kinds of food recommended in the ancient literature must have been based on very rightful observations and are similar to today's balanced diets. Notable is the fact that foods from all groups (cereals, pulses, fruits, vegetables, nuts, sugar, fats, and meat) were recommended. The *Arthashastra* of Kautilya recommended a gentleman's meal to be containing the following: pure unbroken rice—1 prastha (454 g), pulses—1/4 prastha (114 g), *ghee* (clarified butter) —1/6 prastha (77 g), and salt—1/64 prastha (7 g) (Shamashastry, 1967). Except for the higher amount of *ghee*, other recommendations are nutritionally comparable to present recommendations, guidelines for a desirable meal for a man (moderate physical work) suggest an intake of 450 g of cereals, 90 g of pulses, and 30 g of oil/ghee per day (NIN, 2011). A higher amount of ghee prescribed in older document could also be accepted on the fact that the physical activities would have been to a much higher extent allowing higher energy intakes, there was no other source of added fats in diets and foods were unrefined.

6.3.2 Food preparation protocols and etiquettes of eating

The womenfolk of the household were generally responsible for cooking and serving meals, a practice continued even today. The menfolk, elders, and children of the home are served first followed by the women partaking the meal. A meal is always to be taken in a comfortable squatting position (sitting on the floor), which signifies a stress-free environment and consuming the right quantities of food as well as enjoying a meal. Meals are always eaten together emphasizing the family eating together and never in isolation.

There have been certain suggestions of the order of serving dishes in each culture. The sweets are served first or in between the meal followed by other foods. Scientifically, this practice is beneficial because of the sugar being washed off in the mouth with other food; hence, protection from dental caries. It is possible that consuming sugar, in the beginning, raises the blood glucose level quickly giving a feeling of satiety; hence, overeating could be avoided. The meals were to be ended with drinks (water or beverages) and chewing of betel leaves (a practice, which possibly aids in secretion and action of digestive enzymes) (Prabhu et al., 1995). The concept of hygiene and sanitation must have been very well understood, and strict adherence would conform to the standard of modern hazard analysis and critical control point. The person responsible for cooking was required to bathe and wear clean clothes. Only he/she handled entire cooking and serving, with nobody being allowed to touch them in the process or the food thereby limiting any contamination. The cooked food was not carried outside the cooking/dining area. The drinking water was stored in clean copper vessels after filtering making it virtually organism free. The meal had to be prepared afresh every day, and eating of stale foods was not permitted. These practices certainly would have protected the inmates of a home from any foodborne pathogenic organism.

6.4 Cultural influences

6.4.1 Religion

Many dietary practices such as fasting and feasting were routed through religion for better compliance and acceptance without questioning. Certain calendar days were designated as fast days, wherein, eating was totally prohibited or certain types of foods were permitted. These practices differed based on the religious sects, each one laying down specific rules to be followed (Sethi and Jain, 2008). This was one way to rest the digestive organs, lower calorie intake, lower lipid levels, and also to have control over one's mind and body. Feasting was associated with the preparation of special foods on festivals and occasions for celebrations such as weddings, childbirth, and other events. Specifically, sweets were prepared on such occasions; hence, this is another example of dietary diversity signifying the inclusion of foods with different compositions (particularly with high energy and fat density) but only occasionally to avoid excessive intakes. The ritual of offering food to God before eating ensured food quality in terms of using the best of the ingredients available in pure form, and food prepared under hygienic conditions. This, in turn, ensured that the quality of food was maintained by everyone with no knowledge of quality parameters from a scientific point of view. In addition, as the food was prepared fresh every day for such a religious offering, there was no question of stored foods being used. This ensured no nutrient losses in foods due to storage and avoided intake of spoilt or contaminated foods.

6.4.2 Philosophy of life

Food was also a medium to understand the philosophy of life and brace human beings to face all situations in life. The new year as per the Hindu Lunar calendar is celebrated sometime during March/April in Southern Indian states with a mixture of jaggery (unrefined sugar), and neem flowers (*Azadirachta indica*) that are bitter in taste. This bitter + sweet mixture signifies good and bad or happy and sad events, which a person has to face in life on a continuous basis. For example, birth is a joyous occasion and death is a sad occasion, but we need to prepare for both events with equanimity. For every happy occasion, sweets are prepared and offered as human beings primarily like the sweet taste, and hence it enhances the pleasurable feeling. The festival of "*Sankranti*" celebrated during the months of January signifies new harvest season; hence, a nutrient-dense mixture of sesame seeds, jaggery, groundnuts, dry coconut, and chickpea is shared with everyone with a saying—"*Eat this sweet and let your tongue always have good words for everyone.*" Hence food also becomes a driver of good behavior for harmonious living in society.

6.4.3 Harmony with nature

Since all food-related operations utilize natural resources, worshiping nature was integrated into agriculture and food preparation. This manifested as respecting and worshiping all objects, living or nonliving related to food operations. All sources of water, rivers, wells, ponds, lakes, etc. were highly respected and worshiped, and polluting them was a punishable offense. Trees were worshiped as providers of all utility items ranging from wood, fuel, and flowers to food items. Cattle used for agricultural operations such as bullocks were taken care of very well as farmers were dependent on them for their livelihood. Cows were worshiped and respected immensely because of their utility as providers of milk (which was recognized as the most nutritious food product and could be used in many ways). Even today certain rituals demand to worship objects of kitchen use such as pounding or grinding stone, the hearth, storage utensils for water, and pounding staff to express our gratefulness to them for fulfilling the basic need of food.

6.4.4 Concept of sharing and giving

Adequate food at every stage of life is a necessity. We are aware of the hungry populations around the world as well as the shortages or excesses of food. In traditional

Indian culture, the concept of sharing the food was very strongly advocated. Food must be given to every needy person who comes in search of food. No individual was supposed to be sent away without food from the doorstep. All guests were to be treated with the best of sumptuous food at all times of the day (Bajaj and Srinivas, 1996). This practice signified the sharing of food without expecting anything in return and ensured that nobody remained hungry.

6.5 Processed foods and tradition—preserving tradition in a modern context

During the last two decades, the Indian market has seen the entry of foods from other ethnic regions, specifically from Western, European, and Oriental cuisines. Some of these such as Chinese noodles, Manchurian, and Italian pasta are becoming household names and are popular street foods too. However, these are not a replacement for traditional foods but are only additions. Traditional foods routinely prepared in households have moved out to catering facilities and are also available as processed packaged products. Automation has been introduced successfully for many products cutting down on laborious time-consuming preparation processes. Technological upgradation has helped in modernizing the traditional food industry through automation and understanding science behind the tradition handed down from generations as skill. Understanding the principles of the science behind the manufacture of traditional foods has assisted in improving the quality and shelf life of the product. The research sector also paved the way for regulatory compliance.

To summarize, Indian traditional diets are definitely healthy, and vegetarian diets have their own benefits if chosen properly. A diversified diet provides many advantages, whereas an excess of processed refined foods are to be avoided. Certain cultural practices may not have a scientific basis, while others may have provided a good ground for health and freedom from disease. The sense of hygiene and sanitation was very well developed and followed strictly, part of which is lost at present. The science behind the tradition of eating developed by our ancestors was indeed appreciable and based on observations, experience, and wisdom.

References

Achaya, K.T., 1994. Indian Foods – A Historical Companion.. Oxford University Press, New Delhi. India.

ADA, 2009. Position of the American dietetic association: vegetarian diets. J. Am. Diet. Assoc. 109, 1266–1282.

Auboyer, J., 1965. Life in Ancient India. Asia Publishing House, Bombay, p. 98.

Bajaj, J., Srinivas, M.D., 1996. '*Annam Bahu Kurvita*' – Recollecting the Indian Discipline of Growing and Sharing Food in Plenty. Centre for Policy Studies, Madras, India.

Boro, P., Naha, B.C., Saikia, D.P., Prakash, C., 2016. A1 and A2 milk & its impact on human health. Int. J. Sci. Natl. 7 (1), 1–5.

Chapagain, A.K., Hoekstra, A.Y., 2004. Water Footprints of Nations, Value of Water Research Report Series No. 16, UNESCO-IHE, Delft, The Netherlands. <www.waterfootprint.org/Reports/Report16Vol1.pdf>.

Frison, E.A., Smith, I.F., Johns, T., Cherfas, J., Eyzaguirre, P.B., 2006. Agricultural biodiversity, nutrition, and health: making a difference to hunger and nutrition in the developing world. Food. Nutr. Bull. 27 (2), 167–179.

Ghosh, O.K., 1976. The Changing Indian Civilization, vol. 2. South Asia Books – Minerva Associates (Publications) Pvt Ltd, Calcutta, p. 322.

Ghurye, G.S., 1979. Vedic India. Popular Prakashan, Bombay, p. 52.

Gopalan, C., Rama Sastri, B.V., Balasubramanian, S.C., Narasinga Rao, B.S., Deosthale, Y.G., Pant, K. C., 1996. Nutritive Value of Indian Foods. Hyderabad, National Institute of Nutrition, Indian Council of Medical Research, India.

Gupta, S., Lakshmi, J.A., Manjunath, M.N., Prakash, J., 2005. Analysis of nutrient and antinutrient content of underutilized green leafy vegetables. LWT, Food Sci. Technol. 38 (4), 339–345.

Gupta, S., Lakshmi, J.A., Prakash, J., 2006. *In vitro* bioavailability of calcium and iron from selected green leafy vegetables. J. Sci. Food Agric. 86 (13), 2147–2152.

Hoestra, A.Y., 2008. The Water Footprint of Food – Water Footprint Network. <https://waterfootprint.org/media/downloads/Hoekstra-2008-WaterfootprintFood.pdf>.

Horner, I.B., 1945. Early Buddhism and the taking of life. In: Bhandarkar, D.R., Nilakanta Shastri, K.A., Barua, B.M., Gode, P.K. (Eds.), The B.C. Law Volume, vol. 1. The Indian Research Institute, Calcutta, p. 436.

ICMR, 2010. Nutrient Requirements and Recommended Dietary Allowances for Indians. A Report of the Expert Group of the Indian Council of Medical Research. Hyderabad, National Institute of Nutrition, India.

Iyengar, P.T.S., 1912. Life in Ancient India. Srinivasa Varadachari and Co., Madras, pp. 86–91.

Kosambi, D.D., 1975. An Introduction to Study of Indian History. Popular Prakashan, Bombay, 1360-138.

Ksemasarma, 2009. *Ksemakutulaham* (a work on dietetic and well being, translated from original by Scholars of I-AIM). Institute of Ayurveda and Integrative Medicine, Bangalore.

Leitzman, C., 2003. Nutrition ecology: the contribution of vegetarian diets. Am. J. Clin. Nutr. 78 (Suppl.), 657s–659s.

Longvah, T., Ananthan, R., Bhaskarachary, K., Venkaiah, K., 2017. Indian Food Composition Tables. National Institute of Nutrition, Hyderabad.

McEvoy, C.T., Temple, N., Woodside, J.V., 2012. Vegetarian diets, low-meat diets and health: a review. Public Health Nutr. 15 (12), 2287–2294. Available from: https://doi.org/10.1017/S1368980012000936. Available at.

Narasinga Rao, B.S., 2005. Development of Nutrition Science in India. Allied Publishers (P) Ltd, New Delhi.

NIN, 2011. Dietary Guidelines for Indians – A Manual.. National Institute of Nutrition, Hyderabad. India.

Oghbaei, M., Prakash, J., 2013. Effect of fractional milling of wheat on nutritional quality of milled fractions. Trends Carbohydr. Res. 5 (1), 53–58.

Oghbaei, M., Prakash, J., 2016. Effect of primary processing of cereals and legumes on its nutritional quality: a comprehensive review. Cogent: Food Agric. 2, 1–14. Available from: https://doi.org/10.1080/23311932.2015.1136015. 1136015.

Orthoefer, F.T., 2005. Rice bran oil. In: Shahidi, Fereidoon (Ed.), Bailey's Industrial Oil and Fat Products, sixth ed. John Wiley & Sons, Inc, pp. 465–489.

Prabhu, M.S., Platel, K., Saraswathi, G., Srinivasan, K., 1995. Effect of orally administered betel leaf (*Piper betle Linn.*) on digestive enzymes of pancreas and intestinal mucosa and on bile production in rats. Indian J. Exp. Biol. 33, 752–756.

Prasad, M.N.N., Sanjay, K.R., Khatokar, M.S., Vismaya, M.N., Swamy, S.N., 2011. Health benefits of rice bran – a review. J. Nutr. Food Sci. 1, 108. Available from: https://doi.org/10.4172/2155-9600.1000108.

Raghunathsuri, 2012. '*Bhojanakutuhalam*' (Translated from original by Scholars of I-AIM). Institute of Ayurveda and Integrative Medicine, Bangalore.

Raychaudhari, S.P., 1964. Agriculture in Ancient India. Indian Council of Agricultural research, New Delhi, p. 116.

Sethi, M., Jain, B., 2008. Fasting and Feasting – Then and Now. New Age International (P) Ltd. Publishers., New Delhi.

Shamashastry, R., 1967. Kautilya's Arthashastra. Mysore Printing and Publishing House, Mysore. India.

Springmann, M., Godfraya, H.C.J., Raynera, M., Scarborough, P., 2016. Analysis and Valuation of the Health and Climate Change Cobenefits of Dietary Change. Available online at <www.pnas.org/doi:10.1073/pnas.1523119113>.

SRS, 2014. Sample Registration System Baseline Survey. Registrar General of India. Govt. of India., New Delhi.

Wealth of India, 1992. revised ed. A Dictionary of Indian Raw Materials and Industrial Products – Raw Materials, vol. 3. CSIR, New Delhi, pp. 29–59.

CHAPTER 7

Functional foods in Indian tradition and their significance for health

Kalpana Platel
CSIR-Central Food Technological Research Institute, Mysuru, India

Contents

7.1 Introduction

India is known for its rich heritage and cultural diversity. Apart from the latter, India also has vast biodiversity, with a wide variety of cereals, pulses, fruits, vegetables, and spices being grown in different regions of the country. The association of food with health is known since ancient times, with the famous quote of the father of medicine, Hippocrates, "Let thy food be thy medicine and thy medicine be thy food." Many of the traditional foods commonly used in India can be termed as "functional foods," owing to their health beneficial attributes. A variety of spices, herbs, barks, fruits, flowers, and roots from different plants have been used in ancient and traditional medicine (Nadkarni and Nadkarni, 1976).

The daily diet of India contains a wide range of foods drawn from different food categories in various combinations. There are vast regional differences in the type of ingredients used and the dishes prepared and this diversity confers the status of "functional foods" as they are abundant in dietary fiber, antioxidants, and probiotics contributed from whole grains, fruits, vegetables, and fermented foods (Srinivasan, 2010). Thus they are wholesome not only in nutrition but also for their health benefits that range from improving the gastrointestinal health and boosting the immune system to maintaining ideal body weight; attributes that help in the prevention of lifestyle

Nutritional and Health Aspects of Food in South Asian Countries
DOI: https://doi.org/10.1016/B978-0-12-820011-7.00008-3

disorders such as hyperlipidemia, cardiovascular diseases, diabetes, and possibly certain types of cancer (Srinivasan, 2010).

7.2 Traditional Indian food patterns

Traditional dietary patterns in India have evolved basically from available locally grown crops to suit the different climatic conditions. Every region has its own unique choice of foods and combinations. A typical North Indian meal consists of unleavened bread (*chapati*, *paratha*, *nan*, *phulka*, *roti*) as the main course, consumed with accompaniments such as vegetable curries, cooked and seasoned pulse preparations, pickles, chutneys, and curd. South Indian meal consists of rice, served with pulse preparations such as *sambar and rasam* and fried and curried vegetables, accompanied by crispy fried *pappads*, pickles, and curd. These are the daily basic meal patterns. Meals during festivals and other religious functions are much more elaborate, including a wide range of cereal and pulse preparations, vegetables, sweets, and salads, all in one meal.

Chapathi is unleavened bread prepared from a dough of whole wheat flour that is rolled flat on a board and shallow fried with a small amount of oil.

Paratha, roti, and *phulka* are variations of chapathi: paratha being rolled in layers, while roti and phulka are fried without oil.

Nan is prepared from refined wheat flour (maida), and baked in a special kiln called "tandoor."

Chutney is a spicy side dish prepared by frying and grinding together a mixture of spices, tamarind, certain pulses, and vegetables such as onion, cucumber, ridge gourd, and fresh coconut.

Sambar and *rasam* are soups prepared from cooked red gram or masur dhal. The former is a thick soup in which a variety of vegetables are used. Both *sambar* and *rasam* contain tamarind extract and spice powders. *Rasam* is thinner in consistency, usually prepared by adding tomato and pepper powder in addition to the spice powder.

Pappads are round, crispy snacks, usually made from seasoned black gram dough that is flattened and sun dried. The sun-dried *pappads* are stored and deep fried in oil just before use. There are several variations in *pappads*, using ingredients such as potato, tapioca (sabudana), sweet potato, jackfruit, and onion.

Apart from the basic meals, there are a number of dishes prepared from combinations of cereals, pulses, vegetables, and spices, some examples being *biriyani, pulao, bisibele bhath*, khichdi, etc. These are appetizing whole meals by themselves, containing multiingredients in the right proportions to impart desired flavor and texture.

Common South Indian breakfast items include *idli*, *dosa*, *vada*, *pongal*, and *upma*, while North Indians prefer *paratha* or *dhokla* for breakfast.

Biriyani is a main course dish prepared from rice and meat/chicken/vegetables and is heavily spiced.

Pulao is prepared from the aromatic basmati rice and vegetables and is mildly spiced.

Bisibele bhath is a typical south Indian dish prepared from rice, red gram dhal, vegetables, spices, and condiments including tamarind.

Khichidi is a north Indian main course dish prepared from rice, red gram/green gram dhal, vegetables, and seasoned with spices and *ghee*.

Idli is prepared by steaming the fermented batter of rice and black gram dhal. Idli is typically consumed along with *sambar* and coconut *chutney*

Dosa is also prepared from the fermented batter of rice and black gram dhal. In the preparation of dosa, the batter is poured onto a frying pan, flattened, and fried crisp with a small quantity of oil. *Dosa* as well is consumed along with coconut *chutney*, or with cooked and seasoned potato. The proportions of rice and pulse differ between *idli* and *dosa*.

Vada is a deep-fried snack, prepared from the dough of black gram or Bengal gram dhal.

Pongal is prepared by cooking rice and green gram dhal together and seasoning with black pepper, cumin, and *ghee*

Upma is a south Indian breakfast dish prepared by cooking wheat semolina (rava) and seasoning it with onion, curry leaves, tomato, mustard, cumin, etc. Vegetables such as carrot, beans, and potatoes are added to upma.

Dhokla is a north Indian dish prepared using a fermented batter of rice and Bengal gram dhal.

This chapter presents some of the functional components and attributes of foods that are traditionally used in Indian diets.

7.3 Cereals and millets

Cereals and millets form the staple foods of Indian dietary and are the major sources of macronutrients. During the Aryan civilization, around 3000 years ago, barley was the major grain consumed, whereas rice came to prominence a little later (Achaya, 1994). At present, the major cereals and millets commonly consumed are rice, wheat, finger millet (*Eleucine coracana*), and sorghum (*Sorghum bicolor*). Other minor millets such as pearl millet (*Pennisatum glaucum*) are also consumed in various parts of the country, either as a staple or used in addition to the staples.

Apart from being important sources of macronutrients in the Indian context, cereals and millets also contribute micronutrients such as vitamins and minerals (Gopalan et al., 1999), several phytochemicals, as well as dietary fiber (Goufo and Trindade, 2014; Bhaskarachary et al., 2016, Dykes, 2019). The health benefits of whole grains are also attributed to their nondigestible carbohydrate content (Bhaskarachary et al., 2016). Thus cereals and millets are functional foods that are beneficial to health. The bioactive compounds of cereals and millets are presented in Table 7.1.

Rice is a good source of several antioxidant molecules, and colored rice varieties (black, red, purple, and brown) are known to exhibit good antioxidant properties (Goufo and Trindade, 2014). Wheat, which was extensively consumed by the Harappans (Achaya, 1994), is a major staple even today. It is a rich source of fructooligosaccharides, fructans, and other bioactive components that are attributed to several health beneficial properties (Shewry and Hey, 2015). Sorghum also contains a wide array of phytochemicals, most of which are concentrated in the bran layer. These are responsible for a number of health benefits exerted by sorghum (Dykes, 2019). Millets such as finger, pearl, and kodo millet (*Paspalum scrobiculatum*), besides being good sources of micronutrients, are also very rich in several phytochemicals with high antioxidant activity (Palanisamy et al., 2014). This beneficial activity is attributed to their phytate, polyphenol, and dietary fiber contents (Sreeramulu et al., 2009; Vali et al., 2018; Bhaskarachary et al., 2016; Saxena et al., 2007).

Table 7.1 Bioactive components of cereals and millets.

Food	Bioactive components	Health benefits
Rice—white, black, brown, purple, red	γ-Oryzanol, phenolic acids, flavonoids, anthocyanins, tocopherols, tocotrienols, phytic acid	Antioxidant activity
Wheat	Fructooligosaccharides, fructans, dietary fiber, nonstarch polysaccharides—arabinoxylans, cellulose, resistant starch, lignin, chitin, pectins, β-glucans, etc., phenolics, terpenoids	Antidiabetic, cholesterol-lowering, anticancer, antiinflammatory
Sorghum	Phenolic acids, flavonoids, condensed tannins, polycosanols, phytosterols, stilbenes, and phenolamides	
Finger millet; other millets	Benzoic acid, cinnamic acid, other polyphenols	Antidiabetic, antitumerogenic, antiatherosclerogenic, antioxidant, antimicrobial

In India, cereals and millets are consumed in various forms. Rice used to be hand-pounded decades ago in most of the households. Although changing times have seen increased consumption of milled and polished rice, other types of rice, such as par-boiled rice, brown rice, and black rice are also consumed in different regions. Other traditional rice products include flaked rice, puffed rice, and puffed paddy. Whole wheat flour is preferred over the refined wheat flour in the preparation of *chapathi* or *paratha*. Other wheat products such as semolina, vermicelli, and broken wheat are also used almost on a daily basis. Finger millet, sorghum, pearl millet, and other millets are milled into flour before use.

7.4 Pulses and legumes

Pulses and legumes are an integral part of traditional Indian diets and have been so since ancient times; black gram (*Vigna mungo*), green gram (*Vigna radiata*), and lentil (*Lens culinaris*) find a mention in *Vedic* text (Achaya, 1994). At present, along with these, there are many others that are used in whole or dehusked form. These include red gram (*Cajanus cajan*), Bengal gram (*Cicer arietinum*), cowpea (*Vigna unguiculate*), horse gram (*Dolichos biflorus*), and kidney bean (*Phaseolus vulgaris*). These foods are the single most important source of protein in vegetarian diets, especially for the lower economic segments of the population. They also provide significant amounts of micronutrients. Pulses and legumes are rich in dietary fiber, especially when consumed whole. Several studies have documented the antioxidant activity of pulses and legumes (Sreeramlu et al., 2009; Saxena et al., 2007; Kumar and Xu, 2017a, 2017b; Prasad and Singh, 2015). Horse gram was used in traditional medicine to treat ailments such as kidney stones, urinary diseases, piles, common cold, throat infection, and fever (Prasad and Singh, 2015). The antioxidant activity of pulses and legumes is attributed to their rich polyphenol content.

7.5 Milk and milk products

Milk is the only source of complete protein for vegetarians, who form a significant chunk of the Indian population. Indian diets not only include milk, but also its products, the most important being fermented milk, or curd (*dahi*). Curd is consumed on a daily basis in almost all Indian households, particularly in South India. Milk has been reported to be rich in biologically active molecules with demonstrated clinical benefits. Numerous milk-derived compounds have potential applications as clinical therapies in infectious and inflammatory disease, cancer, and other conditions (Hill and Newburg, 2015; Verardo et al., 2017). Curd functions as probiotic on account of lactic acid bacteria with multiple health benefits (Srinivasan, 2010). *Paneer*, or cottage cheese, is another highly nutritious popular milk product used in cooking. Milk and its products find various uses in Indian cuisine. Milk, apart from being consumed as a beverage, is

Table 7.2 Bioactive components of milk and its products.

Food	Bioactive components	Health benefits
Milk	Lactoferrin, transforming growth factor β, cytokine, milk glycans, including human milk oligosaccharides, ω-3 and ω-6 PUFA, short-chain fatty acids, gangliosides, phospholipids	Antiinflammatory, antimicrobial, anticancer
Curd	Probiotics	Cholesterol-lowering, improved lactose intolerance, stimulation of the immune system, cancer prevention
Colostrum	Immune, growth and tissue repair factors, transforming growth factors α and β, insulin-like growth factors 1 and 2	Boosting the immune system, prevention of gastrointestinal infections, muscular and skeletal repair

extensively used in the preparation of a wide variety of traditional sweets. Curd is consumed along with rice and also used in the preparation of various sweets and curries. The bioactive factors of milk and its products are listed in Table 7.2.

The use of bovine colostrum for preparing a sweet dish is a unique feature of Indian cuisine. Colostrum is very rich in immune, growth and tissue repair factors. Bovine colostrum has possible use in the treatment or prevention of gastrointestinal tract infections. It is said to be the only natural source of transforming and insulin-like growth factors. Colostral growth factors have multiple regenerative effects that extend to all structural body cells, such as the gut (Uruakpa et al., 2002).

7.6 Other foods of animal origin

Meat, poultry, and fish are consumed by a large segment of the Indian population. These foods are important sources of complete protein, as well as several micronutrients. Besides this, meat and fish proteins are sources of novel bioactive peptides known to possess several beneficial physiological functions including antihypertensive, antioxidant, immunomodulatory, antimicrobial, prebiotic, antithrombotic, and hypocholesterolemic effects (Ryan et al., 2011). Fish is also an important source of the biologically active fatty acids, docosahexaenoic acid (DHA), and eicosapentaenoic acid (EPA). DHA plays an important role in fetal brain development and the development of motor skills and visual acuity in infants. The other beneficial functions of DHA and EPA include the prevention of atherosclerosis, dementia, rheumatoid arthritis, and Alzheimer's disease (Mohanty et al., 2016). India, being a land of numerous rivers, has abundant biodiversity in fish. Fish is an important food of the population living in coastal regions. A wide variety of freshwater and marine fish is available. The foods of animal origin are consumed in combination with cereals, vegetables, and spices. A wide variety of curries, gravies, and rice dishes are prepared fusing meat and fish. The extensive use of spices adds value to these foods and probably helps in reducing the ill effects of cholesterol, of which these foods are rich sources.

7.7 Vegetables and fruits

India has vast biodiversity of vegetables and fruits that are extensively consumed. Vegetables form a very important part of the daily diet and are consumed in almost all the meals. India is probably the only country where a large variety of vegetables are consumed daily.

Green leafy vegetables (GLV) need a special mention in the Indian context. GLV is extensively and easily grown and is available all through the year. A large variety of GLV, namely amaranth (*Amaranthus gangeticus*), fenugreek (*Trigonella foenum graecum*), spinach (*Spinica oleracea*), drumstick (*Moringa oleifera*), mint (*Mentha spicata*), and coriander (*Coriandrum sativum*), and several local varieties such as mustard leaves (*Brassica campestris var. sarason)*, basale (*Basella rubra*), chakotha (*Rumex vesicarius*), keerai, and kilkeerai (*Amaranthus tricolor*) are a part of the daily diet. There are several hundreds of varieties of GLV, apart from those mentioned here. These greens are prepared as curries, sautéed, shallow fried, boiled, or steamed with other ingredients. GLV is the storehouse of micronutrients, being very rich sources of β-carotene, vitamin C, folic acid, dietary fiber, and several minerals (Krishnaswamy and Rajagopal, 2018). Apart from nutrients, GLV are abundant in several phytochemicals. The consumption of drumstick leaves and mustard leaves is unique to India. Drumstick leaves have been attributed to several medicinal properties (Table 7.3), including stabilizing blood pressure (Motohashi et al., 2017). Mustard leaves as well are a rich source of phytochemicals, which were found to be responsible for the antioxidant and other health beneficial properties (Frazie et al., 2017).

A number of roots and tubers, such as potato, sweet potato, yam, tapioca (cassava), and carrot, are commonly consumed in India. Nutritionally, these vegetables provide energy, while some of them contain protein, vitamin C, and β-carotene. Roots and tubers also contain good amounts of dietary fiber (Chandrasekara and Thamilini Josheph, 2016). In addition to nutrients, roots and tubers are significant sources of a number of bioactive compounds that are responsible for several health beneficial attributes of roots and tubers (Chandrasekara and Thamilini Josheph, 2016).

Several other vegetables such as brinjal, pumpkin, ladies finger (okra), cucumber, *tendli* (coccinia), ridge gourd, snake gourd, bitter gourd, drumstick, and the *brassica* vegetables such as cabbage, cauliflower, knol khol, turnip, and kale are all widely consumed in India. All these vegetables, apart from being good sources of micronutrients,

Table 7.3 Bioactive components of vegetables.

Food	Bioactive components	Health benefits
Green leafy vegetables	Polyphenols, flavonoids, carotenoids, sinigrin and its hydrolysis products (mustard leaves), thiocarbamate glycosides (DSL)	Antimicrobial, antioxidant, antifungal, antihypertensive, antiinflammatory, antihyperglycemic, anticancer
Roots and tubers	Saponins, phenolic compounds, glycoalkaloids, phytic acids, carotenoids, ascorbic acid	Antioxidant, immunomodulatory, antimicrobial, antidiabetic, antiobesity, and hypocholesterolemic
Other vegetables	Gallic acid, protocatechuic acid, catechin, caffeic acid, ferulic acid, sinapic acid, quercetin, resveratrol, and kaempferol	Antioxidant

are also very good providers of phytochemicals with high antioxidant activity (Singh et al., 2016).

India, with its varied agroclimatic conditions, is ideal for growing a wide variety of fruits such as banana, mango, papaya, bael (*Aegle marmelos*), orange, pineapple, guava, custard apple, sapodilla (sapota), jambolan (jamun), pomegranate, and jackfruit. These fruits are rich sources of flavonoids, carotenoids, electrolytes, and other bioactive compounds (Bhaskarachary et al., 2016). They are also very rich sources of minerals and vitamins, especially vitamin C, since they are consumed fresh, without cooking.

Indian cuisine also includes the use of the peels of several vegetables and fruits in preparations such as pickles, chutneys, and preserves, common examples being lime, bitter orange, and mango, being pickled along with the peel. This is an added advantage, as the bioactive components that are localized in the peels would also be included.

Liberal consumption of fruits and vegetables is very well known to promote health and helps in the prevention of diet-related chronic diseases such as cardiovascular disease including stroke, cancer, diabetes mellitus, cataract, age-related maculopathy, gastrointestinal problems, chronic obstructive pulmonary disease, and bone health (Krishnaswamy and Rajagopal, 2018).

7.8 Oilseeds, oils, and fats

Oilseeds are an important part of Indian dietary, being used in the preparation of several powders, sweets, seasoning, etc. The most common oilseeds consumed are peanut, sesame, coconut, and mustard. Peanut (or groundnut, as it is known in India) occupies

Table 7.4 Bioactive components of oilseeds.

Food	Bioactive components	Health benefits
Peanuts	Chlorogenic acid, caffeic acid, coumaric acid, ferulic acid, flavonoids, resveratrol	Antioxidant
Sesame seeds and oil	Sesamin, asarinin, sesamolin	Antioxidant, antiproliferative, antihypertensive, neuroprotective, hypocholesterolemic
Mustard seeds	Sinapic acid, sinapine, sinapoyl glucose, dithiolthiones	Protect against liver toxicity, antimutagenic

a prominent place on the shelf of almost every Indian kitchen. Besides being rich sources of protein, energy, and micronutrients, peanuts have been reported to be rich in phytochemicals (Arya et al., 2016). Apart from containing good amounts of vital minerals, peanuts also contain antioxidant minerals such as selenium, manganese, and copper. Peanuts have a desirable lipid profile, with high unsaturated fatty acid content. The high oleic acid content in peanuts is responsible for their beneficial biological effects (Arya et al., 2016). Sesame seeds and mustard seeds have several health beneficial components (Table 7.4) (Monteiro et al., 2016; Mayengbam et al., 2014; Srinivasan, 2010).

Vegetable oils are most commonly used for cooking in India. Sesame, mustard, groundnut, and coconut oils have been used since ancient times, and continue to dominate even today. Although sesame, groundnut, and coconut oil are used in South India, mustard oil is the most used in the northern parts. In ancient times, cooking oils were not refined, but freshly extracted crude oils were used. It was a common practice for people to go to the traditional oil extracting units to collect oil, which was used for cooking. This practice, however, is no longer common, and refined cooking oils are commercially available. In recent years, sunflower, safflower, and rice bran oils as well have become popular.

Apart from cooking, oils are also used in the preparation of various types of pickles. For this, unrefined oils are preferred, sesame and mustard oils being most commonly used. Sesame seeds were one of the first crops processed for oil. Sesame oil is considered to be more stable than most vegetable oils due to the presence of antioxidants in it; it is also least prone to turn rancid, as it retains its natural structure and does not break down even at very high temperatures (Srinivasan, 2010). Similar to the seeds, sesame oil also has bioactive components with health beneficial effects (Monteiro et al., 2014).

Clarified butter, known as *ghee*, is an important part of the Indian cuisine. Ghee is used as a cooking medium and also added to dishes just before consumption. *Ghee* has been shown to lower blood cholesterol levels by increasing the biliary excretion of cholesterol, bile acids, uronic acid, and phospholipids (Kumar et al., 2000).

7.9 Spices and condiments

Spices, which are used to enhance the flavor of food, form a very important part of traditional Indian cookery. A correct blend of various spices is crucial to every dish. The variety and amount of spices that are used regularly in Indian cuisine is probably the highest, as compared to any country. Spices are used individually as well as in mixes known as *garam masala*, *rasam* powder, *sambar* powder, *chutney* powder, etc. Spices are known to contain several bioactive components such as curcumin, capsaicin, eugenol, gingerone, flavonoids, and essential oils. Exhaustive studies have documented various health beneficial effects of spices (Srinivasan, 2005a; 2005b) (Table 7.5). Spices are known to contain several bioactive components

Condiments used to add a desirable sour taste to many traditional Indian preparations include acidulants such as tamarind (*Tamarindus indica*), kokum (*Garcinia indica*), lime, *amchur* (dried raw mango powder), and *amla* fruit (*Phyllanthus emblica*). The acidulants lime and amchur, by virtue of their organic acid content, have been shown to enhance the in vitro availability of iron and zinc from cereals and pulses (Srinivasan, 2010). These acidulants are known to be good sources of polyphenols. *Amla* fruits are valued highly in the traditional medicinal systems and form the major ingredients in popular Ayurvedic preparations (Srinivasan, 2010). *Kokum*, valued for its nutritive value and medicinal properties, is widely used as an acidulant in the coastal regions of

Table 7.5 Health effects of spices and condiments.

Spices	Health benefits
Garlic, onion, turmeric, fenugreek, red pepper	Hypocholesterolemic
Turmeric, red pepper	Antilithogenic
Fenugreek, onion, garlic, turmeric, cumin	Hypoglycemic
Turmeric, red pepper, clove	Antioxidant, antiarthritic, antiinflammatory
Turmeric, garlic, ginger, mustard	Cancer preventive
Ginger, cumin, ajowan, fennel, coriander, onion, mint, black pepper	Digestive stimulant
Turmeric, garlic, asafetida	Antimicrobial
Amla fruits	Hypolipidemic, antidiabetic, and antiinflammatory, inhibit HIV-1, tumor development, and gastric ulcer
Kokum	Anticarcinogenic, antioxidant, antiinflammatory, antineurodegenerative, antianxiety, antimicrobial, DNA repair activities Reduces obesity and regulates blood cholesterol levels

South India and is a rich source of polyphenols and other bioactive components (Motohashi et al., 2017; Srinivasan, 2010).

Thus almost all the foods that form an integral part of the Indian cuisine are loaded with health beneficial bioactive components, besides being rich in nutritive value. The fact that these ingredients are consumed in ideal combinations enhances their beneficial potency all the more. The variety and ideal combinations of foods in traditional Indian dietary make these diets unique and popular all over the world.

References

Achaya, K.T., 1994. Indian Food: A Historical Companion. Oxford University Press, Delhi.

Arya, S.S., Salve, Akshata R., Chauhan, S., 2016. Peanuts as functional food: a review. J. Food Sci. Technol. 53 (1), 31−41. Available from: https://doi.org/10.1007/s13197-015-2007-9.

Bhaskarachary, K., Vemula, S.R., Subba Rao, M., et al., 2016. Traditional foods, functional foods and nutraceuticals. Proc. Indian Natl. Sci. Acad. 82 (5), 1565−1577. Available from: https://doi.org/10.16943/ptinsa/2016/48888.

Chandrasekara, A., Thamilini Josheph, T.K., 2016. Roots and tuber crops as functional foods: a review on phytochemical constituents and Their potential health benefits. Int. J. Food Sci. 2016, 3631647. Available from: https://doi.org/10.1155/2016/3631647.

Dykes, L., 2019. Sorghum phytochemicals and their potential impact on human health. Methods Mol. Biol. 1931, 121−140. Available from: https://doi.org/10.1007/978-1-4939-9039-9_9.

Frazie, M.D., Kim, M.J., Ku, K.M., 2017. Health-promoting phytochemicals from 11 mustard cultivars at baby leaf and mature stages. Molecules 22 (10), 1749. Available from: https://doi.org/10.3390/molecules22101749.

Gopalan, G., Ramasastri, B.V., Balasubramanian, S.C., 1999. Nutritive Value of Indian Foods. Indian Council of Medical Research, New Delhi.

Goufo, P., Trindade, H., 2014. Rice antioxidants: phenolic acids, flavonoids, anthocyanins, proanthocyanidins, tocopherols, tocotrienols, γ-oryzanol, and phytic acid. Food Sci. Nutr. 2 (2), 75−104. Available from: https://doi.org/10.1002/fsn3.86.

Hill, D.R., Newburg, D.S., 2015. Clinical applications of bioactive milk components. Nutr. Rev. 73 (7), 463−476. Available from: https://doi.org/10.1093/nutrit/nuv009.

Krishnaswamy, K., Rajagopal, G., 2018. Nature's bountiful gift to humankind: vegetables & fruits & their role in cardiovascular disease & diabetes. Indian J. Med. Res. 148 (5), 569−595. Available from: https://doi.org/10.4103/ijmr.IJMR_1780_18.

Kumar, G., Xu, B., 2017a. Polyphenol-rich lentils and their health promoting effects. Int. J. Mol. Sci. 18 (11), 2390. Available from: https://doi.org/10.3390/ijms18112390.

Kumar, G., Xu, B., 2017b. Polyphenol-rich dry common beans (*Phaseolus vulgaris* L.) and their health benefits and their health promoting effects. Int. J. Mol. Sci. 18 (11), 2331. Available from: https://doi.org/10.3390/ijms18112331.

Kumar, M.V., Sambaiah, K., Lokesh, B.R., 2000. Hypocholesterolemic effect of anhydrous milk fat ghee is mediated by increasing the secretion of biliary lipids. J. Nutr. Biochem. 11 (2), 69−75.

Mayengbam, S., Aachary, A., Thiyam-Holländer, U., 2014. Endogenous phenolics in hulls and cotyledons of mustard and canola: a comparative study on its sinapates and antioxidant capacity. Antioxidants (Basel) 3 (3), 544−558. Available from: https://doi.org/10.3390/antiox3030544.

Mohanty, B.P., Ganguly, S., Mahanty, A., et al., 2016. DHA and EPA content and fatty acid profile of 39 food fishes from India. Biomed. Res. Int. 4027437. Available from: https://doi.org/10.1155/2016/4027437.

Monteiro, E.M.H., Chibli, L.A., Yamamotoet, C.H., et al., 2014. Antinociceptive and anti-inflammatory activities of the sesame oil and sesamin. Nutrients 6 (5), 1931−1944.

Motohashi, N., Gallagher, R., Vanam, A., et al., 2017. Functional foods and their importance in geriatric nutrition. J. Clin. Nutr. Metab 1, 1.
Nadkarni, K.M., Nadkarni, A.K., 1976. In Indian Materia Medica. Popular Prakashan, Mumbai.
Uruakpa, F.O., Ismond, M.A.H., Akobundu, E.N.T., 2002. Colostrum and its benefits: a review. Nutr. Res. 22 (6), 755–767.
Palanisamy, B.D., Rajendran, V., Sathyaseelan, S., et al., 2014. Health benefits of finger millet (*Eleusine coracana* L.) polyphenols and dietary fiber: a review. J. Food Sci. Technol. 51 (6), 1021–1040. Available from: https://doi.org/10.1007/s13197-011-0584-9.
Prasad, S.K., Singh, M.K., 2015. Horse gram- an underutilized nutraceutical pulse crop: a review. J. Food Sci. Technol. 52 (5), 2489–2499. Available from: https://doi.org/10.1007/s13197-014-1312-z.
Ryan, J.T., Ross, R.P., Bolton, D., et al., 2011. Bioactive peptides from muscle sources: meat and fish. Nutrients 3 (9), 765–791. Available from: https://doi.org/10.3390/nu3090765.
Saxena, R., Venkaiah, K., Anitha, P., et al., 2007. Antioxidant activity of commonly consumed plant foods of India: contribution of their phenolic content. Int. J. Food. Sci. Nutr. 58 (4), 250–260.
Shewry, P.R., Hey, S.J., 2015. The contribution of wheat to human diet and health. Food Energy Secur 4 (3), 178–202. Available from: https://doi.org/10.1002/fes3.64.
Singh, J.P., Kaur, A., Shevkani, K., et al., 2016. Composition, bioactive compounds and antioxidant activity of common Indian fruits and vegetables. J. Food Sci. Technol. 53 (11), 4056–4066. Available from: https://doi.org/10.1007/s13197-016-2412-8.
Sreeramulu, D., Reddy, C.V., Raghunath, M., 2009. Antioxidant activity of commonly consumed cereals, millets, pulses and legumes in India. Indian J. Biochem. Biophys. 46 (1), 112–115.
Srinivasan, K., 2005a. Spices as influencers of body metabolism: an overview of three decades of research. Food Res. Int. 38, 77–86.
Srinivasan, K., 2005b. Role of spices beyond food flavoring: nutraceuticals with multiple health benefits. Food Rev. Int. 21, 167–188.
Srinivasan, K., 2010. Traditional Indian functional foods. In: Shi, John, Ho, Chi-Tang, Shahidi, Fereidoon (Eds.), Functional Foods of the East. CRC Press, USA, pp. 51–84. (Chapter 3).
Vali, P., Ratnavathi, C.V., Ajani, J., et al., 2018. Proximate, mineral composition and antioxidant activity of traditional small millets cultivated and consumed in Rayalaseema region of south India. J. Sci. Food Agric. 98 (2), 652–660. Available from: https://doi.org/10.1002/jsfa.8510. Epub 2017 Aug 12.
Verardo, V., Gómez-Caravaca, A.M., Arráez-Román, D., et al., 2017. Recent advances in phospholipids from colostrum, milk and dairy by-products. Int. J. Mol. Sci. 18 (1), 173. Available from: https://doi.org/10.3390/ijms18010173.

CHAPTER 8

Traditional foods, Ayurveda, and diet

Ketki Wagh[1] and Supriya Bhalerao[2]
[1]Ayurveda Preventive Medicine & Yoga Consultant, RK University, Rajkot, Gujarat, India
[2]Interactive Research School for Health Affairs, Bharati Vidyapeeth Deemed (to be) University, Pune, India

Contents

8.1 Introduction about Indian traditional foods and Ayurveda

Ayurveda, which is the traditional system of Indian medicine, has originated over almost 3000 years. It provides exhaustive insights related to food, based on concepts unique to the science of life. According to Ayurveda, health can be defined as a state of balance and equilibrium related to one's self (*swastha*). However, it is well linked to the environment, including food. A number of themes are covered throughout various classical Ayurveda texts that give knowledge about food, food-related practices, and principles. The basis for Ayurvedic epistemology on health and nutrition is greatly different from the approach that contemporary life sciences, biomedicine, or modern nutrition takes. Interestingly, healthcare today is advancing toward these concepts of personalized medicine and in a broader context that of a more holistic approach (Payyappallimana and Venkatasubramanian, 2016) thus reinventing the wheels and approaching the Ayurvedic principles again.

8.2 Ayurveda and traditional foods interlink

Ayurveda uses sensory organs and the mind as instruments to understand, theorize, and perceive the fundamentals. The notable features of Ayurveda as a traditional medical system include the individuality of a person, functional aspects of health as well as diseases, multicausality approach, cause-effect method of reasoning, holistic approach

Nutritional and Health Aspects of Food in South Asian Countries
DOI: https://doi.org/10.1016/B978-0-12-820011-7.00016-2

while treating a patient, and host centered treatments. Ayurveda has adopted a top-down, holistic understanding of organisms and their interactions with the environment at a functional level and not so much at the molecular level. The approach of biomedicine, on the other hand, is a bottom-up approach that understands the structural basis and molecular processes of cells, tissues, and organs and not so much of the functional networks within a system and its interactions with the environment (Payyappallimana and Venkatasubramanian, 2016).

8.3 Ayurvedic dietetics

Originated in India, Ayurveda is one of the ancient yet living health traditions. Ayurveda is widely known as "the science of life" owing to the meaning of words *Ayu* (life) and *Veda* (science or knowledge). The main classical treatise of Charaka Samhita, Sushruta Samhita (~400 BC–200 AD), and Ashtanga Hridaya of Vagbhata have given a detailed description of more than 700 herbs and 6000 formulations used for preventive as well as curative purposes. The text of Madhav Nidan (~800 AD) that focuses on diagnostic aspects has provided greater than 5000 signs and symptoms for the diagnosis of a large number of diseases. Ayurveda conceives life as a synergy and union of the body, senses, mind, and soul. The concept of Prakriti or constitution that represents the phenotype of an individual plays a major role in Ayurveda therapeutics (Patwardhan, 2014). As per the great saying of the Roman philosopher Lucretius "One man's meat is another man's poison," each Prakriti requires different food to achieve, maintain, and promote health. Ayurvedic dietetics therefore concentrates on the personalized dietary requirements.

Ahara, the pillar of health: According to Ayurveda, there are three pillars of health, which safeguard the health of an individual from all perspectives. Ahara (food) is one of these, the others being sleep and regulated sexual life. Food is also called "Mahabheshaj," which means "the biggest medicine." There are elaborate references available in the classical texts of Ayurveda from 300 BC to 700 AD that are dedicated to sections on food. The unique principles and descriptions that have been narrated regarding food provide descriptions such as various types of food and beverages, classification of food based on six tastes (*shad rasa*), therapeutic qualities of food, measures for preservation of food, concept of food–food incompatibilities based on different factors like combining different tastes, processing, dose, time, and place; principles of proper eating and guidelines regarding proper food habits; intake based on the digestive capacity of an individual.

The classification of food is primarily based on its appropriateness to an individual's body and mental constitution considering the five elements (*Panchamahabhuta*) and the *Tridosha* theories. The natural transformation of any material, living or nonliving, occurs when the five elements combine and dissociate (Dhyani, 1994).

Food and psychological states: Ayurveda offers another unique taxonomy of foods that is based on the effect that food has on the psychological disposition of any person. A subtle link is observed between the process of manifestation of a disease and the six psychological expressions, namely anger, desire, attachment, lust, greed, and ego. A further discussion of these terms is provided as the three states of being viz. sattva, rajas, and tamas. Sattva is the contented state, rajas an excited state whereas tamas relates to a lethargic disposition, that is, foods can induce these states of mind (Prabhupada, 2002; Murthy, 2001).

Mood affects food benefits: As food can alter the mood, conversely mood can also alter the effect of food. One should eat with utmost concentration on the food, while not talking or laughing. By taking food while talking or laughing or with mind elsewhere, the person cannot ascertain the qualities and taste of the food or even detect any defects in the food. The concept of "mindful eating" that is being propagated these days for health and healthy weight can thus be found in Ayurveda. The mood of the cook and his/her intention while cooking also affects the health benefits of the food and hence outside eating is not favored.

The Shadrasa concept as a health indicator: Rasa of food is one of the ways of classification adopted in Ayurveda. There are six major tastes viz., sweet, sour, salty, pungent, bitter, and astringent. The *guna* (primary and secondary qualities) increases the properties of any material. Further augmentation is achieved by the *veerya* (potency), the *vipaka* (postdigestive effect), and *karma* (therapeutic action). The disease causality of excessive intake of each rasa is described in Charaka Samhita in much detail. The classification based on *rasa*, *guna*, *veerya*, *vipaka*, and *karma* is applied not only to foods but also to medicines, which has been dealt in the Dravyaguna shastra (Ayurvedic Pharmacology) branch of Ayurvedic pharmacology (Dhyani, 1994).

The concept of Agni and its relation to metabolism: Dr. Roger Williams has stated in his book *Biochemical Individuality* "If we continue to try to solve (nutritional) problems on the basis of the average man, we will be continually in a muddle. Such a man (average) does not exist." Ayurveda has described this aspect in great detail and the concept of *Agni* or energy that drives metabolic processes in the body has been described as one of the most important factors that affect health. The digestive process described in Ayurveda is based on the gross form of digestion going deeper to the elemental metabolism. The first stage or gross digestion stage occurs in the gastrointestinal tract, which is then followed by tissue-specific metabolism and lastly the elemental level of metabolism. The postdigestive effect of food has a specific impact on the body in this sequence of events. For materials, which are a combination of multiple tastes, the taste of postmetabolism changes as a postdigestive effect, and this is an important indicator to gauge the impact any food item has on the system. The Indian gooseberry (*amla*) is a good example to explain this concept. The Indian gooseberry has a sour taste as the predominant taste and has been described to have all other tastes except salty as secondary tastes but the postdigestive effect is described as sweet. Hence, in keeping with Ayurvedic principles, even though the sour taste would increase pitta in the body, gooseberry, on the contrary, nullifies pitta due to the sweet postdigestive function (Dwarakanatha, 2003). As per Ayurveda, the digestive capacity of an individual is linked with the physiological constitution of that particular individual, and any diet consumed should be in synergy with these two.

Aharvarga—Morphological features and physiological action-based classification: *Ahar* (food) *varga* (classes) is the categorization of food based on the morphological features and corresponding physiological actions. A total of 12 food categories namely grains and cereals, legumes and pulses, meat and meat-based products, processed foods, leafy vegetables, fruits, salts, various forms of water, milk and milk products, oils, sugarcane-based food group, and alcoholic drinks have been described and their effect on the body has been elaborated (Sharma, 2002). Ayurveda deals with the topic of food processing in detail. The properties of raw, dried, smoked, grilled, pickled, and steamed foods, various additives, and adjuvants find mention based on the five elements theory. The method of processing alters the properties of a substance. For example, puffed rice is light as compared to flaked or cooked rice that is heavier to digest (Sastri, 1997). Curd, which is unwholesome in most situations, becomes a healthy drink when churned and the butter is removed. This sweet-tasting buttermilk kept in an earthen vessel for 2 days develops astringent taste and becomes a wholesome food for the gastrointestinal system especially in conditions such as hyperacidity, irritable bowel syndrome, fissures, and hemorrhoids, and certain types of diarrhea and dysentery (Kukkupuni et al., 2015). The best and worst substance in each food group has also been described. For example, green grams are considered the best among pulses and black grams are the worst in the class (Dutta et al., 2005).

Prakriti-based diet—the concept of individuality: Ayurveda is one of the first ancient sciences to have an intuitive insight into physiological differences according to individual constitutional type and thus the difference in a dietary prescription for different individuals. One of the most important determinants for the effect of food on the system of an individual is their *Prakriti*. This is characterized by a set of physical, physiological, and psychological attributes. For example, based on taste preferences, individuals can be grouped as *vata* (having an affinity for sweet, sour, and salty tastes); pitta (with a liking for sweet, bitter, and astringent taste), and *kapha* (for pungent, bitter, and astringent tastes). Interestingly, these tastes mitigate any negative effects of the inherited constitution, usage of tastes in the reverse order can cause an imbalance in the body. For example, if a *vata* constitution person continuously consumes pungent, bitter, and astringent tasting items, it could lead to rapid aging and degeneration of the body. The concept of Prakriti can also explain the food oxidizer status, viz. fast oxidizer, slow oxidizer, and balanced oxidative state. A person with Pitta dominant type of Prakriti has been described to have a fast oxidizer status and hence should consume foods, which are predominantly sweet in taste, less oily, and should consume multiple small meals. *Prakriti* and its associations with metabolism, chronic diseases, and genotypes open up possibilities of newborn screening and a lifetime of personalized prevention (Dey and Pahwa, 2014; Sharma, 2001).

Viruddha Ahara (incompatible foods): One more distinctive feature of Ayurveda is its understanding of the incompatibilities of food materials and processing. There are descriptions of 18 forms of incompatibilities, which are explained based on the potency of materials, processing, quantity/dose, process of intake, and time/season; combining materials, such as sour fruits and milk or honey and ghee (clarified butter) in equal quantities; milk along with horse gram, jackfruit, or fish, or even heating honey (Sharma, 2001). Although the basis for these incompatibilities has been explained based on Ayurvedic principles, this remains an area of further exploration with the tools of contemporary research available today. One example of an incompatibility most commonly observed is milkshakes described as an incompatibility between milk and fruits.

Pathya and Apathya (wholesome and unwholesome food): The Ayurvedic compendium has several examples described as wholesome and unwholesome foods both as convalescence foods and preventive nutrition. For example, pomegranate, Indian gooseberry, buttermilk, etc. are mentioned as good *pathya ahara* in the management of iron-deficiency anemia. Curd is considered unwholesome. There are specific instructions to consume curd, that it should not be taken at night, or in seasons such as spring, summer, and fall. It should be taken with sugar candy or green gram soup or honey. There are also disease-specific or medicine-specific instructions that should be followed for the consumption of food. A detailed description of convalescence foods is available that is to be consumed during illness and during the recovery period. These foods are particularly indicated in disease management. As an example, a patient suffering from cough is advised to consume vegetables, such as ivy gourd; spices such as garlic and cardamom, long pepper, ginger, and condiments prepared with puffed paddy. It is indicated that certain tastes have a direct correlation with disease manifestation; hence, they are avoided during the treatment of those conditions (Tripati, 1998).

Ashta Aahar Vidhi Vishesh ayatan—eight factors specifically influencing food effects: The following eight factors, which can affect the benefits of food, are described.

1. *Prakriti* (nature of food): The basic nature of food is a consideration when looking at the digestibility of the food. Certain foods by nature are heavy to digest, for example, meat is very heavy for digestion whereas rice and vegetables are much lighter. This basic nature of the food is something to be considered while eating.
2. *Karana* (processing): Different methods are used for processing food such as frying, baking, heating directly on the fire, steaming, barbequed food, drying, and churning. The process used to cook food changes the quality of the food making it

either lighter or heavier to digest for example food cooked on natural wood is lighter to digest and has a better taste than that prepared on electricity or gas.

3. *Samyoga* (combination): The various incompatibilities need to be taken into account when mixing any two ingredients, for example, a combination of sour fruits with milk or curds is described as being incompatible and not at all beneficial.
4. *Rashi* (quantity): One more factor that affects digestibility is the quantity in which food is consumed. This quantity needs to be ascertained based on age, gender, season, digestive capacity, etc. Due consideration is to be given to the quantity of each item (*Parigraha*) and the total of the quantity of food consumed (*Sarvagraha*) as both can affect the digestion. Hence, even if a particular food product is of a lighter nature for digestion, still if consumed in excess quantity can result in vitiation of doshas and reduction in digestive capacity.
5. *Desha* (place): This consideration has two aspects: one where the food is available, that is, types of lands described in Ayurveda viz. marshy, dry, and normal lands. The second aspect is the surrounding. Food should be consumed in a clean space with good and sattvic surroundings. Food consumed in this way has better absorption and a positive effect on the body and mind.
6. *Kala* (time/period/season): Only if the previously consumed food has been properly digested should the next meal be consumed. Kala also refers to the seasonal regimen, and food should be consumed according to different seasonal regimens described.
7. *Upayoga Samstha* (rules for eating): The method for consuming food has been described under this. Rules for proper food consumption include consuming hot food in a relaxed, cheerful, and calm soothing atmosphere. As mood has a direct effect on food and its benefits from the perspective of being healthy, rules like one should not eat if feeling nervous, anxious, or when feeling angry or being in a disturbed state of mind have been described. Among other things to be borne in mind while eating is avoiding eating too slowly or too rapidly, avoiding talking and eating at the same time, excessive laughing, preoccupied mind, or distractions such as watching television is also not advisable. Mindful eating with full concentration on food and with a thought that how it is going to benefit my body and mind is necessary. Eating should be considered a ritual and be practiced with utmost devotion.
8. *Upayokta* (person who takes the food): The last but definitely not the least in considerations is the person consuming food. The person's constitution, their digestive capacity, and their age are all factors that affect the digestion of food and hence consideration needs to be given to this as a factor contributing to proper nourishment.

Effect of Paatra (vessels or medium) used for serving and storing food: Bhoojankutuhalam, a 17th-century culinary text describes the use of various leaves for serving and eating food. Different varieties of leaves have been used in the Indian culture for serving sustenance (Table 8.1).

Table 8.1 Leaves used for serving food (Suri and Balakrishna, 2013).

Leaves	Benefits
Plantain	Improves taste, stimulates the digestive fire, useful in the treatment of toxicity, tiredness, and gout
Bastard teak	Alleviates vata and kapha, treats ascites and abdominal tumor, cures dyspnea, improves taste, and promotes health
Calotropis	Treats abdominal tumor, pain, poisoning, dyspnea, anemia, and skin diseases but aggravates pitta
Castor	Greatly beneficial for eyes and light to digest. Stimulates the digestive fire and alleviates vata
Secrete milky sap	Helps to overcome thirst, burning sensation, and bleeding disorder
Lotus petals	Aphrodisiac removes weariness and is recommended for travelers
Tahitian screw pine	Treats all types of glandular swellings and is beneficial to the eyes

Table 8.2 Vessels and benefits of use (Suri and Balakrishna, 2013).

Vessels	Benefits
Gold	Alleviates doshas, improves sight, and gives wholesome to the body
Silver	Improves sight and alleviates doshas
Bell metal	Imparts intellect, improves appetite, and purifies the blood
Brass	Alleviates kapha and destroys worms but aggravates vata
Iron	Confers success, treats swelling and anemia, imparts strength and is an excellent treatment for jaundice
Earthen	Brings misfortune
Wooden	Improves appetite and aggravates kapha
Leaves	Appetizing, stimulates the digestive fire, removes toxins, and destroys sins
Crystal	Pure and cooling

In Sanskrit, vessels are called paatra (objects help to prepare and store food). Acharya Sushruta has given directions for the storage of food products. For example, ghee should be stored in iron vessels; fruits should be stored in vessels made of leaves, all eatables (snacks); *parishuska* (cooked meat) and *pradigdha* (cooked meat soaked in milk), as well as drinks, are to be stored in silver vessels; stone is the material of choice for storage of sour food items such as various sauces and buttermilk; water should be boiled well and then kept in copper vessels; mud pots should be used to store syrups, and wine should be stored in glass or rock crystal (stone). Suri and Balakrishna (2013) (Table 8.2).

8.4 Regional diversity and its interlaced traditional roots

India is home to a variety of foods and traditions. The origins of geographical diversity in cooking methods, choice of ingredients, and food habits can be traced back to

Ayurvedic classical texts. Ayurveda has described three types of regions (*desha*) namely *Jangala* (dry, arid forestland), *Anupa* (marshy land), and *Sadharan* (normal land). Interestingly, different states of India represent either of the regions, for example, the state of Rajasthan is representative of *Jangala* region, while the state of Kerala is an example of *Anupa* region. The climate of a specific region is an important determinant of the food choices for that particular region. The unsuitability of food with respect to the climate of the region is enlisted as one of the incompatible foods.

There are eight geographically and culturally prominent types of regional cuisines across India: Bengali, Gujarati, Jain, Maharashtrian, Mughlai, Punjabi, Rajasthani, and South Indian. The use of various spices in the preparation of meals across the eight major types of Indian cuisine is the best example of interlaced traditional roots of Ayurveda in Indian cuisine. Trikatu, an Ayurvedic formulation prescribed routinely for a variety of diseases, is a combination of spices viz., black pepper, long pepper, and ginger. The importance of spices in Indian regional cuisines is also highlighted by the fact that these cuisines have many derived ingredients (such as garam masala and ginger garlic paste) that are spice combinations. Spices play a significant role in the Indian diet in the form of spice blends in specific ethnic food preparations.

North Indian cuisine is characterized by high use of dairy products viz. milk, paneer (Indian mild cheese), and ghee (clarified butter). This is in keeping with the principles of Ayurveda, which describes the use of unctuous food ingredients in the area, which are cold and dry. In Northern India, buttermilk is taken as a lassi (sweet and salted buttermilk), generally thicker in consistency and heavy to digest. This is necessary, as people from these regions have been described to have higher digestive power in Ayurveda. As we come to the southern part of India, buttermilk that is sour in taste is consumed in highly diluted form. Similarly, milk preparations thicker in consistency and with cream (*rabdi*) are preferred in North India, whereas in South India they are generally consumed in a thinner paste called kheer with spices that improve digestibility.

Recipes for Eastern Indian cuisine favor poppy seeds, mustard seeds, and mustard oil. This adds pungency to the foods. This is in keeping with the description of food principles for marshy lands described in classical Ayurvedic texts. The western regions of India have geographically drier and hotter climates. The food preferences in these regions have a predominance of spices as an ingredient in most of the recipes, which have antimicrobial and digestion enhancing properties necessary for improving Agni or digestive power.

The staple foods also differ in the different parts of India. Although wheat is the common food grain in the North Indian diet, rice is preferred grain in the south parts. The use of pulses such as kidney beans and chickpea, which are heavy to digest, is common in the north part. The most common pulse used in South India is black gram. The cooking styles also vary region to region mainly influenced by geographical and climatic variance. Methods like cooking in hot clay cove called tandoor and deep-frying are predominantly used in the colder regions of Northern India whereas southern parts of India have a preference of steamed and fermented food. Mustard oil is the most commonly used oil in Northern parts that is again stronger in pungency compared to the coconut oil used in the Southern part of India. Fresh vegetables form a major part of the dietary pattern in the Southern part of India in the form of curries with a variety of spices added.

8.5 Historical overview

8.5.1 Nutritional and dietary intake scenario in ancient India

In the book *Indian Food: A Historical Companion*, the author gives a great overview of the impact that various foreign nations have on the methods of food preparation prevalent in India. The authors state "Ancient Indian literature left a lot of information on extant vegetables, pulses, meat, spices, fruits, cooking methods, and even an occasional recipe or two. The history of Indian cuisine can be divided into several stages or periods. The earliest period is before 1500 BC or the Vedic period."

In the same book, the author explores the ancient civilizations and their culinary practices. In this regard, it is said "The Harappan civilization was known to have rice, barley, wheat, oat, amaranths, great millet, sesame, mustard, chickpeas, red lentil, green gram and horse gram, dates, pomegranates, and perhaps bananas. Bones of numerous animals attest to meat (and fish) eating. The large granaries of Mohenjodaro, Harappa and Lothal attest to a sophisticated, aerated, rodent-free storage practice."

Ayurveda is a part of one of four treatises or Vedas. Traditional foods of India and their scientific study from a nutritional perspective has its roots even in the Vedic era. The author explores the availability of various foods mentioned throughout Rigveda. For the Vedic period, it is commented "Rigveda mentions rice, cereals and pulses, black gram, green gram, red lentil, green leafy vegetables (spinach), melons, pumpkins and gourds and in particular lotus stem, cucumber, bottle gourd, water chestnut, bitter gourd, radish, brinjal, some aquatic plants and fruits such as mangoes, oranges and grapes. Spices such as coriander, turmeric, pepper, cumin, asafoetida, cloves, sesame and mustard were well known, and at least the first four ones are thought to be Indian in origin. Meat eating was prevalent. Pigs, boar, deer, bovines and peacocks were eaten, though chicken (which, though originated in India) was not that desirable. They seem to have been forbidden or discouraged from eating eggs of any kind and in any manner. Turning to Mahabharata, a graphic description of cooking at a picnic has been provided on roasting large pieces of meat on spits, cooked with tamarind, pomegranates and spices with ghee and fragrant leaves. King Yudishtira is said to have fed 10,000 scholars with pork and venison, besides preparation of rice and milk in ghee and honey with fruits and roots.

It was after this time that a change in our food habits occurred. The Dharma Sutras, Manusmriti and related texts of 500–300 BC began forbidding and proscribing food items based on their 'temper' (*sattvik* – peaceful and ascetic, *rajasik* medium, energetic that can be either positive or negative and tamasic or coarse, rough and not all that nice), and prohibiting as *manyas*, 54 items (in particular a variety of animals) from the 'proper' kitchen. The teachings of Buddhism and Jainism against meat eating had taken hold by this time, and a turn towards preferential vegetarianism began to be expressed in Hindu texts as well. These, plus the diktats on *satvik*, *rajasic*, and *tamasic* practices changed the face of Indian gastronomy already around 300 BC." (Achaya, 1998)

8.5.2 Current nutritional and intake scenario

India has a population of 1.35 billion spread across 29 states and 7 union territories (Population of India, 2017). India has more than 2000 ethnic groups with genetically distinct ancestry and diverse lifestyles. The dietary pattern in India is as varied as a nation within a nation since each state has a rich historical background and diverse food and agricultural practices. In the systematic review conducted by Green et al., dietary pattern analysis to study common patterns from a public health nutrition perspective was carried out. This survey identified 29 dietary patterns by predominantly vegetarian food groups, suggesting that vegetarian diets are still prevalent in India. These diets tended to be based on fruits, vegetables, pulses, and cereals (mostly rice), with added dairy products, meat, and eggs in many cases. The most common food groups across all patterns were vegetables (16 out of 41 patterns), cereals (13 patterns) and fruit (10 patterns), meat (9 patterns), pulses (8 patterns), and dairy products (8 patterns). Less common were snacks and sweets, which were found in 6 patterns each (Green et al., 2016).

It is a popular belief that India is predominantly a vegetarian country. However, based on the latest census data, it can be reckoned that a quarter of the population is vegetarian.

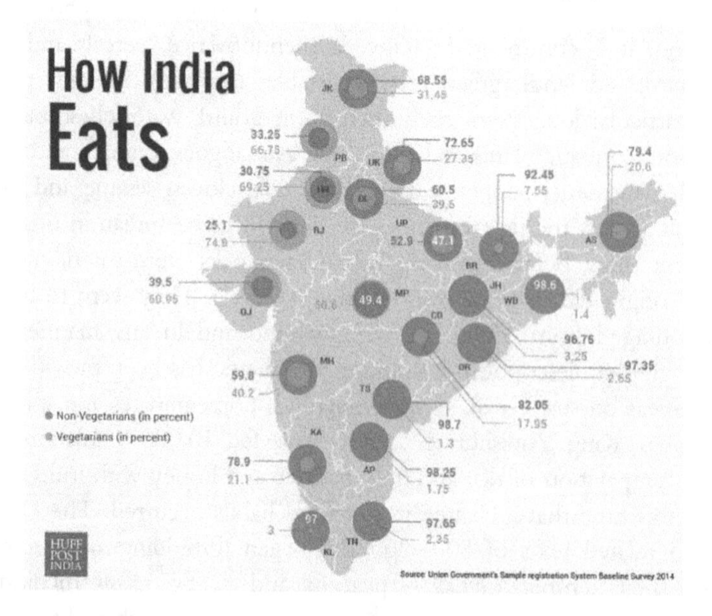

Although economic considerations play a part in this choice, it can be seen that ethical and religious beliefs are a more compelling force, for example, people belonging to the Jain caste avoid meat totally and also many of the Buddhists in India are vegetarians. Among other sects, which avoid meat are several Vaishnavite sects, Brahmins and Saivite nonBrahmins of South India. Interestingly, though it is seen that Brahmins residing in the Eastern part of India, those staying in Kashmir and the Saraswat Brahmins of the Southwest regularly consume fish and some meat (Balasubramanian, 2004).

8.6 Future outlook

Effects of globalization have led to change in the dietary intake pattern throughout the world and similar changes have been seen in India with the disease burden of noncommunicable diseases such as obesity, diabetes, and cancer on the rise in the past decade. The Global Burden of Disease survey conducted in 2017 reported that the number of disability-adjusted life years increased substantially for noncommunicable diseases. The major risk factors for noncommunicable diseases, including high systolic blood pressure, high fasting plasma glucose, high total cholesterol, and high body-mass index, also increased from 1990 to 2016 (Dandona et al., 2017). The role of Ayurvedic dietetics is enhanced in this scenario. The concepts of prakriti-based diet, diets according to desha (region), etc. have a significant role to play in the current dietary situation worldwide. Systematic elucidation can provide new insights to health and nutritional sciences to provide contemporary solutions in healthcare, for instance, how one can modulate the diet and lifestyle to suit one's prakriti, age, and season.

The study by Patwardhan et al. for studying the correlation between specific prakriti and HLA-DRB1 polymorphism (Bhushan et al., 2005). Prasher et al. (2008) and Mukherjee and Prasher (Mukerji and Prasher, 2011) have made the use of classification on the basis of prakriti to demonstrate the genomic and biochemical correlation between specific prakriti types. Ayurgenomics is the term coined by them for this approach, and they have proposed the potential for this approach to be useful in personalized and preventive medicine. Some other studies of note found on going through recent advances in field of Ayurveda and various publications are the study for determining frequency of association of CYP2C19 genotype varying depending on the prakriti (Ghodke et al., 2011) and the differential expression of EGLN1 gene in high-altitude adaptation gene as a response to hypoxia and its correlation to specific prakriti type (Aggarwal et al., 2010). Rotti et al. (2014) have also found there to be a significant correlation between dominant prakriti to place of birth and body mass index.

Another branch of Ayurveda that has the potential to unravel a number of dietary and herbal preventive therapeutic measures is *Rasayana*. This is that branch of Ayurveda, which provides knowledge and methods not only to enhance the quality of life but also to extend lifespan in a healthy way. The use of foods, plants, metals, animal products, and minerals useful in delaying aging to enhance well-being are explored in this branch of Ayurveda. Research using currently available tools for bioassay such as *in vitro* studies and animal models on small organisms such as yeast, Drosophila, and *Caenorhabditis elegans* are now being used to observe the physical, physiological, and behavioral effect of *Rasayanas* and gain insights into the molecular mechanisms of action (Dwivedi et al., 2012). Pomegranate, a *pathya* fruit according to Ayurveda was shown to enhance the lifespan and healthspan in the fruitfly (*Drosophila melanogaster*) model (Balasubramani et al., 2014). Pippali (*Piper longum* L.) and amla (*Phyllanthus emblica*) were shown to be effective bioavailability enhancers due to the inherent ability to increase agni and thereby digestion and absorption. In vitro cell-free and cell (Caco-2 and HepG2)-based models (Venkatasubramanian et al., 2014) were used as bioassay tools. Thus the paradigms for research available in the system of Ayurveda using the references in the Ayurvedic treatise and classical texts in combination with state-of-the-art research tools can unravel solutions to the lifestyle-related diseases of the current era.

References

Achaya, K.T., 1998. Indian Food: A Historical Companion. Oxford University Press, p. 322.

Aggarwal, S., Negi, S., Jha, P., Singh, P.K., Stobdan, T., Pasha, M.A., et al., 2010. EGLN1 involvement in high-altitude adaptation revealed through genetic analysis of extreme constitution types defined in ayurveda. Proc. Natl. Acad. Sci. USA. 107 (44), 18961–18966. Available from: https://doi.org/10.1073/pnas.1006108107.

Balasubramanian, D., 2004. Changes in India Menu Over the Ages, The Hindu, Nov 04.

Balasubramani, S.P., Mohan, J., Chatterjee, A., Patnaik, E., Kukkupuni, S.K., Nongthomba, U., et al., 2014. Pomegranate juice enhances healthy lifespan in *Drosophila melanogaster*: an exploratory study. Front. Public Health 2 (245), 245. Available from: https://doi.org/10.3389/fpubh.2014.00245.

Bhushan, P., Kalpana, J., Arvind, C., 2005. Classification of human population based on HLA gene polymorphism and the concept of Prakriti in Ayurveda. J. Altern. Complement. Med. 11 (2), 349–353.

Dandona, L., Dandona, R., Anil Kumar, G., Shukla, D.K., Paul, V.K., Balakrishnan, K., et al., 2017. Nations Within a Nation: Variations in Epidemiological Transition Across the States of India, 1990–2016 in the Global Burden of Disease Study. Available from: <https://doi.org/10.1016/>.

Dey, S., Pahwa, P., 2014. Prakriti and its associations with metabolism, chronic diseases, and genotypes: possibilities of new-born screening and a lifetime of personalized prevention. J. Ayurveda Integr. Med. 5 (1), 15–24. Available from: https://doi.org/10.4103/0975-9476.128848.

Dhyani, S.C., 1994. Rasapanchaka. Krishnadas Academy, Varanasi, pp. 32–42, 46–60.

Dutta, S.R., Upadhyaya, Y., Pandey, G.S., Gupta, B., 2005. Charaka Samhita. Chaukhambha Bharati Academy, Varanasi.

Dwarakanatha, C., 2003. Digestion and Metabolism in Ayurveda. Chaukhambha Krishnadas Academy, Varanasi, pp. 48–53, 59–61.

Dwivedi, V., Anandan, E.M., Mony, R.S., Muraleedharan, T.S., Valiathan, M.S., Mutsuddi, M., et al., 2012. In vivo effects of traditional ayurvedic formulations in *Drosophila melanogaster* model relate with therapeutic applications. PLoS ONE 7 (5), e37113. Available from: https://doi.org/10.1371/journal.pone.0037113.

Ghodke, Y., Joshi, K., Patwardhan, B., 2011. Traditional medicine to modern pharmacogenomics: ayurveda prakriti type and CYP2C19 gene polymorphism associated with the metabolic variability. Evid. Based Complement. Alternat. Med. 2011, 249528. Available from: https://doi.org/10.1093/ecam/nep206.

Green, R., Milner, J., Joy, E.J.M., Agrawal, S., Dangour, A.D., 2016 Public Health Foundation of India, Delhi NCR, Plot No. 47, Sector 44, Institutional Area Gurgaon 122002. Available from: <http://sustaininghealth.lshtm.ac.uk/sahdi/>. (accessed 30.07.19.).

Hegde, S., Nair, L.P., Chandran, H., Irshad, H., 2018. Traditional Indian way of eating - an overview. Journal of Ethnic Foods, 5 (1), 20–23. Available from: <https://doi.org/10.1016/j.jef.2018.02.001>.

Kukkupuni, S.K., Shashikumar, A., Venkatasubramanian, P., 2015. Fermented milk products: probiotics of ayurveda. J. Med. Nutr. Nutraceut. 4, 14–21. Available from: https://doi.org/10.4103/2278-019X.146149.

Mukerji, M., Prasher, B., 2011. Ayurgenomics: a new approach in personalized and preventive medicine. Sci Cult. 77 (1–2), 10–17.

fifth ed. Murthy, K.R.S. (Ed.), 2001. Vagbhata's Astanga Hrdayam, vol. 1. Chaukhambha Orientalia, Varanasi, pp. 53–57.

Patwardhan, B., 2014. Bridging Ayurveda with evidence-based scientific approaches in medicine. EPMA J.

Payyappallimana, U., Venkatasubramanian, P., 2016. Exploring Ayurvedic knowledge on food and health for providing innovative solutions to contemporary healthcare. Front Public Heal. 4.

Population of India, 2017. IndiaOnlinePages. <http://www.indiaonlinepages.com/population/india-current-population.html>. (accessed 29.07.19.).

Prabhupada, B.S. (Ed.), 2002. Bhagavad Gita Yatharupa. nineteenth ed. ISKCON, Bangalore [Kannada Language translation].

Prasher, B., Negi, S., Aggarwal, S., Mandal, A.K., Sethi, T.P., Deshmukh, S.R., et al., 2008. Whole genome expression and biochemical correlates of extreme constitutional types defined in ayurveda. J. Transl. Med. 6, 48. Available from: https://doi.org/10.1186/1479-5876-6-48.

Rotti, H., Raval, R., Anchan, S., Bellampalli, R., Bhale, S., Bharadwaj, R., et al., 2014. Determinants of prakriti, the human constitution types of Indian traditional medicine and its correlation with contemporary science. J. Ayurveda Integr. Med. 5 (3), 167–175. Available from: https://doi.org/10.4103/0975-9476.140478.

Sastri, K. (Ed.), 1997. Caraka Samhita, Part-1. fifth ed. Chaukhambha Sanskrit Sansthan, Varanasi, pp. 555–558.

Sharma, P.V. (Ed.), 2001. Caraka Samhita, vol. 1. Chaukhambha Orientalia, Varanasi, pp. 5–9. , 190,228,375–6.

Sharma, P.V. (Ed.), 2002. Astanga Samgraha of Vagbhata, vol. 1. sixth ed. Chaukhambha Orientalia, Varanasi, pp. 81–114.

Suri, R., Balakrishna, A., 2013. Bhojankutuhalam, first ed. Divya Prakashan, Haridwar, pp. 1–373.

Tripati, B., 1998. Pathyapathyanirnayah. Chaukhambha Sanskrit Pratishtan, Delhi, pp. 2–4, 39.

Venkatasubramanian, P., Koul, I.B., Varghese, R.K., Koyyala, S., Shivakumar, A., 2014. Amla (*Phyllanthus emblica* L.) enhances iron dialysability and uptake in in vitro models. Curr. Sci. 107, 1859–1866.

CHAPTER 9

Foods from the ocean for nutrition, health, and wellness

T.K. Srinivasa Gopal
Centre of Excellence in Food Processing Technology, Kerala University of Fisheries and Ocean Studies, Cochin, India

Contents

9.1 Introduction

Various organizations in the world have emphasized the importance of a varied diet to meet nutritional requirements for achieving the ideal body weight. These varied diets are related among others, to limited intake of saturated fats and cholesterol, and regulation of intake of sodium. In this context, fish and seafood can play a great role in the nutritional picture. Fish provides a good source of protein, vitamins, minerals and relatively low caloric content. In addition, fish are excellent sources of ω-3 polyunsaturated fatty acids (PUFAs) that appear to have beneficial effects in reducing the risk of cardiovascular diseases and are linked with positive benefits in many other pathological conditions, particularly, certain types of cancer and arthritis.

As far as India is concerned, the successful outcome of green revolution has answered the challenges of food security due to rapid growth in population. However, the fact that 35% of the Indian population still falls below the poverty line emphasizes the need to recognize fisheries as an important sector of the National economy for meeting the food and nutritional security. In the days ahead, "blue revolution" will be the buzzword to meet the challenges of food and nutritional security.

Fish and fishery products form an important food component for a large section of the world population. They represent 15.6% of animal protein supply and 5.6% of the total protein supply on a worldwide basis. Fish is the primary source of animal protein

Nutritional and Health Aspects of Food in South Asian Countries
DOI: https://doi.org/10.1016/B978-0-12-820011-7.00017-4

for over one billion people in developing countries. It is estimated that 60% of people in developing countries obtain 40%–100% of the animal protein in their diets from fish (Lowe et al., 1998). Protein, lipids, and bioactive compounds from seafood have unique features that differ from those of land animals. The uniqueness of fish protein is due to its excellent nutritive value, high digestibility, and presence of all essential amino acids. In general, fish flesh contains 60%–84% water, 15%–24% protein, 0.1%–22% fat, and 1%–2% minerals. It is a good source of PUFAs, especially ω-3 PUFAs, minerals, and vitamins (Fierens and Corthout, 2007).

9.2 Indian fish market—production and consumption

India's economy is the seventh-largest in the world and in the last quarter of 2014, it became the fastest-growing major economy. India made a paradigm shift in food availability by transforming from a begging bowl to breadbasket during the course of seven decades. Its fisheries sector has registered a sustainable growth of over 10% and has contributed over 1% of India's annual gross domestic product during the last decade. The vibrancy of the sector can be visualized by its tremendous growth in recent years.

India's coastline (8129 km) of the exclusive economic zone (2.02 million sq. km) and continental shelf (0.506 million sq. km) contributed to an estimated possible exploitable resource of 4.41 million tons of seafood in 2017–2018, of which approximately 3.40 million tons are being currently exploited. Rivers, canals, reservoirs, ponds, tanks, oxbow lakes, derelict waters, brackish water, and estuaries also contribute to the Indian fish industry. The brackish waters (14%) contribute mainly to shrimp farming. India enjoys the seventh position regarding marine fish production in the world and exported 1,377,244 MT of seafood worth US$ 7.08 billion during the financial year 2017–18, which is considerably higher (21.35% growth) than 1,134,948 MT and US$ 5.77 billion in the preceding fiscal year, with frozen shrimp and fish continuing to dominate the export basket. The Indian seafood industry is known for quality seafood and has become a leading supplier to major markets of the world. Recently, frozen cephalopods also registered a growth and added to the landings of the country. In recent years, dried, chilled, and live fish are also showing an upward trend. Indian aquaculture industry (fresh water and brackish water) currently holds the second position in aquaculture production (7.21 MMT from the inland sector and 3.58 MMT from the marine sector in 2016–17). The freshwater aquaculture sector contributed about 85% of the inland share. The recent improvements in the marine and inland sectors contribute to domestic food security. Nevertheless, the future production and consumption challenges, industrial uses, wastages/discards, and other industrial applications need to be streamlined and price difference based on geographical disparity needs to be controlled.

The fisheries sector offers an attractive and promising future for employment, livelihood, and food security. The fisheries and aquaculture production contribute around 1% to India's gross domestic product (GDP) and over 5% to the agricultural GDP. According to the Food and Agriculture Organization (FAO) report "The State of World Fisheries and Aquaculture 2018" apparent per capita fish consumption in India [average (2013–15)] lies between 5 and 10 kg. Fish has become an integral constituent in the Indian food basket as a healthy food with a high level of edible protein and availability across the states. It is considered as poor man's protein (low-value fishes) ensuring food security and delicacy. It has been estimated that 60% of the Indian populace consume fish and the consumption varies spatiotemporally and across the different social fabric. Indian Council of Medical Research recommends annual per capita consumption to be 12 kg per annum. Sardine and mackerel are the most often consumed fish in the domestic market.

9.3 Fish as healthy food

Fish is a health food, with relatively lesser taboos connected to it, unlike meat. World over fish is considered as a delicious item and from a nutritional point of view, it balances the cereal-based diets. A health food should contain all the principal constituents, viz. carbohydrates, proteins, lipids, minerals and vitamins in the right proportions. Detailed biochemical composition of all-important Indian food fishes (including proximate composition, fatty acid composition of body and liver oils, mineral content, and amino acid composition of muscle proteins) from fresh water, brackish water, and marine and deep-sea waters have been compiled and reported by the Central Institute of Fisheries Technology (Gopakumar, 1997). People are now more health conscious. Diets low in fat and cholesterol with high vitamin and mineral contents are often preferred, especially in the affluent west. For a healthy lifestyle, fish is a good starting point. The importance of fish as a source of high quality, balanced and easily digestible protein is now well understood. For the affluent, it is the best health food with curative properties, whereas for the less privileged section in developing nations, it is the only source of high-quality protein available at affordable cost and in sufficient quantity.

Fish plays a major role in human nutrition. Fish and shellfish form an important part of the human diet, both of the poor and of the wealthy. Good quality fish is an extremely safe food. Meat products are viewed as unsafe after the incidences of illnesses like mad cow disease. Fish is a versatile, tasty, and easy to prepare food. Consumers are increasingly demanding natural foods, which contain no chemical residues and are not genetically manipulated. Fish is organic and is considered as wild, and for the same reason safer, though late farmed fish has posed minor problems of harmful residues. For thousands of years, fish has been an important part of the human diet.

The ancient Assyrians, Romans and Chinese were famous for their fish farming. During the past decades, per capita consumption of fish has gone up globally. Fish is the diet of the poor fishermen and meets most of their nutritional requirements.

Researchers worldwide have repeatedly emphasized the beneficial effect of eating fish, after conducting systematic research for many years. In recent years, the link between fish oil and heart disease has been the subject of thousands of scientific papers. The whole story began following the discovery that coronary heart disease while being one of the biggest killers in the world is practically unknown among the Eskimos. The investigators found that their diet is mostly fish-based and rich in long-chain n-3 PUFAs (Lee and Lip, 2003; von Schacky and Dyerberg, 2001). Eskimos also have a reduced tendency to blood clotting and longer bleeding times compared to other people. Medical researchers carried out detailed investigations and showed that men who ate fish once or twice per week were protected against coronary heart disease (He et. al., 2004: Heikkila et al., 2004). An increase in fish oils in the diet results in a marked reduction in blood cholesterol and triglyceride levels and also prevents thrombosis (Bjerregaard et al., 2004).

9.4 Dietary lipids and disease management

The lipid content in fish varies between species as also within the species depending on many factors. Fish with a fat content as low as 0.5% and as high as 18%–20% is common. Squalene and wax esters are other components found in unusually high concentrations in certain fish. The fatty acid composition of marine lipids is much more complex than others. Lipids of fish and other aquatic animals contain a high proportion of highly unsaturated long-chain fatty acids. Fatty acids with carbon chains varying from 10 to 22 and unsaturation varying from 0 to 6 double bonds are common. Among the saturated acids, palmitic and stearic acids are the important ones, and in the monounsaturated group, palmitoleic and oleic acids are the major constituents. Among the polyunsaturated acids, arachidonic acid, eicosapentaenoic acid (EPA), and docosahexaenoic acid (DHA) are the major components (Mathew et al., 1998).

Fish oils have no effect on the levels of low-density lipoprotein cholesterol but they do raise high-density lipoprotein (HDL) by about 10%. HDL is a protective type of lipoprotein as it takes excess cholesterol away from the tissue and returns it to the liver. Diseased heart muscle is susceptible to bouts of irregular electrical activity (arrhythmias), which are potentially lethal and often cause sudden cardiac arrests. There is evidence from animal studies that increasing fish oil in the diet helps to reduce cardiac arrhythmias (Sellmayer et al., 2004; Covington, 2004). Fish oils improve the functionality of cell membranes, which helps in proper signal transmission. Fish oil inhibits platelet aggregation, which also reduces the risk of heart disease (Vanschoonbeek et al., 2004). Raised blood pressure is known to be a major risk factor in coronary heart disease. Most studies on the effects of fish oil given as dietary supplements have shown modest reductions in blood pressure, especially in hypertensive people (Aguilera et al., 2004; Wilburn et al., 2004; Mano et al., 1995).

The lipid composition of fish is unique having long long-chain PUFAs in the form of arachidonic and eicosapentaenoic acids with many potential effects of adult health and child development. Among fish species that are cheaper and often traded in developing countries, small pelagic fish such as anchovy and sardine are perhaps some of the richest sources of long-chain PUFAs. The amount of PUFAs in large fresh water fish such as carp and tilapia is lower. EPA and DHA reduce vasoconstriction by competing with arachidonic acid for the enzyme cyclo-oxygenase (Sametz et al., 2000). EPA, the main n-3 acid is converted by platelet cyclooxygenase to thromboxane A3, which is a very weak vasoconstrictor, unlike thromboxane A2, which is formed by the action of cyclooxygenase on arachidonic, the n-6 acid, and is a strong vasoconstrictor (Tapiero et al., 2002; Akiba et al., 2000). The American Heart Association recommends including fatty fish at least twice a week in the diet (Kris-Etherton et al., 2002; Krauss et al., 2000). Institute of Human Nutrition in New York also recommends eating plenty of fish. Italian study involving 985 people who survived heart attacks, also proved the beneficial effect of fish oil (Tavani et al., 2001). The new slogan in the west is that a tuna sandwich a day keeps heart problems at bay (Mozaffarian et al., 2004; O'Neill, 2002). It is also stated that if a person wants to reduce the risk of heart attack by more than 20%, he has to eat a tuna sandwich just once a month. No wonder they say, "Seafood is heartfood."

Recently, the inhibitory role of n-3 PUFAs in the development and progression of a range of human cancers has been established by researchers worldwide. Studies have found that the antitumor effect of EPA is mainly related to its suppression of cell proliferation (Pham and Ziboh, 2002; Yuri et al., 2003). The effect of DHA appears to be related to its ability to induce apoptosis or cell death (Baumgartner et al., 2004; Chiu et al., 2004). The dietary n-3/n-6 fatty acid ratio, rather than the quantity administered, appears to be the principal factor in the antitumor effect of n-3 PUFAs.

Apart from heart disease and cancer, fish oil is proved to be effective for preventing a wide variety of diseases. In several observational studies, low concentrations of n-3 PUFAs were predictive of impulsive behaviors and severe mental depression (Ruxton, 2004; Freeman et al., 2004). The importance of PUFAs in the maintenance of insulin in the blood has also been proven experimentally (Holness et al., 2004). Clinical and biochemical studies have shown that fish oil and to a lesser extent fish can be used as a source of n-3 fatty acids in the treatment of rheumatoid arthritis (Ruxton, 2004; Remans et al., 2004). Supplementations with fish oils can markedly reduce interleukin-1β production and result in a significant reduction in morning stiffness and the number of painful joints in arthritis patients. Studies have shown fish oil to be effective in the treatment of acute respiratory distress syndrome (Pacht et al., 2003), psoriasis (Mayser et al., 2002), and also in multiple sclerosis (Nordvik et al., 2000). Older people who eat fish at least once a week may reduce their risk of Alzheimer's disease by more than half (Yazawa, 2004; Morris et al., 2003). Other diseases that are reduced due to the consumption of PUFAs include primary Raynaud's disease (Di Giacomo, 1989; Swanson, 1986), gastric ulcer (Olafsson et al., 2000; Manjari and Das, 2000), and Crohn's disease (Geerling et al., 2000).

Along with fish oils, proteins in fish also have a positive role in reducing blood cholesterol (Ait Yahia et al., 2004). Studies have shown that fish proteins have a clear protective effect in diabetic renal diseases (Mollsten et al., 2001). Fish proteins are of high biological value, as they contain all essential amino acids in the right proportion. Plant proteins, although rich in certain essential amino acids, do not always offer all essential amino acids in a single food. Legumes lack methionine, while grains lack lysine. Fish protein is also an excellent source of lysine as well as the sulfur-containing amino acids, methionine and cysteine. Amino acid scores of fish protein agree well with the FAO reference pattern. In the studies conducted in the Central Institute of Fisheries Technology, Kochi, it was seen that the amino acid composition of the protein is crucial in determining its hypocholesterolemic properties. The alanine/proline ratio in a protein was found to be a significant factor determining its hypocholesterolemic properties (Ammu et al., 1994).

9.5 Other dietary components and their health significance

The protein content of fish muscle ranges between 16% and 20% depending on the species, the nutritional condition, and the type of muscle. The crude protein calculated on the basis of the total nitrogen content represents proteins and other nitrogenous compounds, such as nucleic acids, nucleotides, trimethylamine and trimethylamine oxide, free amino acids, and urea. Protein from fish is easily digested, with most species showing a protein digestibility greater than 90%. Chemical score or amino acid score of fish compares very well with that of whole egg protein. The chemical score of finfish is 70, an indication of its high quality, beef is 69, and cow's milk is 60. The protein efficiency ratio, another measure of protein quality of fish is around 3.5, which is much higher than beef (2.30) and milk proteins (2.5) and close to that of an egg (3.92). Fish is a good dietary source of taurine, a nonprotein amino acid with multiple functions like neurotransmission in the brain, stabilization of cell membranes and in the transport of ions such as sodium, potassium, calcium, and magnesium (Franconi et al., 2004; Birdsall, 1998; Del Olmo et al., 2000). Nutritional quality of protein is generally determined by factors such as essential amino acid composition, digestibility, and biological value. Fish protein is rated high in all the above qualities and is considered as a good dietary protein in all respects.

In general, both water-soluble and fat-soluble vitamins are present in fish. Fat-soluble vitamins A, D, K, and E are present in fish in varying amounts—often in higher concentrations than in land animals. The content of vitamins and minerals is species-specific and can vary with season. Fish compared to other foods is known to be an important source of essential micronutrients and minerals such as calcium, copper, phosphorus, iodine, zinc, iron, and selenium. Salt-water fish are rich in iodine. The iodine in marine fish ranges from 300 to 3000 μg/kg. Fish is a good source of almost all the minerals present in seawater (Nair and Mathew, 2000). The total content of minerals in the raw flesh of fish and aquatic invertebrates is in the range of 0.6%−1.5% of wet weight. Certain seafood such as snails and tuna are a good source of the macromineral magnesium. Seafood, especially tuna, is an important source of the essential antioxidant trace element selenium, which provides protection against heavy metal poisonings and a variety of carcinogens. As it contains vitamin E, selenium is a vital factor in the protection of lipids from oxidation as part of the enzyme glutathione peroxidase, which detoxifies products of rancid fat. The carbohydrate content of finfish is insignificant, but certain shellfish store some of their energy reserves as glycogen, which contributes to the characteristic sweet taste of these products.

The flesh of lean white fish, such as cod, haddock, and pollock, contains from 25 to 50 IU of vitamin A per 100 g, while in the fatty species such as herring, the amount ranges from 100 to about 4500 IU per 100 g. The content of vitamin D in sardines and pilchards and in tuna is in the range of 530−5400 and 700−2000 IU per 100 g, respectively. The contents of vitamin E in the edible parts of fish and marine invertebrates range from about 0.2 to 270 mg/100 g. Fish is a good source of B vitamins. The red meat has a higher content of vitamin B than white meat. Fish liver, eggs, milk, and skin are good sources of thiamine (B_1), riboflavin (B_2), pyridoxine (B_6), folic acid, biotin, and cyanocobalamine (B_{12}).

9.6 Nutritional superiority of fish in Indian scenario

Fish is highly favored in West Bengal, Assam, Kerala, and the coastal regions of India. It is included in almost every meal as it is one of the healthiest foods. Fish has a unique flavor and taste, which is specific to each variety. It is easy to cook, and the flesh becomes really soft upon cooking. It can be grilled, poached, steamed, baked, or boiled, and it pairs well with every Indian staple, whether rice or wheat.

Different from other meat sources, it contributes greatly to human health by improving metabolism, sleep quality, skin quality, and concentration and prevents inflammation. Fish contains components such as protein, which is healthy, cheap, and readily available; hence, it will help in curtailing malnutrition and prevent noncommunicable diseases. Indian coastal lines can provide apt nutritional security to the Indian population, specifically in the coastal areas. Fatty fishes such as salmon, trout, sardines, tuna, and mackerel are rich sources of ω-3 fatty acids, which are extremely important for the proper functioning of the brain and eyes. It is also recommended for pregnant women. The absence of saturated fatty acids makes fish apt heart food. It keeps cholesterol at bay and reduces the risk of cardiovascular diseases. The abundance of vitamins specifically vitamin D in fish aids in the absorption of other nutrients during metabolism. Consequently, fish becomes a necessary food that has a superior place and is inevitable in our daily diet. ω-3 fatty acids (DHA) and vitamin D help in maintaining mental health and act as an antidepressant. Further, it reduces the risk of autoimmune diseases such as diabetes and rheumatoid arthritis. Hence, fish could be considered as a one-stop source of all vital nutrients that maintain a healthy balance in the human system and curb all major diseases.

When the beneficial effects of dietary fish are considered, vegetarianism in dietary habits does not seem to be wise. When one decides to become an obligate vegetarian and cuts out meat/dairy/fish out of the diet, he/she decides to cut out some of the major nutrients body needs on a daily basis for effective functioning. The argument that fish lives in unhygienic habitat and polluted waters is also not valid, as pollution is a universal phenomenon, affecting air, land, and water. Fish is the heart food that gives you both satisfaction and health and it is the word for nutritional security.

References

Aguilera, A.A., Diaz, G.H., Barcelata, M.L., Guerrero, O.A., Ros, R.M., 2004. Effects of fish oil on hypertension, plasma lipids, and tumor necrosis factor-alpha in rats with sucrose-induced metabolic syndrome. J. Nutr. Biochem. 15 (6), 350–357.

Ait Yahia, D., Madani, S., Prost, J., Bouchenak, M., Belleville, J., 2004. Fish protein improves blood pressure but alters HDL(2) and HDL(3) composition and tissue lipoprotein lipase activities in spontaneously hypertensive rats. Eur. J. Nutr. 10, 1–8.

Akiba, S., Murata, T., Kitatani, K., Sato, T., 2000. Involvement of lipoxygenase pathway in docosapentaenoic acid-induced inhibition of platelet aggregation. Biol. Pharm. Bull. 23 (11), 1293–1297.

Ammu, K., Devadasan, K., Stephen, J., 1994. Influence of alanine/proline ratio of dietary fish proteins on serum cholesterol level of albino rats. In: Devadasan, K., Mukundan, M.K., Antony, P.D., Viswanathan Nair, P.G., Perigreen, P.A. Joseph, J. (Eds.), Proceedings, 'Nutrients and Bioactive substances in aquatic organisms'. SOFT(I), Cochin, pp. 67–75.

Baumgartner, M., Sturlan, S., Roth, E., Wessner, B., Bachleitner-Hofmann, T., 2004. Enhancement of arsenic trioxide-mediated apoptosis using docosahexaenoic acid in arsenic trioxide-resistant solid tumor cells. Int. J. Cancer 112 (4), 707. 20.

Birdsall, T.C., 1998. Therapeutic applications of taurine. Altern. Med. Rev. 3 (2), 128–136.

Bjerregaard, L.J., Aardestrup, I.V., Christensen, J.H., Schmidt, E.B., 2004. The effect of adhesion to recommendations for fish intake on adipose tissue composition and plasma lipids. Asia. Pac. J. Clin. Nutr. 13 (Suppl), S95.

Chiu, L.C., Wong, E.Y., Ooi, V.E., 2004. Docosahexaenoic acid modulates different genes in cell cycle and apoptosis to control growth of human leukemia HL-60 cells. Int. J. Oncol. 25 (3), 737–744.

Covington, M.B., 2004. Omega-3 fatty acids. Am. Fam. Physician. 70 (1), 133–140. 1.

Del Olmo, N.D., Galarreta, M., Bustamante, J., Martin del Rio, R., Solis, J.M., 2000. Taurine-induced synaptic potentiation: dependence on extra- and intracellular calcium sources. Adv. Exp. Med. Biol. 483, 283–292.

Di Giacomo, R.A., Kremer, J.M., Shah, D.M., 1989. Fish-oil dietary supplementation in patients with Raynaud's phenomenon: a double-blind, controlled, prospective study. Am. J. Med. 86 (2), 158–164.

Fierens, C., Corthout, J., 2007. Omega-3 fatty acid preparations--a comparative study. J. Pharm. Belg. 62 (4), 115–119.

Franconi, F., Diana, G., Fortuna, A., Galietta, G., Trombetta, G., Valentini, G., et al., 2004. Taurine administration during lactation modifies hippocampal CA1 neurotransmission and behavioural programming in adult male mice. Brain Res. Bull. 63 (6), 491–497.

Freeman, M.P., Helgason, C., Hill, R.A., 2004. Selected integrative medicine treatments for depression: considerations for women. J. Am. Med. Womens Assoc. 59 (3), 216–224.

Geerling, B.J., Badart-Smook, A., van, Deursen, C., van, Houwelingen, A.C., Russel, M.G., Stockbrugger, R.W., et al., 2000. Nutritional supplementation with N-3 fatty acids and antioxidants in patients with Crohn's disease in remission: effects on antioxidant status and fatty acid profile. Inflamm. Bowel Dis. 6 (2), 77–84.

Gopakumar, K., 1997. Biochemical Composition of Indian Food Fish. Central Institute of Fisheries Technology, Cochin.

He, K., Song, Y., Daviglus, M.L., Liu, K., Van Horn, L., Dyer, A.R., et al., 2004. Accumulated evidence on fish consumption and coronary heart disease mortality: a meta-analysis of cohort studies. Circulation 109 (22), 2705–2711.

Heikkila, A.T., Lichtenstein, A.H., Mozaffarian, D., Herrington, D.M., 2004. Fish intake is associated with a reduced progression of coronary artery atherosclerosis in postmenopausal women with coronary artery disease. Am. J. Clin. Nutr. 80 (3), 626–632.

Holness, M., Smith, N., Greenwood, G., Sugden, M., 2004. Acute omega-3 fatty acid enrichment selectively reverses high saturated fat feeding induced insulin hyper secretion but does not improve insulin resistance. Diabetes 53, S166–S171.

Krauss, R.M., Eckel, R.H., Howard, B., Appel, L.J., Daniels, S.R., Deckelbaum, R.J., et al., 2000. AHA Dietary Guidelines: revision 2000: a statement for healthcare professionals from the Nutrition Committee of the American Heart Association. Circulation. 102 (18), 2284–2299. 31.

Kris-Etherton, P.M., Harris, W.S., Appel, L.J., American Heart Association, Nutrition Committee, 2002. Fish consumption, fish oil, omega-3 fatty acids, and cardiovascular disease. Circulation. 106 (21), 2747–2757.

Lee, K.W., Lip, G.Y., 2003. The role of omega-3 fatty acids in the secondary prevention of cardiovascular disease. QJM 96 (7), 465–480.

Lowe, T.E., Brill, R.W., Cousins, K.L., 1998. Responses of the red blood cells from two high-energy-demand teleosts, yellowfin tuna (*Thunnus albacares*) and skipjack tuna (Katsuwonus pelamis), to catecholamines. J. Comp. Physiol. [B] 168 (6), 405–418.

Manjari, V., Das, U.N., 2000. Effect of polyunsaturated fatty acids on dexamethasone-induced gastric mucosal damage. Prostaglandins Leukot. Essent. Fatty Acids 62 (2), 85–96.

Mano, M.T., Bexis, S., Abeywardena, M.Y., McMurchie, E.J., King, R.A., Smith, R.M., et al., 1995. Fish oils modulate blood pressure and vascular contractility in the rat and vascular contractility in the primate. Blood. Press. 3, 177–186.

Mathew, S., Ammu, K., Nair, P.G.V., Devadasan, K., 1998. Cholesterol content of Indian fish and shellfish. Food. Chem. 66, 455–461.

Mayser, P., Grimm, H., Grimminger, F., 2002. n-3 fatty acids in psoriasis. Br. J. Nutr. 87 (Suppl 1), S77–S82.

Mollsten, A.V., Dahlquist, G.G., Stattin, E.L., Rudberg, S., 2001. Higher intakes of fish protein are related to a lower risk of microalbuminuria in young Swedish type 1 diabetic patients. Diabetes Care 24 (5), 805–810.

Morris, M.C., Evans, D.A., Bienias, J.L., Tangney, C.C., Bennett, D.A., Wilson, R.S., et al., 2003. Consumption of fish and n-3 fatty acids and risk of incident Alzheimer disease. Arch. Neurol. 60 (7), 940–946.

Mozaffarian, D., Psaty, B.M., Rimm, E.B., Lemaitre, R.N., Burke, G.L., Lyles, M.F., et al., 2004. Fish intake and risk of incident atrial fibrillation. Circulation 110 (4), 368–373.

Nair, P.G.V., Mathew, S., 2000. Biochemical composition of fish & shellfish. CIFT Technology Advisory Series. Central Institute of Fisheries Technology, Cochin.
Nordvik, I., Myhr, K.M., Nyland, H., Bjerve, K.S., 2000. Effect of dietary advice and n-3 supplementation in newly diagnosed MS patients. Acta Neurol. Scand. 102 (3), 143–149.
Olafsson, S.O., Hallgrimsson, J., Gudbjarnason, S., 2000. Dietary cod liver oil decreases arachidonic acid in rat gastric mucosa and increases stress-induced gastric erosions. Lipids 35 (6), 601–605.
O'Neill, S., 2002. Cardiac Ca(2+) regulation and the tuna fish sandwich. News Physiol. Sci. 17, 162–165.
Pacht, E.R., DeMichele, S.J., Nelson, J.L., Hart, J., Wennberg, A.K., Gadek, J.E., 2003. Enteral nutrition with eicosapentaenoic acid, gamma-linolenic acid, and antioxidants reduces alveolar inflammatory mediators and protein influx in patients with acute respiratory distress syndrome. Crit. Care Med. 31 (2), 491–500.
Pham, H., Ziboh, V.A., 2002. 5 alpha-reductase-catalyzed conversion of testosterone to dihydrotestosterone is increased in prostatic adenocarcinoma cells: suppression by 15-lipoxygenase metabolites of gamma-linolenic and eicosapentaenoic acids. J. Steroid. Biochem. Mol. Biol. 82 (4-5), 393–400.
Remans, P.H., Sont, J.K., Wagenaar, L.W., Wouters-Wesseling, W., Zuijderduin, W.M., Jongma, A., et al., 2004. Nutrient supplementation with polyunsaturated fatty acids and micronutrients in rheumatoid arthritis: clinical and biochemical effects. Eur. J. Clin. Nutr. 58 (6), 839–845.
Ruxton, C., 2004. Health benefits of omega-3 fatty acids. Nurs. Stand. 18 (48), 38–42.
Sametz, W., Jeschek, M., Juan, H., Wintersteiger, R., 2000. Influence of polyunsaturated fatty acids on vasoconstrictions induced by 8-iso-PGF(2alpha) and 8-iso-PGE(2). Pharmacology. 60 (3), 155–160.
Sellmayer, A., Schrepf, R., Theisen, K., Weber, P.C., 2004. Role of omega-3 fatty acids in cardiovascular prevention. Dtsch. Med. Wochenschr. 129 (38), 1993–1996.
Swanson, D.R., 1986. Fish oil, Raynaud's syndrome, and undiscovered public knowledge. Perspect. Biol. Med. 30 (1), 7–18.
Tapiero, H., Ba, G.N., Couvreur, P., Tew, K.D., 2002. Polyunsaturated fatty acids (PUFA) and eicosanoids in human health and pathologies. Biomed Pharmacother. 56 (5), 215–222.
Tavani, A., Pelucchi, C., Negri, E., Bertuzzi, M., La Vecchia, C., 2001. n-3 Polyunsaturated fatty acids, fish, and nonfatal acute myocardial infarction. Circulation 104 (19), 2269–2272.
Vanschoonbeek, K., Feijge, M.A., Paquay, M., Rosing, J., Saris, W., Kluft, C., et al., 2004. Variable hypocoagulant effect of fish oil intake in humans: modulation of fibrinogen level and thrombin generation. Arterioscler. Thromb. Vasc. Biol. 24 (9), 1734–1740.
von Schacky, C., Dyerberg, J., 2001. omega 3 fatty acids. From eskimos to clinical cardiology--what took us so long? World Rev. Nutr. Diet. 88, 90–99.
Wilburn, A.J., King, D.S., Glisson, J., Rockhold, R.W., Wofford, M.R., 2004. The natural treatment of hypertension. J. Clin. Hypertens. (Greenwich) 6 (5), 242–248.
Yazawa, K., 2004. Importance of "health foods", EPA and DHA, for preventive medicine. Rinsho Byori 52 (3), 249–253.
Yuri, T., Danbara, N., Tsujita-Kyutoku, M., Fukunaga, K., Takada, H., Inoue, Y., et al., 2003. Dietary docosahexaenoic acid suppresses N-methyl-N-nitrosourea-induced mammary carcinogenesis in rats more effectively than eicosapentaenoic acid. Nutr. Cancer 45 (2), 211–217.

PART 3

Food, Nutrition, and Health in Sri Lanka

CHAPTER 1

Introduction

Viduranga Y. Waisundara
Australian College of Business & Technology - Kandy Campus, Sri Lanka

Sri Lanka is a low-middle income country that is currently undergoing a rapid epidemiological and nutritional transition. Nevertheless, as a whole, the country still remains very much an agricultural nation. The staple food of Sri Lankan is rice, and it is not an uncommon sight to see paddy plantations alongside roads and hillsides when driving through the country.

Sri Lanka's commercial agriculture is nevertheless dominated by its tea industry. This is especially true for the sloping hill-country and mid-country regions. Tea is one of the major sources of foreign exchange for the country, moreover, because Sri Lanka supplies about 18% of the tea traded in world markets.

The typical diet of Sri Lanka composes mainly of rice with some vegetables and a small portion of meat or fish, or a chicken egg. The bulk of the food consumed by the average Sri Lankan can be considered as composed of rice with a few vegetables. In particular, the diet of the rural populations in Sri Lanka is high in cereals with a low intake of foods of animal origin. Cereals are the main sources of protein in the Sri Lankan diet, and most of these are consumed for breakfast. On top of that, herbs and leafy greens incorporated into rice broth is becoming a popular food item in the country as well. Consuming herbal porridges or *kola kanda* for breakfast has become a trend in modern Sri Lanka to keep up good health as well as to obtain necessary phytonutrients. The younger generation finds the habit of consuming herbal porridge more palatable, as some of the herbs and leafy greens help to prevent the occurrence of diseases. When rice gruel is incorporated with minced leaves and consumed as a broth, the bitterness and grassy note present in many of the leaves is masked, and the resulting food product is more appetizing. Additionally, drinking one glass of herbal porridge is considered an all-in-one breakfast among Sri Lankans, and given the presence of fibers contributed by the broth, it offers a feeling of satiety. This is very important for the urban population of Sri Lanka who leads high-powered corporate-level careers but is nevertheless keen on incorporating a healthy diet and exercise as part of their lifestyle.

Sri Lanka offers a variety of traditional sweets that are especially prepared during festive occasions. These products are primarily made of rice flour, and traditional preparations of these food items do not use sugar. Instead, treacle obtained from the sap of the

Nutritional and Health Aspects of Food in South Asian Countries
DOI: https://doi.org/10.1016/B978-0-12-820011-7.00018-6

tree *Caryota urens* or *kitul* as called in the Sinhala language is utilized. Kitul treacle offers body the food product as well as fiber and several other minerals and nutrients. Other than rice flour, the flour obtained from pulverizing the mung bean (*Vigna radiata*) is also used in the preparation of some of the traditional sweets, especially *Mung Kavum*.

Sri Lanka is part of the Western Ghats biodiversity hot spot that extends southward from Western India. This honor is bestowed upon the country due to the wide variety of flora and fauna. As a result of this diversity, the region as a whole has a high level of endemism in the animal species as well. It is important therefore for Sri Lanka to balance agricultural development and conservation efforts to meet sustainable development goals for biodiversity conservation while at the same time meeting demands to increase the national production of food. Several traditional Sri Lankan farming systems are based on diversified farms and landscapes that provide a series of benefits for both humans and wildlife. Traditional practices such as deep water and stepped rice production that adapt to natural water regimes and use minimal inputs are recognized as potentially sustainable food production systems. However, the environmental and socioeconomic sustainability of traditional agricultural systems has received relatively little research attention compared with intensified and commercialized production systems. Traditional agricultural systems are often the result of centuries of experience in farming under local environmental and climatic conditions. Efforts to modernize such systems can sometimes result in reduced environmental sustainability and degradation of land or water, with consequent abandonment of farming or a return to original, traditional methods. Thus all efforts to produce sustainable food production systems via agriculture should bear in mind that the flora, fauna, and wildlife of Sri Lanka does not get destroyed as a result.

CHAPTER 2

Traditional and ethnic foods of Sri Lanka—safety aspects

Chathudina J. Liyanage
Department of Food Science and Technology, Faculty of Applied Sciences, Sabaragamuwa University of Sri Lanka, Belihuloya, Sri Lanka

Contents

2.1 Introduction

It has been estimated that 600 million people fall ill after eating contaminated food and 420,000 die every year (World Health Organization, 2017). Food safety has therefore gained the status of a key global concern related to public health.

Today, there is a growing interest in traditional and ethnic food throughout the world. In Sri Lanka as well, foods that are produced according to the gastronomic traditions hold a prominent place in the local cuisine and diet. The ethnic diversity of Sri Lanka has contributed significantly to the wide variety of traditional and ethnic foods consumed in the country. The nutritional and microbiological profiles of many traditional and ethnic food types in Sri Lanka are relatively well described, but the safety aspects of these foods are not to be undermined as they are yet to be well researched and documented.

Even though many of the traditional and ethnic food items are rich in functional (bioactive) ingredients that lead to improved nutrition and health status, some key food safety challenges have been identified in studies conducted elsewhere in the world regarding microbiological and chemical risk factors (Cagri-Mehmetoglu, 2017; Lücke and Zangerl, 2014; Tajkarimi et al., 2013). Addressing the specific food safety challenges associated with traditional and ethnic food therefore is a key demand from

Nutritional and Health Aspects of Food in South Asian Countries
DOI: https://doi.org/10.1016/B978-0-12-820011-7.00019-8

the perspective of consumers as well as food producers. As the local food culture places an important emphasis on traditional and ethnic food dishes, providing wholesome and safe food is a key challenge associated with domestic- and commercial-level food preparations with traditional ingredients and/or traditional types of food processing and production methods. Chemical and microbiological aspects are the top priorities when the safety of raw materials and production processes of these foods are addressed with respect to the food safety standards and regulations (Prakash, 2016).

This chapter presents an overview of the key food safety issues and concerns associated with the traditional and ethnic foods in Sri Lanka emphasizing on the chemical (toxicological) and microbiological safety aspects of the raw materials and processing/preparation methods. The local regulations pertaining to food safety are also briefly described with a discussion on the specific strategies to address the key food safety issues and how they can be integrated into and addressed under the existing regulatory frameworks.

2.2 Historical overview, culture, and traditions associated with traditional and ethnic food in Sri Lanka

Traditional and ethnic foods constitute an important part in the heritage and culture of Sri Lankan people. Being a tropical country of immense indigenous floral and faunal diversity, the Sri Lankan diet remained largely plant-based for centuries. As documented by writers such as Robert Knox (1681) and Emerson Tennet (1860), plenty of naturally growing food commodities were available for consumption by the locals and a wide variety of gastronomic delights were prepared from them, thereby ensuring food security. According to the ancient legends and chronicles, the traditional Sri Lankan diet used to be mainly plant-based, rich in indigenous cereals and grains, roots, tubers and indigenous yams, legumes, vegetables, oil seeds, and fruits, with little or no animal products, meticulously selected for their specific nutritional as well as therapeutic properties (Perera, 2008; Weerasekara et al., 2018).

Contemporary culinary traditions of Sri Lanka are largely influenced by the different ethnicities of the country, namely Sinahala, Tamil, Sri Lankan Moor, Burgher, and Malay. In addition, colonization periods have also contributed significantly to shape the present culinary traditions of Sri Lanka. In particular, the shift from rice flour-based food items to wheat flour-based items was largely influenced by the colonization of the Dutch, Portuguese, and the English. A large number of ethnic and traditional Sri Lankan dishes are influenced by the Malay, Arabic, and South Indian culinary flavors and characteristics.

2.3 Major traditional and ethnic food categories consumed in Sri Lanka

Sri Lankans predominantly consume rice and curry-based diets for the main meals of lunch and dinner. A typical meal comprises a large portion of steamed/cooked rice served with two or three vegetable dishes in the form of curries (mostly coconut milk–based and seasoned with local spices and condiments) and leafy vegetables (green leaves). Fish, meat, or dried fish (anchovy is the most widely consumed type) may also be included. Tubers, local yams, and local pulses are also a popular choice. Local fruits are eaten as dessert along with traditional sweets. A variety of traditional and ethnic food items exist in Sri Lanka to supplement the main meals, and in some cases they are chosen as a main item in breakfast or dinner (e.g., *pittu*, hoppers, string hoopers, *roti*). Traditional sweets are usually served with tea, and they are the typical choice for any special occasion and celebration such as the Sri Lankan New Year celebration. All forms of new beginnings and auspicious occasions in Sri Lanka are marked with the consumption of milk rice along with traditional sweets. A summary of the most important traditional and ethnic food categories in Sri Lanka is presented in Table 2.1.

2.4 Safety of traditional and ethnic food in Sri Lanka

2.4.1 Safety of raw materials

Quality and safety of raw materials are of paramount importance when it comes to food preparation and processing. As many traditional food preparations rely on locally or regionally sourced unique raw materials, their safety aspects should be assessed systematically, in terms of potential hazards.

Rice, the staple food of the Sri Lankan traditional diet, can be easily contaminated from agrochemicals, insects, molds, mycotoxins, and bacteria. As traditional Sri Lankan cuisine has evolved around rice and due to the high level of consumption of rice flour-based traditional foods in Sri Lanka, there may be a possible overexposure to some toxic elements such as lead, chromium, and arsenic that may accumulate in rice. The metalloid arsenic (As) has gained much attention recently due to its chronic health effects. As soil in rice paddy fields can contain naturally occurring arsenic and also can be polluted by irrigation water that is contaminated with arsenic from anthropogenic sources such as agrochemicals, rice and rice flour-based foods can be potential dietary sources of arsenic. The Codex Alimentarius Commission has established a maximum allowable limit of 200 μg/kg for inorganic arsenic (iAs) in rice (Codex Alimentarius Commission, 2014; Carbonell-Barrachina et al., 2015, Jallad, 2015). The presence of arsenic in rice cultivated in Sri Lanka has been investigated in recent studies. Jayasumana et al. reported As levels in the range of 20.6–540.4 μg/kg in polished rice obtained from agrochemical dependent newly improved varieties of rice cultivated in seven different locations in Sri Lanka (Jayasumana et al., 2015). As reported in studies conducted elsewhere, there also exists a high potential for the occurrence of other toxic elements such as Cd, Cr, Hg, and Pb (Shraim, 2017). As rice is produced in Sri Lanka under environmental conditions favorable for the growth of fungi such as

Table 2.1 Main categories of traditional Sri Lankan food.

Food category	Examples
Cereal and grain-based food	Fermented: *hoppers* (crispy rice flour pancakes: plain flour and egg are the most common forms, and treacle is added sometimes to produce a sweet version), *dosa/thosé* (a type of pancake made from black gram flour with many local variations), *idli* (a type of savory rice flour cake) Nonfermented: boiled or steamed rice (a fragrant variation is known as Sri Lankan yellow rice), *kiribath* (milk rice: sometimes mixed with green gram, jaggery, raisins, cashew nut, etc. and also prepared with sweetened coconut stuffing—*imbul kiribath*), *string hoppers* (rice flour, finger millet flour, wheat flour), pittu (rice flour, odiyal flour-ground palmyrah root, finger millet, foxtail millet flour, or sorghum flour mixed with grated coconut and steamed), *upma* (dry roasted semolina or coarse rice flour porridge), *rotti* (a type of round flatbread, made from wheat flour, rice flour, finger millet flour, or a mix of them and usually mixed with grated coconut and sometimes with grated vegetables), *paratha/godamba roti* (a type of wheat flour flatbread), *kurrakkan thalapa* (a thick ball of dough made of finger millet flour), *habala pethi* (rice flakes—a traditional breakfast cereal)
Flour (from rice, wheat and other cereals, grains, and pulses) and sugar syrup/ treacle-based confectionery and other confectionery, snacks, and desserts	Traditional sweets: *aggala* (sweet roasted rice balls), *aluwa*, *welithalapa (sau dodol)*, *kevum* (deep-fried oil cakes-lots of regional varieties exist such as *konda kevum*, *pethi kevum*, *athirasa*, *naran kevum*, *mung kevum*—a mixture of green gram and rice flour is used), *aasmi*, *unduwel/päni*—walalu (deep-fried coils of black gram flour and rice flour mixture), *kokis* (crispy cookies), *hälapa* (finger millet steamed cake), *wandu appa* (a sweet steamed hopper), *lävariya* (sweet dumpling string hoppers), *rulang aluwa* (semolina toffees), *thala guli/ thala bola* (sesame rolls/balls), *kalu dodol* (a sticky, gel-like candy), *bibikkan* (Sri Lankan coconut cake), *pol dosi* (coconut toffees), *päni-kaju* (sweet toffee slices from ground nut or cashew nut), *ala dosi* (potato fudge), *inguru dosi* (sweet and spicy ginger toffee) Traditional snacks/appetizers: *wadai* (lentil fritters), *murukku* (spicy batter or sugar-coated diamond cuts), fried cassava chips and sweet potato chips, fried ash plantain chips, *papadam* (crispy black gram flour appetizer), odiyal (from palmyrah palm tubers/palmyrah sprouts) Traditional desserts: *watallapan* (cardamom-spiced coconut custard pudding), fishtail palm flour pudding, sago pudding

(*Continued*)

Table 2.1 (Continued)

Food category	Examples
Vegetable-based	Fermented: *Lunu dehi* Sinhala *achcharu* (traditional Sri Lankan pickle), *wambatu moju* (eggplant/brinjal pickle) Nonfermented: vegetable curries (with coconut milk), *Seeni sambol* (sweet onion relish or spicy caramelized onion relish), *kochchi sambol* (chili pepper)
Root crops and tuber-based	Boiled cassava tubers, boiled sweet potato tubers, cassava curry, sweet potato curry
Fruit-based	Fermented: *Polos achcahru* (pickle with baby jackfruit pickle) Nonfermented: *puhul dosi* (ash pumpkin preserves), pineapple curry, baby jackfruit curry, raw mango curry, amabrella curry, boiled jack bulbs, mango chutney, ambarella chutney, *atu kos* (jackfruit bulbs dehydrated on the hearth)
Milk-based	*Mee kiri* (buffalo curd)
Fish-based	Fish curry (with coconut milk), *Ambul Thiyal* (sour fish), *Jaadi* (cured fish), Maldive fish (boiled, smoked, and dried tuna fish)
Herbal plant-based	*Kola kända* (a creamy herbal porridge/gruel—prepared with the extracts of a variety of local fresh herbs and/or green leaves, mixed with raw rice and coconut milk)
Other traditional dishes	*Aanama, hath maluwa* (a mixed vegetable curry with seven ingredients), *niyabalawa. kos äta kalu pol maluwa* (Sri Lanka jackfruit seed curry), *lunu miris* (onions ground with dried red chili powder and lime), *coconut sambol* (grated coconut, onions, red chili powder, lemon, salt, and Maldive fish), *mallung* (shredded leafy vegetables, grated coconut, and various spices), coconut milk gravy

Aspergillus spp, there is a high potential for the contamination of rice form mycotoxins such as aflatoxin B_1, especially after harvest (Elzupir et al., 2015). Besides rice, the occurrence of As and Cd was detected in cereals and legumes such as finger millet, sesame, cowpea/black-eyed pea, urad dal/split bean, foxtail millet, long bean, and green gram that are commonly used as raw materials for traditional food preparations (Edirisinghe and Jinadasa, 2019).

From a safety point of view, the spices used in traditional food preparations should be free of undeclared contaminants and adulterants, such as toxic botanicals, pathogenic microorganisms, and excessive levels of microbial toxins, pesticide residues, or residues of fumigation agents (Salgueiro et al., 2010). The prevailing climatic conditions in Sri Lanka are highly favorable for mold infestations in spices leading to subsequent contamination with mycotoxins. Chilli and black pepper are perhaps the two most widely used spices in traditional Sri Lankan cuisine. A recent study reports the occurrence of multiple mycotoxins such as aflatoxins, ochratoxin A, toxic sterigmatocystin, citrinin, and fumonisin B1 in Sri Lankan black peppers regardless of their low water activity and strong antimicrobial property (Yogendrarajah et al., 2014a). Similarly, aflatoxin B1 was found to be the predominant mycotoxin contaminating Sri Lankan dry chilli followed by ochratoxin A, sterigmatocystin, fumonisin, and citrinin (Yogendrarajah et al., 2014b).

As rice is accompanied by an assortment of vegetable curries in the typical Sri Lankan diet, vegetables are abundantly consumed in Sri Lanka. Vegetable farming is one of the most intensive cultivated farming systems in Sri Lanka that consumes a high volume of pesticides and fertilizers, leading to the accumulation of pesticide residues. Recent studies report the presence of diazinon, chlorpyrifos, phenthoate, prothiofos, oxyfluorfen, and tebuconazole in tomato, capsicum, and cabbage cultivated in major agricultural regions in Sri Lanka (Rajapakse et al., 2018; Lakshani et al., 2017). Residues of chlorpyrifos, captan, profenofos, diazinon, permethrin, and oxyfluorfen were detected in *Mukunuwenna* (*Alternanthera sessilis*), the most widely produced and consumed leafy vegetable in Sri Lanka (De Alwis et al., 2006). Green leafy vegetables can also be a source of foodborne pathogens. A study reports the presence of pathogenic bacteria such as *Salmonella* spp., *Listeria monocytogenes* in *Mukunuwenna*, *Gotukola* (*Centella asiatica*), and lettuce in local markets (De Silva et al., 2014). Cytotoxicity of the widely consumed green leafy vegetables in the Sri Lankan diet and the ones commonly used for preparing traditional types of herbal porridge (*kola kända*) were also reported (Balasuriya and Dharmaratne, 2007).

Marine foods are a common source of food poisoning worldwide. Although traditional dishes like *ambul thiyal* prepared from local fish such as tuna are highly popular in Sri Lankan cuisine, they are also linked to the prevalence of scromboid fish poisoning. Histamine is produced in high levels during the storage of Sri Lankan yellow fin tuna, and this may lead to acute toxicity in some sensitive individuals when consumed (Jinadasa et al., 2015). Traditional fish dishes can also be a major route of exposure for toxic heavy metals such as Hg, Cd, and Pb (Jinadasa et al., 2014; Jinadasa et al., 2018). Some local fish species could also be vectors of ciguatera toxin that leads to ciguatera fish poisoning—one of the most common foodborne illnesses related to seafood consumption (Deepananda et al., 2016). Crustacean shellfish and molluscan shellfish consumed in the form of traditional dishes can also be sources of seafood allergy and paralytic shellfish poisoning, although cases are not well reported (Taylor, 2008). Predominant presence of pathogenic species such as *Aeromonas hydrophila*, *Vibrio parahaemolyticus*, *Vibrio carchariae*, *Vibrio harveyi*, and *Plesiomonas shigelloides* in marine shrimp harvested in Sri Lanka was also reported (Jayasinghe et al., 2010).

Milk-based traditional foods such as curd are widely consumed in Sri Lanka. Contamination of cow's and buffalo milk used for the production of such traditional food by residues of veterinary drugs could be a significant food safety issue since bearing a risk to human health, as they can cause allergic reactions in hypersensitive individuals (Vishnuraj et al., 2016). In addition, the incidence of aflatoxin M1, a common contaminant in cow's milk, was reported in locally produced raw milk (Pathirana et al., 2010). The potential IgE-mediated food allergenicity of cow's milk has also been widely recognized, although specific cases are not well documented regarding Sri Lanka (Arakali et al., 2017).

Coconut oil, traditionally extracted from dried coconut kernels, is the most widely used vegetable oil in Sri Lankan cuisine. It has been a key source of fat in the local diet for ages. A recent study reports aflatoxin contamination in locally produced coconut oil in the ranges of 2.25–72.70 μg/kg for total aflatoxins and 1.76–60.92 μg/kg for aflatoxin B1 (Karunarathna et al., 2019).

Nuts such as peanuts and cashew nuts used commonly for traditional food preparations can also pose food safety concerns with the presence of allergenic substances and mycotoxins. Moderate contamination (12.5 ppb) of local peanut with aflatoxins was reported in studies (Dissanayake and Manage, 2010).

Adulterants have been detected in many market food commodities resulting in the production of inferior quality raw materials for traditional food, rendering it a significant food safety concern. Routine inspections by public health inspectors have found adulteration by unapproved flavors, preservatives, and coloring and addition of unpermitted organic substitutes. As revealed by such inspections, spices have been adulterated with wheat or rice flour, paddy husk, poonac, sawdust, salt, and a variety of synthetic colors/fabric dyes. Coconut oil is adulterated with cheaper oils such as palm oil. Coconut vinegar is adulterated with acetic acid (The Sunday Times, 2017).

Central to any food processing is the availability of potable water. Lack of municipal water in many rural areas compels the use of water from dug wells and other sources such as streams for traditional food preparations that may pose food safety hazards through the presence of microbial pathogens such as *Escherichia coli*.

2.4.2 Safety during processing, handling/serving, and storage

Many traditional and ethnic foods in Sri Lanka are characterized by the use of unsophisticated, informal, and low-cost food processing techniques.

Heat treatment, being one of the most ancient technologies used for traditional food processing, significantly improves the raw material quality features such as digestibility, taste, mouth feel, and consistency. From a food safety perspective, heat treatment can effectively eliminate many pathogenic microorganisms. Boiling is perhaps the most common heat treatment in Sri Lankan traditional food that gives rise to microbiological safety. However, widely used heat treatment options for traditional food at the household level such as boiling (rice, caasava, most vegetable curries), steaming (*pittu, wandu appa, string hoppers*), simmering in hot water and coconut milk (vegetable curries), deep and shallow frying (traditional sweets and snacks) that lacks precise control of the temperature and holding time, and total inactivation of pathogenic microorganisms may not be achieved therefore. The growth of Gram-positive food poisoning bacteria such as *Bacillus cereus* that can also cause spoilage of cooked rice was reported from studies (Waduwawara and Manage, 2009). Intensive thermal processing of traditional food especially the starch-based food items also generates carcinogenic process contaminants such as acrylamide (Arvanitoyannis and Dionisopoulou, 2014). Recycling of frying oils or repeatedly heating oil is a regular practice at domestic-level traditional food preparations that can lead to the generation of carcinogenic free radicals. In addition, repeated heating of oils at high temperatures (160°C−190°C) over a long period of time causes the conversion of fatty acid from *cis* to *trans* isomers, which can pose a significant health hazard (Perumalla Venkata and Subramanyam, 2016). Burning of locally sourced wood for food preparations is still common in many rural areas in Sri Lanka. Besides the environmental impact, it can also contribute to the deposition of ash and other toxic emanates to deposit on food. A common practice after frying food at a domestic level is to drain the oil through leaflets of newspapers. This can lead to the transfer of toxic metals such as Pb, which are normally used in printing ink. The same happens when food items are wrapped in such leaflets.

Sun drying and other traditional dehydration methods used in Sri Lanka, such as placing in the surroundings of the hearth in the kitchen (used for dehydrating jackfruit bulbs and seeds), are economical means of reducing the water content in food matrices that lead to the retardation of microbial growth. Such dried food may nevertheless subject to spoilage by fungi (particularly yeasts and molds) if they are processed and stored under unhygienic conditions. Sun-dried local raw materials are also prone to the accumulation of dust and other environmental contaminants and pest attacks.

Fermentation is a highly useful food processing technique applied to traditional food such as fermented fish and curd. The incorporation of spices for their antimicrobial effect (garcinia, black pepper, ginger, and cinnamon leaves) and natural preservatives such as salt help in preventing major food safety issues due to the growth of pathogenic bacteria (Ekanayake, 2016). Fermentation in buffalo curd is controlled mainly by the growth of microorganisms belonging to the genera of *Lactobacillus and Streptococcus*. The fermentation process comes with the additional benefit of the preservative effect from lactic acid synthesized during the process. Beneficial *Lactobacillus* strains (some of them are regarded as probiotics) in curd can effectively retard the growth of harmful bacteria and common foodborne pathogens, such as *E. coli* and *Salmonella* spp., through a competitive inhibition mechanism (Lievin-Le Moal and Servin, 2014). However, inadequate fermentation conditions and/or contamination during processing may lead to the occurrence foodborne pathogens in all fermented products. To produce safer traditional foods with consistent quality, the fermentation process must therefore be controlled and carefully selected raw materials should be used so that contamination by pathogenic microorganisms can be eliminated.

Low-cost traditional techniques such as burial in dry sand (lime fruits, yams, tubers, jackfruit seeds), immersing in honey (meat), sun drying (fish, vegetables, and mushroom), and fermentation (fruit- and vegetable-based pickles, milk) used in traditional food preservation are intended to have a significant impact on food safety by controlling the growth of foodborne pathogens. Salting and addition of sugar syrup and/or treacle and bee honey aid in controlling the water activity in many traditional food preparations that impart a significant controlling effect on the growth of microorganisms.

There are also some equipment and raw material handling-related aspects that may contribute to food safety issues such as the absence of mechanized grinding and milling tools (milling and grinding in domestic food preparations are done manually using mortar and pestle) and issues regarding improper cleaning. Such practices may give rise to cross contamination and allow the harboring of foodborne pathogens and their subsequent growth.

Some food items such as the traditional sweets are specially prepared for some occasions and consumed within a short period before any food safety issue arises due to ambient storage. However, the potential for cross contamination is still high due to manual handling.

Some fermented fruit and vegetable products are also regarded as integral elements in traditional Sri Lankan cuisine. Lime pickle, perhaps the most popular traditional pickle, benefits largely by the incorporation of salt crystals during its production for its extended shelf life owing to the natural preservative effect of salt. In other types of pickles, vinegar is used as an additive, which imparts natural preservative effect.

Domestic-level traditional food preparations followed by the exposure to household flies, ants, rodents, and cockroaches in most cases lead to cross contamination and may shorten the expected shelf life. In some cases, when the traditional confectionery items are sold in mass food markets, they are usually stored in open containers, leading to possible contamination by microorganisms and environment pollutants.

The use of aluminum ware for cooking traditional food instead of food-grade stainless steel or traditional clay pots may lead to the leaching of aluminum into the food.

Food poisoning at a household level is not often reported in Sri Lanka. Hence, there is not much evidence to believe that there are hygiene concerns in homemade foods. Furthermore, incidences of food poisoning of people who regularly eat food prepared outside such as in hotels, food stalls, and restaurants are rare. Sri Lankan food habits mostly consist of well-cooked food items instead of raw food items, and this may be a possible reason for lesser number of food poisoning incidents. One reason

Table 2.2 Major food safety issues and concerns associated with Sri Lankan traditional food.

Food category	Safety issues and concerns
Fermented fish products	Histamine food poisoning Growth of food poisoning bacteria (e.g., Clostridium) Heavy metal poisoning (e.g., Pb, Hg) Unpermitted food additives used in the curing process Yeast and mold infestations Insects and mice infestations
Fermented dairy food products	Residues of antibiotics in other veterinary drugs in milk Yeast and mold infestations Use of unpermitted preservatives (e.g., formalin) Contaminated packaging (clay pots)
Vegetable and fruit-based food items	Pesticide residues in raw commodities Presence of microbial pathogens
Cereal and legume-based foods/baked and confectionery items	Adulterated raw materials (rice flour, treacle, jaggery) Pesticide residues and heavy metal residues Yeast and mold infestations Presence of mycotoxins Repeated use of frying oil Food allergies (e.g., nut allergies) Unsafe packaging materials (e.g., newspapers and printed material)

for low number of recorded incidences may be due to nonserious nature or personal treatments using easily accessible medicines and other traditional home remedies.

A summary of some general food safety issues and concerns associated with traditional food is given in Table 2.2.

2.4.3 Regulations governing food safety in Sri Lanka

Food Act No. 26 of 1980 (amendment No. 20 of 1991 and amendment No. 29 of 2011) is the apex national regulation governing food safety in Sri Lanka with the primary purpose of regulating and controlling the manufacture, importation, sale, and distribution of food within the country (Parliament of the Democratic Socialist Republic of Sri Lanka, Food Act, No. 26 of 1980). There are some other supportive acts, such as Food Supplies Ordinance Act 30 of 1957, The Consumer Affairs Authority Act, 2003, Food Production (Estates) Act No. 40 of 1954, that aid in the governance of overall food quality and safety. Although there are no special provisions for traditional and ethnic foods under the existing regulations, the generic principles pertaining to food preparation, storage, handling, serving, and distribution are applicable.

Some of the raw materials used in the production of the popular traditional food items are covered by Sri Lanka Standards (SLS), issued by the national authority responsible for issuing food standards (e.g., Wheat flour SLS 144, White Sugar SLS 191, Cashew nuts SLS 245, Sesame seeds (gingelly seeds) SLS 386, Rice flour SLS 913).

Industrial producers (large scale) frequently use certification schemes and standardizations such as good manufacturing practices (GMP) and hazard analysis and critical control point (HACCP), ISO22000. However, there are several small-scale entrepreneurs who produce traditional food products such as pickles, snacks, and confectioneries in the household and distribute it to the consumers in the same area. These products are not subjected to any test or certification procedures, and therefore food safety concerns may arise. The nonavailability or inadequacy of standards for assuring the quality and safety of local produced spices and condiments is perhaps one of the key issues when using such raw material for traditional food preparations.

2.4.4 Strategies to address the food safety issues of traditional and ethnic food

Given their significance in the local food culture, there is a dire need of robust prevention and control strategies to assess and mitigate the microbiological and chemical (toxicological) risks associated with Sri Lankan traditional and ethnic foods. In this context, it is imperative that basic food safety principles and practices are applied throughout the entire food supply chain to ensure the safety of the final product.

There are however some inherent techniques in the traditional food preparations that can evade some of the common chemical and microbiological food safety issues. Traditional Sri Lankan dishes contain a lot of spices that render a lot of additional benefits in addition to their effect on the taste profile. Antibacterial and antifungal activities of widely used spices in traditional food preparations against food spoilage bacteria such as *Bacillus subtilis* and *Pseudomonas fluorescens*, pathogens such as *Staphylococcus aureus* and *Vibrio parahaemolyticus*, and harmful fungi such as *Aspergillus flavus* have been reported (Liu et al., 2017). Spices and condiments such as cloves, nutmeg, cinnamon, black pepper, cucurmin, ginger, and garlic containing natural bacteriocins are frequently associated with traditional food preparations. Acidification using natural agents such as tamarind (tartaric acid) and garcinia (hydrocitric acid) also aids in controlling the growth of foodborne pathogens while curry leaves/pandan leaves can absorb some of toxic elements present. Cooking rice in excess water, pressure cooking, and the use of clay pots are identified as effective strategies to reduce the level of aflatoxin in rice grains (Reddy et al., 2008).

Different solutions for the reduction of arsenic and other toxic element intake are proposed at different levels: (1) during the plant-growing process through agronomic practices, (2) pretreatment of rice before its use in the food industry, (3) optimization of the conditions of unit operations during processing, and (4) by cooking (Carbonell-Barrachina et al., 2015).

Reliable and unsophisticated indices/indicators are required to circumvent certain issues such as the repeated use of oil for frying that can be used for traditional food preparations at household level as well as commercial level. Postharvest conditions, especially the storage conditions, for raw materials should be strictly controlled and monitored, as they have a direct impact on the quality and safety of the final product. Environmental factors (light, humidity, oxygen, and temperature) and the presence of living organisms (bacteria, yeasts and molds, mites and nematode worms, insects/moths) should be taken into consideration when designing storage systems for raw materials such as spices (Salgueiro et al., 2010). Given that Sri Lankan ambient storage conditions are in the ranges of 30°C ± 2°C in terms of the temperature and relative humidity of 75% ± 5%, proper attention must be placed on using the correct storage techniques for raw materials used for traditional food processing procedures, especially cereals, grains, and spices that are highly susceptible for mycotoxigenic fungal contamination. Cultivation of such crops under Good Agricultural Practices would be one strategy to especially address the issue of pesticide residues resulting from the indiscriminate use of pesticides on plant material used for traditional food preparations. The Sri Lankan Good Agricultural Practices has been launched recently to achieve this objective.

Although there may be technological and financial constraints regarding the implementation of recommended food safety strategies such as HACCP, at least basic GMP Good Hygiene Practices can be adopted regarding traditional and ethnic food preparation even at the household level, storage, handling, serving, and distribution. Therefore adequate quality control measures should be applied along the food chain to circumvent the common food safety issues.

Sun drying in open air is the traditional method of drying spices in Sri Lanka. As this method potentially exposes them to the risk of contamination by a wide range of mycotoxigenic fungi, emerging techniques such as irradiation can be applied as a surface decontamination treatment for spices. Incorporation of an aflatoxin contamination monitoring system into the regulatory scope for dried coconut kernels (copra) would also be an important step toward ensuring consumer safety in that aspect.

Food service establishments such as restaurants and the household or private residences are identified as the most common venues for foodborne illnesses (Gormley et al., 2012). The small-scale food processing plants and food service establishments such as small eateries and groceries producing and serving the traditional and ethnic foods in Sri Lanka can possibly ignore basic sanitation and hygiene rules. Street food vending outlets could also contribute to a higher incidence of foodborne pathogens, probably due to the lack of safe food handling, improper packaging, and poor storage facilities. Therefore regular inspections should be carried out by the relevant authorities to avoid any risk for public health in traditional food prepared and served in such places.

2.5 Future outlook

Any future strategy to address the safety of traditional and ethnic food should be based on a risk analysis approach, and any national food regulatory standards for them should be aligned according to the Codex principles. It should also be emphasized that food safety is not the responsibility of a single stakeholder but is a shared responsibility between all involved in the value chain.

The existing national regulatory frameworks should be strengthened by integrating prevention and control strategies to address the microbiological and chemical risks associated with traditional and ethnic foods. Food safety regulations and standards for traditional and ethnic food should only be established based on a comprehensive risk assessment, and they should be based on a holistic approach that extends from farm-to-fork and involves all the relevant stakeholders in the agri-food chain.

As traditional and ethnic food preparation practices are informal and mostly transferred from generation to generation, basic food safety education should be an integral component of the public school curriculum to ensure that all citizens are equally well educated on food safety issues and concerns, particularly those associated with traditional and ethnic food.

References

Arakali, S.R., Green, T.D., Dinakar, C., 2017. Prevalence of food allergies in South Asia. Ann. Allergy Asthma Immunol. 118 (1), 16–20. Available from: https://doi.org/10.1016/j.anai.2016.09.441.

Arvanitoyannis, I.S., Dionisopoulou, N., 2014. Acrylamide: formation, occurrence in food products, detection methods, and legislation. Crit. Rev. Food. Sci. Nutr. 54 (6), 708–733. Available from: https://doi.org/10.1080/10408398.2011.606378.

Balasuriya, B.M.G.K., Dharmaratne, H.R.W., 2007. Cytotoxicity and antioxidant activity studies of green leafy vegetables consumed in Sri Lanka. J. Nat. Sci. Found. Sri Lanka 35 (4), 255–258.

Cagri-Mehmetoglu, A., 2017. Food safety challenges associated with traditional foods of Turkey. Food Sci. Technol. (Campinas) 38 (1), 1–12. Available from: https://doi.org/10.1590/1678-457X.36916.

Carbonell-Barrachina, Á., Munera-Picazo, S., Cano-Lamadrid, M., Burló, F., Castaño-Iglesias, M.C., 2015. Arsenic in your food: potential health hazards from arsenic found in rice. Nutr. Diet. Suppl. 1. Available from: https://doi.org/10.2147/nds.s52027.

Codex Alimentarius Commission, 2014. Joint FAO/WHO Food Standards Programme. 37th Session. Distribution of the Report of the Eighth Session of the Codex Committee on Contaminants in Foods. <http://www.fao.org/input/download/report/906/REP14_CFe.pdf> (accessed 19.01.03.).

De Alwis, G.K.H., Wijesekera, R.D., Jayasekera, T.A.D.N.A.K., 2006. Use patterns and residue levels of pesticides on Mukunuwenna, a leafy vegetable grown in Sri Lanka. Bull. Environ. Contam. Toxicol. 76 (1), 119–125. Available from: https://doi.org/10.1007/s00128-005-0897-3.

Deepananda, K.H.M.A., Amarasinghe, U.S., Jayasinghe-Mudalige, U.K., 2016. *Herklotsichthys quadrimaculatus* Korumburuwa in the stilt fishery in Southern Sri Lanka: are they really poisonous? Sri Lanka J. Aquat. Sci. 21 (1), 73–75.

De Silva, A., Abayasekara, C., Dissanayake, D., 2014. Freshly eaten leafy vegetables: a source of food borne pathogens? Ceylon J. Sci. (Biol. Sci.) 42 (2), 95–99. Available from: https://doi.org/10.4038/cjsbs.v42i2.6613.

Dissanayake, D., Manage, P.M., 2010. Aflatoxin contamination in peanuts commercially available in Sri Lanka. Vidyodaya J. Sci. 14 (1), 151–159.

Edirisinghe, E.M.R.K.B., Jinadasa, B.K.K.K., 2019. Arsenic and cadmium concentrations in legumes and cereals grown in the North Central Province, Sri Lanka and assessment of their health risk. Int. J. Food Contam. 6 (1). Available from: https://doi.org/10.1186/s40550-019-0073-x.

Ekanayake, S., 2016. Ethnic fermented food and beverages of Sri Lanka. In: Tamang, J.P. (Ed.), Ethnic Fermented Foods and Alcoholic Beverages of Asia. Springer, New Delhi, pp. 139–150. Available from: https://doi.org/10.1007/978-81-322-2800-4.

Elzupir, A.O., Alamer, A.S., Dutton, M.F., 2015. The occurrence of aflatoxin in rice worldwide: a review. Toxin Rev. 34 (1), 37–42. Available from: https://doi.org/10.3109/15569543.2014.984229.

Gormley, F.J., Rawal, N., Little, C.L., 2012. Choose your menu wisely: cuisine-associated food-poisoning risks in restaurants in England and Wales. Epidemiol. Infect. 140, 997–1007. Available from: https://doi.org/10.1017/S0950268811001567.

Jallad, K.N., 2015. Heavy metal exposure from ingesting rice and its related potential hazardous health risks to humans. Environ. Sci. Pollut. Res. 15449–15458. Available from: https://doi.org/10.1007/s11356-015-4753-7.

Jayasinghe, C., Ahmed, S., Kariyawasam, M., 2010. The isolation and identification of Vibrio Species in Marine Shrimps of Sri Lanka. J. Food Agric. 1 (1), 36–44. Available from: https://doi.org/10.4038/jfa.v1i1.1838.

Jayasumana, C., Paranagama, P., Fonseka, S., Amarasinghe, M., Gunatilake, S., Siribaddana, S., 2015. Presence of arsenic in Sri Lankan rice. Int. J. Food Contam. 2 (1). Available from: https://doi.org/10.1186/s40550-015-0007-1.

Jinadasa, B.K.K.K., Edirisinghe, E.M.R.K.B., Wickramasinghe, I., 2014. Total mercury, cadmium and lead levels in main export fish of Sri Lanka. Food Addit. Contam. B 7 (4), 309–314. Available from: https://doi.org/10.1080/19393210.2014.938131.

Jinadasa, B.K.K.K., Galhena, C.K., Liyanage, N.P.P., 2015. Histamine formation and the freshness of yellowfin tuna (*Thunnus albacares*) stored at different temperatures. Cogent Food Agric. 1 (1). Available from: https://doi.org/10.1080/23311932.2015.1028735.

Jinadasa, B.K.K.K., Chathurika, G.S., Jayaweera, C.D., Jayasinghe, G.D.T.M., 2018. Mercury and cadmium in swordfish and yellowfin tuna and health risk assessment for Sri Lankan consumers. Food Addit. Contam. B 1–6. Available from: https://doi.org/10.1080/19393210.2018.1551247.

Karunarathna, N.B., Fernando, C.J., Munasinghe, D.M.S., Fernando, R., 2019. Occurrence of aflatoxins in edible vegetable oils in Sri Lanka. Food Control 101, 97–103. Available from: https://doi.org/10.1016/j.foodcont.2019.02.017.

Lakshani, P.W.Y., Rajapakse, M.K.L.K., Sendthuran, K., 2017. Pesticide residues in selected vegetables in several growing areas by GC/MS using QuEChERS technique. Ann. Sri Lanka Dep. Agric. 19 (2), 188–208.

Lievin-Le Moal, V., Servin, A.L., 2014. Anti-infective activities of *Lactobacillus* strains in the human intestinal microbiota: from probiotics to gastrointestinal anti-infectious biotherapeutic agents. Clin. Microbiol. Rev. 27 (2), 167–199. Available from: https://doi.org/10.1128/cmr.00080-13.

Liu, Q., Meng, X., Li, Y., Zhao, C.-N., Tang, G.-Y., Li, H.-B., 2017. Antibacterial and antifungal activities of spices. Int. J. Mol. Sci. 18 (6), 1283. Available from: https://doi.org/10.3390/ijms18061283.

Lücke, F.K., Zangerl, P., 2014. Food safety challenges associated with traditional foods in German-speaking regions. Food Control 43, 217–230. Available from: https://doi.org/10.1016/j.foodcont.2014.03.014.

Parliament of the Democratic Socialist Republic of Sri Lanka, Food Act, No. 26 of 1980. <http://www.health.gov.lk/en/FOODWEB/files/regulations.html> (accessed 12.02.19.).

Pathirana, U.P.D., Wimalasiri, K.M.S., Silva, K.F.S.T., Gunarathne, S.P., 2010. Investigation of farm gate cow milk for Aflatoxin M1. Trop. Agric. Res. 21 (2), 119–125.

Perera, A.N.F., 2008. Sri Lankan traditional food cultures, and food security. Econ. Rev. 34 (7–8), 40–43.

Perumalla Venkata, R., Subramanyam, R., 2016. Evaluation of the deleterious health effects of consumption of repeatedly heated vegetable oil. Toxicol. Rep. 3, 636–643. Available from: https://doi.org/10.1016/j.toxrep.2016.08.003.

Prakash, V., 2016. Introduction: the importance of traditional and ethnic food in the context of food safety, harmonization, and regulations. In: Prakash, V., Martín-Belloso, O., Keener, L., Astley, S., Braun, S., McMahon, H., et al.,Regulating Safety of Traditional and Ethnic Foods. Academic Press Elsevier, Waltham, MA, pp. 1–6. Available from: https://doi.org/10.1016/B978-0-12-800605-4.00023-2.

Rajapakse, M.K.L.K., Weerakkody, N.S., Lakshani, P.W.Y., 2018. Quantification of pesticide residues in selected vegetables using the QuEChERS method. OUSL J. 13 (1), 29–42. Available from: https://doi.org/10.4038/ouslj.v13i1.7427.

Reddy, K.R.N., Reddy, C.S., Abbas, H.K., Abel, C.A., Muralidharan, K., 2008. Mycotoxigenic fungi, mycotoxins, and management of rice grains. Toxin Rev. 27 (3–4), 287–317. Available from: https://doi.org/10.1080/15569540802432308.

Salgueiro, L., Martins, A.P., Correia, H., 2010. Raw materials: the importance of quality and safety. A review. Flav. Frag. J. 25 (5), 253–271. Available from: https://doi.org/10.1002/ffj.1973.

Shraim, A.M., 2017. Rice is a potential dietary source of not only arsenic but also other toxic elements like lead and chromium. Arab. J. Chem. 10, S3434–S3443. Available from: https://doi.org/10.1016/j.arabjc.2014.02.004.

Tajkarimi, M., Ibrahim, S.A., Fraser, A.M., 2013. Food safety challenges associated with traditional foods in Arabic speaking countries of the Middle East. Trends Food Sci. Technol. 29, 116–123. Available from: https://doi.org/10.1016/j.tifs.2012.10.002.

Taylor, S.L., 2008. Molluscan shellfish allergy. In: Taylor, S. (Ed.), Adv. Food Nutr. Res.. Academic Press, New York, pp. 139–177. Available from: https://doi.org/10.1016/s1043-4526(07)00004-6.

The Sunday Times., 2017. Tainted food, fruit, veggies, and cooking oil galore. <http://www.sundaytimes.lk/171022/news/tainted-food-fruit-veggies-and-cooking-oil-galore-265175.html> (accessed 19.04.20.).

Vishnuraj, M.R., Kandeepan, G., Rao, K.H., Chand, S., Kumbhar, V., 2016. Occurrence, public health hazards and detection methods of antibiotic residues in foods of animal origin: a comprehensive review. Cogent Food Agric. 2 (1). Available from: https://doi.org/10.1080/23311932.2016.1235458.

Waduwawara, S., Manage, P.M., 2009. Spoilage after cooking of some rice varieties commonly consumed in Sri Lanka. Vidyodaya J. Sci. 14 (1), 131–141.

Weerasekara, P., Withanachchi, C., Ginigaddara, G., Ploeger, A., 2018. Nutrition transition and traditional food cultural changes in Sri Lanka during colonization and post-colonization. Foods 7 (7), 111. Available from: https://doi.org/10.3390/foods7070111.

World Health Organization, 2017.Food Safety Fact Sheet. <https://www.who.int/en/news-room/fact-sheets/detail/food-safety> (accessed 19.01.20.).

Yogendrarajah, P., Deschuyffeleer, N., Jacxsens, L., Sneyers, P.-J., Maene, P., De Saeger, S., et al., 2014a. Mycological quality and mycotoxin contamination of Sri Lankan peppers (*Piper nigrum* L.) and subsequent exposure assessment. Food Control 41, 219–230. Available from: https://doi.org/10.1016/j.foodcont.2014.01.025.

Yogendrarajah, P., Jacxsens, L., De Saeger, S., De Meulenaer, B., 2014b. Co-occurrence of multiple mycotoxins in dry chilli (*Capsicum annum* L.) samples from the markets of Sri Lanka and Belgium. Food Control 46, 26–34. Available from: https://doi.org/10.1016/j.foodcont.2014.04.043.

CHAPTER 3

Traditional functional food of Sri Lanka and their health significance

Viduranga Y. Waisundara
Australian College of Business & Technology - Kandy Campus, Sri Lanka

Contents

3.1 Background of Sri Lanka and its diversity of food

Sri Lanka is an island country in South Asia, located in the Indian Ocean to the southwest of the Bay of Bengal and to the southeast of the Arabian Sea. As shown in Fig. 3.1, the country is historically and culturally intertwined with the Indian subcontinent, but it is geographically separated by the Gulf of Mannar and the Palk Strait. The climate of Sri Lanka is tropical and warm, due to the moderating effects of ocean winds. It has an ancient cultural heritage spanning of 3000 years, with evidence of prehistoric human settlements dating back over 125,000 years. Sri Lanka is very similar to many of the other tropical countries possessing a wide range of plant species as well as a significant variability of climatic zones. Although the country is relatively small in size, it has the highest biodiversity density in Asia. In fact, Sri Lanka is part of the Western Ghats biodiversity hot spot that extends southward from Western India (Myers et al., 2000). Between 27 and 33 of Sri Lanka's 453 bird species (Weerakoon and Gunawardena, 2012), 50 of 91 freshwater fish species (De Alwis Goonatilake, 2012) and 95 of 111 amphibian species are endemic (Manamendra-Arachchi and Meegaskumbura, 2012); the existence of such biodiversity is evidence to an abundant natural food supply in the country to cater to all the animal species of diverse diets. The country consists mostly of flat lands with mountains existing only in the south-central part of the island. There is a

Nutritional and Health Aspects of Food in South Asian Countries
DOI: https://doi.org/10.1016/B978-0-12-820011-7.00020-4

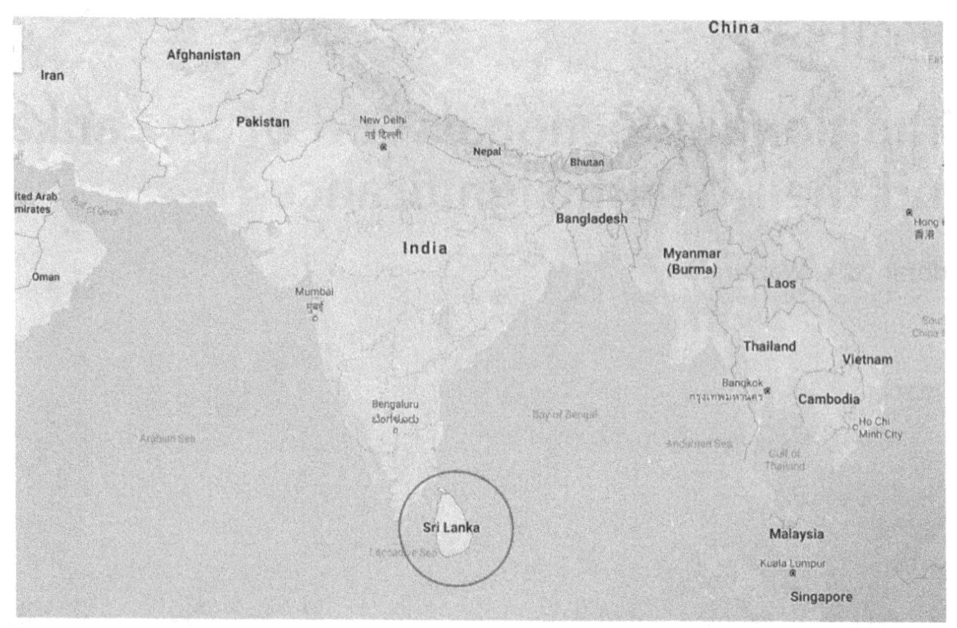

Figure 3.1 Location of Sri Lanka relative to India in the South Asian region.

significant diversity of flora and fauna owing to these geographical and climatic landscapes. It is important therefore for Sri Lanka to balance agricultural development and conservation efforts to meet sustainable development goals while at the same time meeting demands to increase national food production (Horgan et al., 2017).

Being a small country, there is easy access to many of the plant-based food material across the island from wherever the population is located. Despite attempts of deforestation and disappearance of habitat in both the lowlands and hill-country, the country still boasts of luscious greenery and dense forests that provide accommodation for many unique species of plants. For generations, many of the plants of Sri Lanka have been consumed for the purposes of disease prevention, cures for ailments, or for maintaining health and wellness (Waisundara and Watawana, 2014a). Owing to the diversity in the flora and fauna in Sri Lanka, the range of diseases that were treated through administration of plants has been numerous as well. Due to the familiarity of widely available medicinal plants, many Sri Lankans can identify the varieties and types of plants growing within their area of residence that are good in preventing disease conditions. In fact, the local people have the habit of growing at least one or two medicinal plants in their backyards, or any available space within their area of residence. It is this age-old habit coupled with the easy access to diverse plant sources that has led Sri Lankans to be more health conscious even in modern times.

The staple diet of Sri Lanka primarily comprises rice (about 300–400 g) (FBDG, 2011) with some vegetables and typically a small portion (about 15 g) of meat or fish

(Jayawardena et al., 2012), or a chicken egg (whole or half) (Karunaratne, 2012). Although the intake of specific quantities from a variety of food is recommended for Sri Lankans (FBDG, 2011), the bulk of the food consumed by the average Sri Lankan can be considered as rice, vegetables, and fruits (Jayawardena et al., 2012). A well-balanced Sri Lankan diet consisting of rice, spicy vegetable curries, and protein sources (pulses or food of animal origin) at recommended portion sizes (FBDG, 2011) could be considered as enriched with dietary fiber and antioxidants and hence has the potential of being a healthy meal. With the growing rate of urbanization in Sri Lanka as well as the increased awareness on nutrition in playing a crucial role in the prevention of chronic diseases, the population of the country have become very concerned about the functional properties of locally available food products. In this aspect, functional food within a Sri Lankan context is considered as not only food necessary for living but also as a source of mental and physical well-being. A food product can truly be regarded as functional, only if it is satisfactorily demonstrated to affect one or more target functions in the body beyond adequate nutritional effects, in a way that is relevant to either the state of well-being and health or reduction of the risk of a disease (Perera and Li, 2012). The increasing interest in functional food in Sri Lanka reflects the fact that epidemiological studies indicating a specific diet or component of the diet is associated with a lower risk for a disease conditions, especially those that are noncommunicable.

It is imperative to mention herein that almost all of the Sri Lankan functional food have had a traditional stance and therefore have been "clinically tested" for years, with their recipes fine-tuned across the generations (Lee et al., 2014); these food products require minimal processing, easing their incorporation into the fast-paced modern lifestyle of urban populations, where diseases related to the diet seem to be comparatively more prevalent. The Sri Lankan functional foods are also mostly plant-based, owing to the geographical features mentioned in the first few paragraphs. There are several categories of traditional food products in Sri Lanka that may be considered as functional. The major types are collectively discussed in this chapter along with their nutritive properties and ability to prevent diseases.

3.2 Rice

Rice is the most commonly consumed cereal and is a staple food by over one-half of the world's population including Sri Lanka. The country holds a rich treasure of agro-biodiversity that harbors many traditional, indigenous, and improved rice varieties containing health benefits (Rajapakse et al., 2000). According to FAOSTAT (2009), in 2008, China was the major rice producer with 187.4 Mio tonnes, followed by Thailand with 32.1 Mio tonnes and Sri Lanka with 3.1 Mio tonnes. Although widely consumed as white rice, there are many special cultivars of rice that contain color pigments, such as black rice, red rice, and brown rice (Sompong et al., 2011). Their names refer to the kernel color (black, red, or purple) that is formed by deposits of anthocyanins in different layers of the pericarp, seed coat, and aleurone (Chaudhary, 2003). Plant pigments as well as other phytochemicals in grains are constantly being attributed to positive nutritional properties, such as prevention of cardiovascular diseases and cancer. In this context, the phytochemical content in Sri Lankan rice varieties is deemed an important aspect of investigation. Premakumara et al. (2013) analyzed the brans of 23 traditional and 12 improved (both red and white) rice varieties in Sri Lanka for antiamylase and antiglycation activities in vitro. It was heartening to observe that the traditional red rice varieties of "Masuran," "Sudu Heeneti," "Dik Wee," and "Goda Heeneti" exhibited significant and dose-dependent antiamylase, antiglycation, and glycation-reversing activities. These varieties had also shown marked antioxidant properties. Studies such as those by Premakumara et al. (2013) could help rice producers in Sri Lanka or food technologists to promote the consumption of rice products by increasing consumer awareness of the health benefits of grains. In this respect, further research could also be directed to the alteration of functional properties through food processing and help find recommended areas for their application in food.

3.3 Leafy greens

Most of the leafy greens that are consumed in vegetable form in Sri Lanka have functional properties. In fact, they have been used in the traditional medicinal system of Sri Lanka for several thousands of years. The traditional medicinal system of Sri Lanka itself, which has more than 3000 years of tested and proven efficacy, is still in use and generally the first approach for disease control by the locals, especially those who have been contracted with the stated diseases (Waisundara and Watawana, 2014b). Recent scientific studies such as that by Lee et al. (2014) have analyzed the antioxidant and starch hydrolase inhibitory properties of many of these leafy vegetables that are also medicinal ingredients of the traditional medicinal system of the country. The contents of antioxidants present in some of the leafy vegetables are shown in Table 3.1. Functional foods are viewed as a novel therapeutic intervention in the West, although food has been viewed as medicine in many of the traditional medicinal systems of the East (Madsen, 2007). Thus many of the leafy vegetables that are presently considered as functional food by definition have in fact been associated with disease prevention for many years in Sri Lanka.

Some of the leafy greens in Sri Lanka are consumed as herbal beverages. Examples of such plants include *Acacia arabica*, *Aegle marmelos*, *Aerva lanata*, *Asteracantha longifolia*, *Cassia auriculata*, *Hemidesmus indicus*, *Hordeum vulgare*, *Phyllanthus emblica*, and *Tinospora cordifolia*. These plants in particular were in fact tested recently by Jayawardena et al. (2015)

Table 3.1 Antioxidant compounds present in 18 selected commonly consumed leafy vegetables in Sri Lanka.

Scientific name of leafy green	Total phenolics content (mg GAE/g FW)	Neoxanthin (μg/g FW)	Viola xanthin (μg/g FW)	Lutein (μg/g FW)	Zea xanthin (μg/g FW)	Lycopene (μg/g FW)	Carotene (μg/g FW)		Tocopherol (μg/g FW)		
							α	β	α	δ	γ
Coccinia grandis	125.1 ± 13.5	39.63	5.95	13.65	7.31	1.12	0.06	0.25	0.08	0.06	0.05
Asparagus racemosus	118.3 ± 13.6	2.61	1.55	5.26	1.32	ND[b]	0.06	3.58	0.45	0.08	6.55
Costus specious	99.8 ± 14.6	32.25	6.21	12.95	6.18	0.95	0.08	0.38	0.19	0.15	0.18
Amaranthus viridis	90.6 ± 9.8	14.81	5.94	3.46	5.49	1.05	1.15	1.16	2.06	1.95	1.88
Annona muricata	86.5 ± 14.8	20.46	6.51	ND	3.54	ND	0.65	0.28	0.41	0.07	0.34
Sesbania grandiflora	82.6 ± 6.5	12.95	12.66	3.44	3.68	ND	0.54	1.68	0.55	0.52	0.41
Desmodium gangeticum	83.4 ± 5.5	10.84	1.29	0.90	0.29	0.05	0.22	0.28	0.09	0.08	0.06
Mimosa pudica	70.2 ± 5.5	9.86	6.57	7.75	ND	0.62	0.19	0.25	0.25	ND	ND
Momordica charantia	69.6 ± 9.6	18.65	2.58	17.64	0.55	0.36	0.21	0.25	0.08	0.06	0.06
Alternanthera sessilis	56.8 ± 5.9	3.69	4.58	4.20	0.69	0.49	0.35	0.47	0.28	0.04	0.06
Artocarpus heterophyllus	54.3 ± 6.9	4.55	6.48	ND	ND	0.61	0.58	0.34	0.07	0.06	0.06
Adhathoda vasica	52.3 ± 8.6	3.19	3.54	6.58	6.47	0.94	0.64	0.85	0.07	0.06	0.05
Psidium guava	51.3 ± 9.2	8.64	3.67	5.50	6.35	0.84	0.38	0.81	0.07	ND	ND
Solanum americanum	48.1 ± 6.9	5.87	4.31	3.84	0.90	0.55	0.20	0.80	0.10	0.08	ND
Gymnema sylvestre	46.1 ± 7.5	14.38	5.64	2.80	1.24	0.47	0.14	0.61	0.84	0.39	0.41
Centella asiatica	40.6 ± 5.9	17.96	3.22	3.64	1.58	1.47	0.26	0.24	0.81	0.37	0.54
Wattakaka volubilis	40.7 ± 6.8	11.38	10.55	4.28	4.20	1.28	1.24	0.34	0.83	0.71	0.69
Ipomoea aquatica	36.4 ± 6.1	9.64	11.68	2.65	ND	0.82	0.34	0.57	0.88	0.24	0.75

Source: Modified from Lee, Y.H., Choo, C., Watawana, M.I., Jayawardena, N., Waisundara, V.Y., 2014. An appraisal of eighteen commonly consumed edible plants as functional food based on their antioxidant and starch hydrolase inhibitory activities. J. Sci. Food. Agric. 95, 2956–2964.

for their antioxidant capacity and the starch hydrolase inhibitory activities as well as their stability of these two parameters in an in vitro digestion model. These herbal beverages demonstrated noteworthy functional properties in this particular study. Another more common form of consuming leafy greens in Sri Lanka nowadays is to incorporate them into porridge. This is a trend of increasing popularity for health and wellness purposes, especially among the younger generation of the country who tend to find the habit of consuming herbal porridge more palatable. When rice gruel is incorporated with minced leaves of the leafy greens, the bitterness and grassy note present in many of the leaves is concealed. Drinking one glass of herbal porridge is considered as an all-in-one breakfast among Sri Lankans as well. Some of the leafy greens that are consumed in porridge form and their purported therapeutic effects are shown in Table 3.2.

Table 3.2 Selected health benefits of some of the most popular leafy greens that are used to prepare porridges in Sri Lanka.

Scientific name of leafy green	Health benefits elucidated through scientific studies
Aerva lanata Linn	Antioxidant (Hara et al., 2018), antiproliferative and apoptotic activity (Anusha et al., 2016), antidiabetic (Akanji, Olukolu and Kazeem, 2018)
Alternanthera sessilis Linn	Antioxidant (Lee et al., 2014), antiinflammatory (Muniandy et al., 2018)
Asparagus racemosus Wild	Antioxidant and starch hydrolase inhibitory activity (Lee et al., 2014)
Astercantha longifolia	Antioxidant (Jayawardena et al., 2015), starch hydrolase inhibitory activity (Jayawardena et al., 2015), and antidiabetic (Fernando et al., 1991; Ediriweera and Ratnasooriya, 2009)
Atlantia ceylanica Linn	Hepatoprotective (Oh et al., 2002), antidiabetic (Senadheera and Ekanayake, 2012)
Centella asiatica Urb	Antioxidant (Lee et al., 2014; Waisundara and Watawana, 2014), starch hydrolase inhibitory activity (Lee et al., 2014), antidiabetic (Ullah et al., 2009), anticancer (Ullah et al., 2009)
Hemidesmus indicus Linn	Antioxidant and starch hydrolase inhibitory activity (Jayawardena et al., 2015)
Lasia spinosa Linn	Antiinflammatory (Deb et al., 2010)
Murraya koenigi Spreng	Antioxidant (Tachibana et al., 2003), hepatoprotective (Gupta and Singh, 2007), anticancer (Kok et al., 2012)
Sesbania grandiflora Pers	Antidiabetic (Ediriweera and Ratnasooriya, 2009; Kumar et al., 2015), antioxidant (Lee et al., 2014; Waisundara and Watawana, 2014), starch hydrolase inhibitory activity (Lee et al., 2014), anticancer (Pajaniradje et al., 2014)

3.4 Spices

Sri Lanka is well known for its plethora of spices—a trade that commenced by their sale to merchants traveling along the ancient Silk Road (Siriweera, 1994). There was great commercial importance placed upon spices as a trade commodity, and Sri Lanka has been identified since ancient times as a hub of high quality spices that carry medicinal value. The key spices, which were traded during the days of the ancient Silk Road were cinnamon, cardamom, and cloves, while pepper, nutmeg, and gamboge were also sold to overseas merchants. These spices were used as flavoring agents both locally as well as overseas, and they also carried therapeutic properties. Pictures of these major spices are shown in Fig. 3.2. The medicinal properties of the Sri Lankan spices are an aspect that was known to the traditional medicinal practitioners of the country since ancient times. However, it should be noted that the establishment and popularity of the traditional medicinal system of Sri Lanka since ancient times was independent from the commercial exchanges made during the ancient Silk Road days, although it is possible that the recognition of certain spices with medicinal value as an agricultural crop was imparted due to the influence of international traders visiting the country. In the present day, in terms of foreign exchange earnings to the country, spice exports reached US$ 214 million in 2011 indicating a 11.73% growth within the next decade or so. Some of the therapeutic properties of the major spices being exported by Sri Lanka are summarized in Table 3.3.

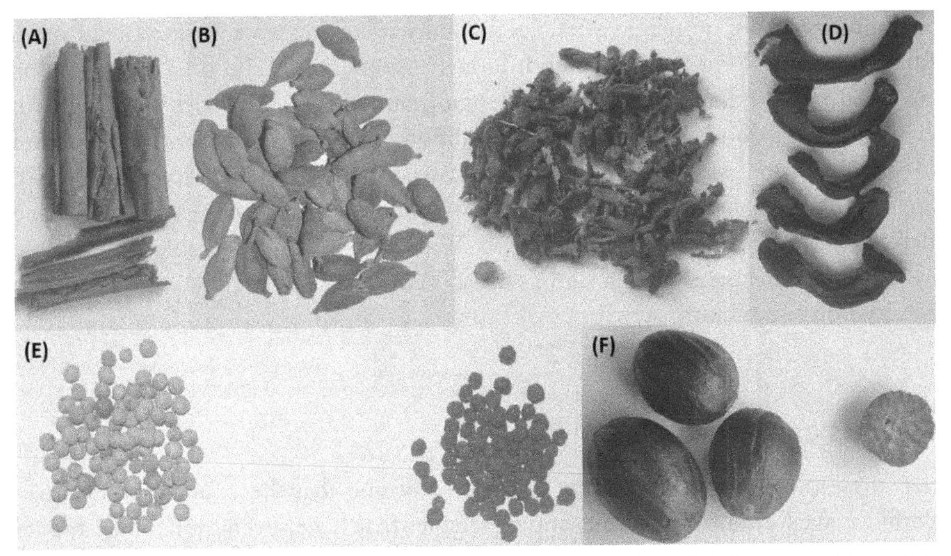

Figure 3.2 Some of the major Sri Lankan spices in the local as well as global market with medicinal properties: (A) cinnamon, (B) cardamom, (C) cloves, (D) gamboge, (E) black and white pepper, and (F) nutmeg.

Table 3.3 Therapeutic properties and selected studies demonstrating the beneficial effects of the commonly consumed spices in Sri Lanka.

Common name of spice	Scientific name of the spice variety with a higher commercial value	Therapeutic property
Cinnamon	*Cinnamomum zelanicum* Blume	Anticancer (Lu et al., 2010), antidiabetic (Cao et al., 2007), antiinflammatory (Yu et al., 2012), antioxidant (Dhuley, 1999)
Cloves	*Syzygium aromaticum*	Antimicrobial (Sofia et al., 2007), antioxidant (Pérez-Jiménez et al., 2010)
Cardamom	*Elettaria cardamomum*	Antibacterial (Kaushik et al., 2010), antioxidant (Badei et al., 1991), antiinflammatory (Sharma et al., 2011)
Black pepper	*Piper nigrum*	Thermonutrient and bioavailability enhancer (Srinivasan, 2009)
Nutmeg	*Myristica fragrans*	Antioxidant, antiinflammatory analgesic, antidiabetic (Asgarpanah and Kazemivash, 2012), anticancer (Piras et al., 2012)
Gamboge	*Gambogia morella*	Antioxidant and anticancer (Choudhury et al., 2016)

Waisundara (2018) mentions the evaluation of antioxidant and starch hydrolase inhibitory activities of cardamom, cloves, coriander, cumin seeds, curry leaves, fenugreek, mustard seeds, nutmeg, sweet cumin, and star anise extracts in an in vitro model of digestion mimicking the gastric and duodenal conditions. The total phenolic contents in all spice extracts had statistically significantly ($P < .05$) increased following both gastric and duodenal digestion. In addition, with the exception of the cumin seed extract, none of the spice extracts showed statistically significant ($P < .05$) changes in the initial starch hydrolase enzyme inhibitory values before gastric and duodenal digestion. In conclusion, the study by Waisundara (2018) was able to prove that the 10 Sri Lankan spices were a significant source of total phenolics, antioxidant, and starch hydrolase inhibitory activities.

3.5 Fruits and vegetables

Given the biodiversity of Sri Lanka, it is not surprising that the country houses many endemic as well as nutritious fruits and vegetables that have several functional properties. These health benefits are mostly seen in the ethnobotanical uses of these fruits and vegetables. In the ethnobotanical survey conducted by Marwat et al. (2014), the following fruits that are readily available in Sri Lanka were found to be used for antidiabetic effects: *Benincasa hispida, Psidium guajava, Xanthium strumarium, Averrhoa bilimbi* L., *Artocarpus heterophyllus* Lam., *A. marmelos, Anacardium occidentale* L. *Citrullus lanatus* (Thunb.) Mats. & Nakai, *Lycopersicon esculentum* Miller, *Pyrus malus* L. *Spondias dulcis*. The following vegetables were also seen to be administered to diabetics according to this survey: *Allium sepa, Allium sativum, Cucumis sativus* L. Bittergourd is a popular vegetable in Sri Lanka that is typically consumed by those with diabetes. It has also been known to possess antioxidant effects (Choo et al., 2014). As a tropical country, Sri Lanka has been gifted with a myriad of fruits: some of which are rare and endemic and consumed by locals for generations for their associated therapeutic properties. Given their extensive and historical usage as traditional medicines, it is to be expected that many of these fruits are considered as "superfoods." Waisundara (2018) reported the stability of the antioxidant and starch hydrolase inhibitory activities of the following endemic fruits when subjected to pancreatic and duodenal digestion: *Elaeocarpus serratus, Flacourtia indica, Flacourtia inermis, Pouteria campechiana,* and *Solanum nigrum*. These two functional properties were found to be noteworthy in these fruits. It must be mentioned that the antioxidant and starch hydrolase inhibitory activities of these five endemic Sri Lankan fruits were reported in this study for the first time.

3.6 Roots and tuber crops

Starchy roots and tuber crops are an important source of carbohydrates in the Sri Lankan diet, apart from rice. They provide a substantial part of the country's food supply and are also an important source of animal feed and processed products for human consumption and industrial use. Tubers and root crops are generally considered as a significant source of a number of compounds, namely saponins, phenolic compounds, glycoalkaloids, phytic acids, carotenoids, and ascorbic acid (Chandrasekara and Kumar, 2016). Additionally, they provide a variety of nutrients as shown in Table 3.4. Several bioactivities, namely antioxidant, immunomodulatory, antimicrobial, antidiabetic, anti-obesity, and hypocholesterolemic activities, among others, are reported for tubers and root crops (Chandrasekara and Kumar, 2016). Although processing methods used for the preparation of these starches may affect the overall bioactive components, flavonols such as rutin that are not heat-labile may remain in the roots and tubers during the cooking process (Navarre et al., 2010). Many of the starchy tuber crops in Sri Lanka, except the common potatoes, sweet potatoes, and cassava, are not yet fully explored for their nutritional and health benefits (FAO, 1990). This is a significant void given that some of these edible tubers have also been used as medicines in the Sri Lankan traditional medicinal system. For instance, *Ipomoea batatas* (L.) Lam. or sweet potato has been administered to diabetics by local traditional medicinal practitioners (Marwat et al., 2014).

Table 3.4 Chemical composition of some of the commonly consumed roots and tubers in Sri Lanka.

Root/tuber	Chemical properties	Composition	References
Cassava	Moisture content	9.40% ± 0.48%	Emmanuel et al. (2012)
	Protein	2.93% ± 0.45%	
	Fat	0.74% ± 0.27%	
	Crude fiber	2.22% ± 0.63%	
	Ash	2.26% ± 0.24%	
	Carbohydrate	84.67% ± 0.81%	
	Energy	1491 kJ/100 g DM	
Sweet potato	Moisture content	70.0%	Antonio et al. (2011)
	Protein	1 g/100 g	
	Total lipids	0.3–0.8 g/100 g	
	Cholesterol	0.0 g/100 g	
	Carbohydrates	28.0 g/100 g	
	Dietary fiber	2.6 g/100 g	
	Ash	0.9 g/100 g	
	Energy	114.0 kcal/100 g	
Yam	Moisture	82.19 ± 0.41 g/100 g	Shajeela et al. (2011)
		9.47% ± 0.12%	Obadina et al. (2014)
	Crude protein	7.57% ± 0.11 g/100 g	Shajeela et al. (2011)
		1.51% ± 0.01%	Obadina et al. (2014)
	Crude lipids	5.28 ± 0.18 g/100 g	Shajeela et al. (2011)
	Crude fiber	3.96 ± 0.11 g/100 g	Shajeela et al. (2011)
		1.93% ± 0.21%	Obadina et al. (2014)
	Ash	3.56 ± 0.02 g/100 g	Shajeela et al. (2011)
		1.67% ± 1.15%	Obadina et al. (2014)
	Energy	1655.30 kJ/100 g (dry matter)	Shajeela et al. (2011)
	Fat	1.77% ± 0.20%	Obadina et al. (2014)
	Carbohydrates	83.96% ± 0.21%	Obadina et al. (2014)

Source: Modified from Waisundara, V.Y., & Obadina, A.O., 2018. Asian and African starches: health properties and food applications. Niger. Food J. 36, 109–123.

3.7 Other traditional functional food of Sri Lanka

Cereals play a vital role in the human diet as an important source of energy, protein, and micronutrients among others for most people in the world. This is so for the Sri Lankan diet as well. Recommendations in Sri Lanka as well as worldwide emphasize the significance of cereals in a balanced diet. Furthermore, cereals have been proven to provide additional health benefits while satisfying the energy and nutritional needs of humans (Kumari et al., 2016). Several studies have demonstrated that the regular consumption of whole grains and whole grain products are helpful to prevent and to reduce the prevalence of noncommunicable diseases (Okarter and Liu, 2010). Millet is a commonly consumed grain in Sri Lanka, and its chemical composition is shown in Table 3.5.

Table 3.5 Chemical composition of some of the commonly used Sri Lankan starches with a low GI.

Type of starch	Chemical properties	Composition	References
Kithul	Moisture	10.1% ± 2.1%	Wijesinghe et al. (2015a,b,c)
	Crude protein	1.0 ± 0.2 g/100 g	
	Total fat	0.33 ± 0.08 g/100 g	
	Crude fiber	1.0 ± 0.5 g/100 g	
	Ash content	0.8 ± 0.6 g/100 g	
Finger millet	Protein	7.3%	Devi et al. (2014)
		5%–12.7%	Singh and Rajhuvanshi (2012)
	Fat	1.3%	Devi et al. (2014)
	Crude fiber	3.6%	Devi et al. (2014)
		12%	Ramulu and Udayaekhara Rao (1997)
	Total dietary fiber	19.1%	Devi et al. (2014)
		18.6%	Singh and Rajhuvanshi (2012)
	Ash	3%	Devi et al. (2014)
		1.7%–4.13%	Singh and Rajhuvanshi (2012)
	Starch	59%	Devi et al. (2014)
	Total carbohydrates	72%–79.5%	Singh and Rajhuvanshi (2012)
	Dietary fiber	18.6%	Singh and Rajhuvanshi (2012)
		18%	Thapliyal and Singh (2015)
Chickpea	Moisture	10.35% ± 0.31%	Chandrasekara (2002)
	Protein	23.64 ± 0.50 g/100 g	
	Nonprotein nitrogen	1.82 ± 0.10 g/100 g	
	Fat	6.48 ± 0.08 g/100 g	
	Crude fiber	3.82 ± 0.13 g/100 g	
	Ash	3.72 ± 0.04 g/100 g	
Lotus root (cooked)	Protein	1.58 g/100 g	Sheikh (2014)
	Fat	0.07 g/100 g	
	Dietary fiber	3.1 g/100 g	
	Carbohydrates	16.02 g/100 g	
	Sugars	0.52 g/100 g	
	Energy	278 kJ/100 g	
Sorghum	Moisture	8–12 g/100 g	Dicko et al. (2006)
	Proteins	7–15 g/100 g	
	Fat	1.5–6 g/100 g	
	Ash	1–4 g/100 g	
	Carbohydrates	65–80 g/100 g	

Source: Modified from Waisundara, V.Y., 2018. Assessment of bioaccessibility: a vital aspect for determining the efficacy of superfoods. In: Shiomi, N. (Ed.), Current Topics in Superfoods. InTech Open, Rijeka, Croatia.

Kumari et al. (2016) analyzed the soluble and bound phenolic compounds from different varieties of millet types, namely finger millet, foxtail, and proso millet cultivated at dry and intermediate climatic zones in Sri Lanka. Finger millet showed the highest phenolic content and antioxidant activities compared to proso and foxtail millets. The phenolic content as well as antioxidant activities of soluble and bound phenolic extracts of millets were affected by variety and cultivated location. The highest phenolic content and antioxidant activities were reported for millet samples cultivated in areas belonging to the dry zone in Sri Lanka.

Although the most popular source of starch in the world is corn, there are many other types of starches such as potato, cassava, rice, sweet potato, and yam that are produced largely throughout the world for human consumption. The production of a specific starch depends on the geographical location and availability. Starches do have functional properties; although they vary in physicochemical properties (such as retrogradation, gelation and viscosity), their potential health benefits (such as preventing gastrointestinal cancer and arthritis) could be promoted among consumers as healthier choices, especially for those who are obese and/or diabetic. Some of the commonly consumed Sri Lankan starches and their chemical compositions are shown in Table 3.5. These starches are low in their glycemic index as well (GI).

There are lots of traditional foods in Sri Lanka that are being improved through incorporation of functional ingredients, for instance through addition of soybean flour. Soybeans (*Glycine max*) are native to Asia, although this plant is cultivated and consumed worldwide. It is a popular food item in Sri Lanka as well. Soybean flour has many important nutritious components, such as protein (29.8 g%), including all essential amino acids, fats (19.5 g%), carbohydrates (36.1 g%), fibers (3.8 g%), water-soluble vitamins particularly B1 (0.45 g%), B2 (0.21 g%), and minerals particularly calcium (189 mg%), phosphorus (540 mg%), and iron (7.5 mg%) (Food Composition Tables for South East Asia, 1972). Perera et al. (2013) conducted an initial study to evaluate the feasibility of incorporating soy flour into traditional Sri Lankan breakfast foods such as roti, pittu, wandu, thosai, hoppers, and string hoppers. That way, the food products could be used as a vehicle to impart protein, fiber, and polyunsaturated fat in addition to being low in the GI. Except string hoppers, all the other preparations with soy flour had not changed the sensory attributes of these tested products, and thus could be seen as an alternative flour to be used in the preparation of these items.

3.8 Conclusions

Sri Lanka has much to offer in terms of functional food. It has lots of endemic plants that may be considered as unexplored territories of bioactive compounds with a multitude of disease-preventing properties. When conducting studies on these traditional food products though, it is important to simulate the customary methods of preparation, especially the temperature and processing conditions. There have been instances where the preparation methods have deviated or were modified owing to the usage of modern laboratory and culinary equipment, resulting in the complete destruction of the bioactivity of the phytochemicals and leading to inaccurate conclusions. Although they may appear primeval, the traditional processing methods have been tested and made perfect across generations through inadvertent "clinical trials," making it virtually impossible to match the level of optimization and accuracy through modern scientific interpretations. Additionally, it has to be borne in mind that many of the Sri Lankan food products that are consumed for disease prevention have not been traditionally used in isolation. They were combined with food products and ingredients of the like, hinting at the synergistic effects of bioactive compounds that may exist in these items. Nevertheless, the gap existing between the traditional knowledge of Sri Lanka and scientific proof is a matter that requires resolution before propagation and promotion of the traditional and functional food of Sri Lanka to the global consumer market.

References

Akanji, M.A., Olukolu, S.O., Kazeem, M.I., 2018. Leaf extracts of *Aerva lanata* inhibit the activities of type 2 diabetes-related enzymes and possess antioxidant properties. Oxid. Med. Cell Longev. Available from: https://doi.org/10.1155/2018/3439048.

Antonio, G.C., Takeiti, C.Y., De Oliveira, R.A., Park, K.J., 2011. Sweet potato: production, morphological and physicochemical characteristics and technological process. Fruit Veg. Cereal Sci. Biotechnol. 5, 1–18.

Anusha, C.S., Kumar, B.P., Sini, H., Nevin, K.G., 2016. Antioxidant *Aerva lanata* extract supresses proliferation and induce mitochondria mediated apoptosis in human hepatocelluar carcinoma cell line. J. Exp. Integr. Med. 6, 71–81.

Asgarpanah, J., Kazemivash, N., 2012. Phytochemistry and pharmacologic properties of *Myristica fragrans* Hoyutt: a review. Afr. J. Biotechnol. 11, 12787–12793.

Badei, A.Z.M., Morsi, H.H.H., El-Akel, A.T.M., 1991. Chemical composition and antioxidant properties of cardamom essential oil. Bull. Fac. Agric. Univ. Cairo 42, 199–215.

Cao, H., Polansky, M.M., Anderson, R.A., 2007. Cinnamon extract and polyphenols affect the expression of tristetraprolin, insulin receptor, and glucose transporter 4 in mouse 3T3-L1 adipocytes. Arch. Biochem. Biophys. 459, 214–222.

Chandrasekara, S.R., 2002. Traditional Sri Lankan diet. Diabetes Care 25, 14–16.

Chandrasekara, A., Kumar, T.J., 2016. Roots and tuber crops as functional foods: a review on phytochemical constituents and their potential health benefits. Int. J. Food Sci. Available from: https://doi.org/10.1155/2016/3631647.

Chaudhary, R.C., 2003. Speciality rices of the world: effect of WTO and IPR on its production trend and marketing. J. Food Agric. Environ. 1, 34–41.

Choo, C., Waisundara, V.Y., Lee, Y.H., 2014. Bittergourd (*Momordica charantia*) scavenges free radicals by enhancing the expression of superoxide dismutase in *in vitro* models of diabetes and cancer. CyTA – J. Food 12, 378–382.

Choudhury, B., Kandimalla, R., Bharali, R., Monisha, J., Kunnumakara, A.B., Kalita, K., et al., 2016. Anticancer activity of *Garcinia morella* on T-cell murine lymphoma via apoptotic induction. Front. Pharmacol. Available from: https://doi.org/10.3389/fphar.2016.00003.

De Alwis Goonatilake, S., 2012. The taxonomy and conservation status of freshwater fishes in Sri Lanka. In: Weerakoon, D.K., Wijesundara, S. (Eds.), The National Red List 2012 of Sri Lanka:

Conservation Status of the Fauna and Flora. Ministry of Environment, Colombo, Sri Lanka, pp. 77–81.

Deb, D., Dev, S., Das, A.K., Khanam, D., Banu, H., Shahriar, M., et al., 2010. Antinociceptive, anti-inflammatory and anti-diarrheal activities of the hydroalcoholic extract of *Lasia spinosa* Linn. (Araceae) roots. Lat. Am. J. Pharm. 29, 1269–1276.

Devi, P.B., Vijayabharathi, R., Sathyabama, S., Malleshi, N.G., Priyadarisini, V.B., 2014. Health benefits of finger millet (*Eleusine coracana* L.) polyphenols and dietary fiber: a review. J. Food Sci. Technol. 51, 1021–1040.

Dhuley, J.N., 1999. Anti-oxidant effects of cinnamon (*Cinnamomum verum*) bark and greater cardamon (*Amomum subulatum*) seeds in rats fed high fat diet. Indian J. Exp. Biol. 37, 238–242.

Dicko, M.H., Gruppen, H., Voragen, A.G.J., van Berkel, W.J.H., 2006. Sorghum grain as human food in Africa: relevance of starch content and amylase activities (review). J. Biotechnol. 5, 384–395.

Ediriweera, E.R.H.S.S., Ratnasooriya, W.D., 2009. A review on herbs used in treatment of diabetes mellitus by Sri Lankan Ayurvedic and traditional physicians. Ayu 30, 373–391.

Emmanuel, O.A., Clement, A., Agnes, S.B., 2012. Chemical composition and cyanogenic potential of traditional and high yielding CMD resistant cassava (*Manihot esculenta* Crantz) varieties. Int. Food Res. J. 19, 175–181.

FAOSTAT, 2009. FAO Statistics Division 2009. <http://faostat.fao.org> (accessed 22.01.19.).

FBDG, 2011. Food Based Dietary Guidelines for Sri Lankans, second ed. A Publication by Nutrition Division of Ministry of Health of Sri Lanka in collaboration with the World Health Organization. <http://www.fao.org/3/a-as886e.pdf> (accessed 01.01.19.).

Fernando, M.R., Wickramasinghe, S.M.D.N., Thabrew, M.I., Ariyananda, P.L., Karunanayake, E.H., 1991. Effect of *Artocarpus heterophyllus* and *Asteracanthus longifolia* on glucose tolerance in normal human subjects and in maturity onset diabetic patients. J. Ethnopharmacol. 31, 277–282.

Food and Agriculture Organization (FAO), 1990. Roots, Tubers, Plantains and Bananas in Human Nutrition, vol. 24 of Food and Nutrition Series. Food and Agriculture Organization, Rome, Italy.

Food Composition Tables for South Asia, 1972. FAO, Manila, Philippine.

Gupta, R.S., Singh, D., 2007. Protective nature of *Murraya koenigii* leaves against hepatosupression through antioxidant status in experimental rats. Pharmacologyonline 1, 232–242.

Hara, K., Someya, T., Sano, K., Sagane, Y., Watanabe, T., Wijesekara, R.G.S., 2018. Antioxidant activities of traditional plants in Sri Lanka by DPPH free radical-scavenging assay. Data Brief 17, 870–875.

Horagan, F.G., Kudavidanage, E.P., Weragodaarachchi, A., Ramp, D., 2017. Traditional 'maavee' rice production in Sri Lanka: environmental, economic and social pressures revealed through stakeholder interviews. Paddy Water Environ. Available from: https://doi.org/10.1007/s10333-017-0604-0.

Jayawardena, R., Byrne, N.M., Soares, M.J., Katulanda, P., Hills, A.P., 2012. Food consumption of Sri Lankan adults: an appraisal of serving characteristics. Public Health Nutr. 16, 653–658.

Jayawardena, N., Watawana, M.I., Waisundara, V.Y., 2015. Evaluation of the total antioxidant capacity, polyphenol contents and starch hydrolase inhibitory activity of ten edible plants in an *in vitro* model of digestion. Plant Foods Hum. Nutr. 70, 71–76.

Karunaratne, A.M., 2012. Probiotic foods: benefits to the cereal based Sri Lankan diet. Ceylon J. Sci. 47, 105–123.

Kaushik, P., Goyal, P., Chauhan, A., Chauhan, G., 2010. *In vitro* evaluation of antibacterial potential of dry fruit extract of *Ellatria cardamom* Maton (chhoti elaichi). Iran. J. Pharm. Res. 9, 287–297.

Kok, S.Y.Y., Mooi, S.Y., Ahmad, K., Sukari, M.A., 2012. Antitumour promoting activity and antioxidant properties of girinimbine isolated from the stem bark of *Murraya koenigii*. Molecules 17, 4651–4660.

Kumari, D., Madhujith, T., Chandrasekara, A., 2016. Comparison of phenolic content and antioxidant activities of millet varieties grown in different locations in Sri Lanka. Food Sci. Nutr. 5, 474–485.

Lee, Y.H., Choo, C., Watawana, M.I., Jayawardena, N., Waisundara, V.Y., 2014. An appraisal of eighteen commonly consumed edible plants as functional food based on their antioxidant and starch hydrolase inhibitory activities. J. Sci. Food. Agric. 95, 2956–2964.

Lu, J., Zhang, K., Nam, S., Anderson, R.A., Jove, R., Wen, W., 2010. Novel angiogenesis inhibitory activity in cinnamon extract blocks VEGFR2 kinase and downstream signaling. Carcinogenesis 31, 481–488.

Madsen, C., 2007. Functional foods in Europe. Ann. Nutr. Metabol. 51, 298–299.

Manamendra-Arachchi, K., Meegaskumbura, M., 2012. The taxonomy and conservation status of freshwater fishes in Sri Lanka. In: Weerakoon, D.K., Wijesundara, S. (Eds.), The National Red List 2012 of Sri Lanka: Conservation Status of the Fauna and Flora. Ministry of Environment, Colombo, Sri Lanka, pp. 88–91.

Marwat, S.K., Rehman, F.U., Khan, E.A., Khakwani, A.A., Ullah, I., Khan, K.U., et al., 2014. Useful ethnophytomedicinal recipes of angiosperms used against diabetes in South East Asian Countries (India, Pakistan & Sri Lanka). Pak. J. Pharm. Sci. 27, 1333–1358.

Muniandy, K., Gothai, S., Badran, K.M.H., Kumar, S.S., Esa, N.M., Arulsevlan, P., 2018. Suppression of proinflammatory cytokines and mediators in LPS-induced RAW 264.7 macrophages by stem extract of *Alternanthera sessilis* via the inhibition of the NF-κB pathway. J. Immunol. Res. Available from: https://doi.org/10.1155/2018/3430684.

Myers, N., Mittermeier, R.A., Mittermeler, C.G., da Fonseca, G.A.B., Kents, J., 2000. Biodiversity hotspots for conservation priorities. Nature 403, 853–858.

Navarre, D.A., Shakya, R., Holden, J., Kumar, S., 2010. The effect of different cooking methods on phenolics and vitamin C in developmentally young potato tubers. Am. J. Potato Res. 87, 350–359.

Obadina, A.O., Babatunde, B.O., Olotu, I., 2014. Changes in nutritional composition, functional, and sensory properties of yam flour as a result of pre-soaking. Food Nutr.Sci. 2, 676–681.

Oh, H., Lee, S.H., Kim, T., Chai, K.Y., Chung, H.T., Kwon, T.O., et al., 2002. Furocoumarins from *Angelica dahurica* with hepatoprotective activity on tacrine-induced cytotoxicity in Hep G2 cells. Planta Med. 68, 463–464.

Okarter, N., Liu, R.H., 2010. Health benefits of whole grain phytochemicals. Crit. Rev. Food. Sci. Nutr. 50, 193–208.

Pajaniradje, S., Kumaravel, M., Pamidimukkala, R., Subramanian, S., Rajagopalan, S., 2014. Antiproliferative and apoptotic effects of *Sesbania grandiflora* leaves in human. cancer cells. BioMed Res. Int . Available from: https://doi.org/10.1155/2014/474953.

Perera, P.K., Li, Y., 2012. Functional herbal food ingredients used in type 2 diabetes mellitus. Pharmacogn. Rev. 6, 37–45.

Perera, M.P.M.S.S., Sivakanesan, R., Abeysekara, D.T.D.J., Sarananda, K.H., 2013. Sensory evaluation, proximate analysis and available carbohydrate content of soy flour incorporated cereal based traditional Sri Lankan breakfast foods. Int. J. Res. Agric. Food Sci. 1, 10–19.

Pérez-Jiménez, J., Neveu, V., Vos, F., Scalbert, A., 2010. Identification of the 100 richest dietary sources of polyphenols: an application of the phenol-explorer database. Eur. J. Clin. Nutr. 64, S112–S120.

Piras, A., Rosa, A., Marongiu, B., Atzeri, A., Dessì, M.A., Falconieri, D., et al., 2012. Extraction and separation of volatile and fixed oils from seeds of *Myristica fragrans* by supercritical CO_2: chemical composition and cytotoxic activity on Caco-2 cancer cells. J. Food. Sci. 77, C448–C453.

Premakumara, G.A.S., Abeysekara, W.K.S.M., Ratnasooriya, W.D., Chandrasekharan, R.V., Bentota, A.P., 2013. Antioxidant, anti-amylase and anti-glycation potential of brans of some Sri Lankan traditional and improved rice (*Oryza sativa* L.) varieties. J. Cereal Sci. 58, 451–456.

Rajapakse, R.M.T., Sandanayake, C.A., Pathinayake, B.D., 2000. Foot prints in rice variety improvement and its impact on rice production in Sri Lanka. In: Annual Symposium of the Department of Agriculture, Sri Lanka, vol. 2, pp. 423–433.

Ramulu, P., Udayaekhara Rao, P., 1997. Effect of processing on dietary fibre content of cereals and pulses. Plant Foods Hum. Nutr. 50, 249–257.

Senadheera, S.P.A.S., Ekanayake, S., 2012. Green leafy porridges: how good are they in controlling glycaemic response? Int. J. Food Sci. Nutr. 64, 169–174.

Shajeela, P.S., Mohan, V.R., Jesudas, L.L., Tresina Soris, P., 2011. Nutritional and anti-nutritional evaluation of wild yam (*Dioscorea* spp.). Trop. Subtrop. Agroecosyst. 14, 723–730.

Sharma, S., Sharma, J., Kaur, G., 2011. Therapeutic uses of *Elettaria cardomum*. Int. J. Drug Formul. Res. 2, 102–108.

Sheikh, S.A., 2014. Ethno-medicinal uses and pharmacological activities of Lotus (*Nelumbo nucifera*). J. Med. Plant Stud. 2, 42–46.

Singh, P., Rajhuvanshi, R.S., 2012. Finger-millet for food and nutritional security. Afr. J. Food Sci. 6, 77–84.

Siriweera, W.I., 1994. A Study of the Economic History of Pre Modern Sri Lanka. Vikas Publishing House, India, ISBN 978-0-7069-7621-2.

Sofia, P.K., Prasad, R., Vijay, V.K., Srivastava, A.K., 2007. Evaluation of antibacterial activity of Indian spices against common foodborne pathogens. Int. J. Food Sci. Technol. 42, 910–915.

Sompong, R., Siebenhandl-Ehn, S., Linsberger-Martin, G., Berghofer, E., 2011. Physicochemical and antioxidative properties of red and black rice varieties from Thailand, China and Sri Lanka. Food Chem. 124, 132–140.

Srinivasan, K., 2009. Black pepper (*Piper nigrum*) and its bioactive compound, piperine. Molecular Targets and Therapeutic Uses of Spices . Available from: https://doi.org/10.1142/9789812837912_0002.

Tachibana, Y., Kikuzaki, H., Lajis, N.H., Nakatani, N., 2003. Comparison of anti oxidative properties of carbazole alkaloids from *Murraya koenigii* leaves. J. Agric. Food. Chem. 51, 6461–6467.

Thapliyal, V., Singh, K., 2015. Finger millet: potential millet for food security and power house of nutrients, Int. J. Res. Agric. Forest., 2. pp. 22–33.

Ullah, M.O., Sultana, S., Haque, A., 2009. Antimicrobial, cytotoxic and antioxidant activity of *Centella asiatica*. Eur. J. Sci. Res. 30, 260–264.

Waisundara, V.Y., 2018. Assessment of bioaccessibility: a vital aspect for determining the efficacy of superfoods. In: Shiomi, N. (Ed.), Current Topics in Superfoods. InTech Open, Rijeka, Croatia.

Waisundara, V.Y., Watawana, M.I., 2014a. Evaluation of the antioxidant activity and additive effects of traditional medicinal herbs from Sri Lanka. Austr. J. Herb. Med. 26, 22–28.

Waisundara, V.Y., Watawana, M.I., 2014b. The classification of Sri Lankan medicinal herbs: an extensive comparison of the antioxidant activities. J. Tradit. Complement. Med. 4, 196–202.

Waisundara, V.Y., Obadina, A.O., 2018. Asian and African starches: health properties and food applications. Niger. Food J. 36, 109–123.

Weerakoon, D.K., Gunawardena, K., 2012. The taxonomy and conservation status of birds in Sri Lanka. In: Weerakoon, D.K., Wijesundara, S. (Eds.), The National Red List 2012 of Sri Lanka: Conservation Status of the Fauna and Flora. Ministry of Environment, Colombo, Sri Lanka, pp. 114–117.

Wijesinghe, J.A.A.C., Wickramasinghe, I., Saranandha, K.H., 2015a. Deviation of chemical properties of kithul (*Caryota urens*) flour obtained from five different growing areas in Sri Lanka. Int. J. Innov. Res. Technol. 2, 67–76.

Wijesinghe, J.A.A.C., Wickramasinghe, I., Saranandha, K.H., 2015b. Kithul flour (*Caryota urens*) as a potential flour source for food industry. Am. J. Food Sci. Technol. 3, 10–18.

Wijesinghe, J.A.A.C., Wickramasinghe, I., Saranandha, K.H., 2015c. Kithul flour (*Caryota urens)* as new plant origin gelatinizing agent with a product development of fruit-based dessert. Eng. Technol. 2, 72–78.

Yu, T., Lee, S., Yang, W.S., Jang, H.J., Lee, Y.J., Kim, T.W., et al., 2012. The ability of an ethanol extract of *Cinnamomum cassia* to inhibit Src and spleen tyrosine kinase activity contributes to its anti-inflammatory action. J. Ethnopharmacol. 139, 566–573.

PART 4

Food, Nutrition, and Health in Nepal

CHAPTER 1

Introduction

Jiwan Prava Lama
Nepal Agribusiness Innovation Centre, Kathmandu, Nepal

Contents

1.1 Introduction

Nepal is a land of diversity in terms of ethnicity, tradition, socioculture, topography, and agroclimate. This diversity is reflected in the variety of traditional foods and beverages with respect to the methods of preparation, ethnic origination, consumption pattern, organoleptic perception, and shelf life. It has over a hundred ethnicities with each major ethnicity celebrating their own indigenous customs, beliefs, foods, and traditions. The locals live under diverse geographical and environmental orientations, from the low plains (*Terai*), northward through the middle hills and up to the high plains of the mountain region. The customs and traditions are heavily influenced by the ethnicity, climate, land, and resources of these regions. The mountain region consists of *Sherpas*, *Dolpa-pas*, and *Lopas*, where the cuisine and culture are influenced by the Tibetan culture. The hilly region consists of mixed ethnicities such as *Magars*, *Gurungs*, *Tamangs*, *Sunuwars*, *Newars*, *Thakalis*, *Chepangs*, *Brahmins*, *Kshetris*, and *Thakuris*. It is a hub of diversity rich in culture, arts, and traditions. It holds half of the population of the country including the capital, Kathmandu. The major ethnic groups found in the *Terai* regions are diverse, such as *Brahmin*, *Kshetri*, *Rajput*, *Tharus*, *Dalai*, *Kumal*, and *Majhi*. These regions, specifically the regions adjacent toward the Indian borders, follow the Indo sociocultural traditions.

With such diversity, there is an abundance of varied indigenous foods within the country. They have distinctive characteristics, unique processing techniques, and high nutritive value. These foods are the representatives of the ideas and technologies that have been passed down for generations keeping the history, culture, and traditions of the country intact.

Nutritional and Health Aspects of Food in South Asian Countries
DOI: https://doi.org/10.1016/B978-0-12-820011-7.00021-6

1.2 Food habits

The Nepalese food habit has adopted rice as its staple, as it is the most widely consumed food in the country. The main course is collectively known as *Dal–Bhat–Tarkari* (rice–pulse–vegetable) with a pickle of seasonal vegetables or fruits, and meat as a non-vegetarian option is commonly consumed twice a day. *Dal–Bhat–Tarkari* is synonymous with lunch or dinner; this signifies the ingrained influence of the cuisine in society. In the high hills and mountain regions where there is an insufficiency of rice, *Dhindo* (boiled maize/millet flour) is consumed as a staple as well as *roti* made up of wheat or other grains. In the *Terai* region the people consume *Dal–Bhat–Tarkari* and/or *roti*. Most Nepali cuisines consist of dairy products (curd, whey, ghee) in their serving. Some ethnic groups also consume fermented alcoholic drinks made from millet or rice as a beverage with respect to their cultures and traditions.

The food habits of the people have been changing over the years. The consumption of indigenous foods has decreased, seemingly playing an important role only during the festive seasons or religious rituals rather than an everyday diet. Eating out has become less of a novelty and more of a necessity, and fast foods seem to have more appeal to the general consumer, especially in the urban regions. Some foods have been adapted commercially into the mainstream such as *Newari* food, which has become one of the more popular cuisines and has been gaining cross-cultural popularity over the years. Especially, *Momo* (dumpling) has been a cultural phenomenon in the country, and most other foods have been considered as a lunch staple in the city areas.

1.3 Categorization of traditional foods

Each ethnicity has its own versions of indigenous foods consisting of cereals, pseudo-cereals, pulses and legumes, vegetables, fruits, milk, meat, etc. Table 1.1 categorizes some common Nepali traditional food and beverages (NTFBs) by the raw materials being used.

1.4 Challenges and opportunities

The production of NTFBs is limited to the household level and/or cottage scale. There is a lack of recorded methods of preparation and processing techniques that are verbally handed down from generations. However, these foods are now receiving renewed interest in the scientific community to respect the local wisdom, improvising the process for enhanced safety and nutritional properties. Although some of the traditional foods such as *achar, chiura, churpi, sukuti,* and *selroti* have been found to be commercialized, it still requires extensive research and innovation on the pre- and postharvest operations of the raw materials and postproduction storage and distribution.

Table 1.1 Nepali traditional food and beverages.

Raw materials	Traditional foods
Cereals	*Anarasa, Bhakka, Chatamari, Chiura, Dhido, Golphuki, Hakuwa, Jand, Kasar, Khajuri, Khapsa, Khatte, Lunghakcha, Malpuri, Phiniroti, Selroti, Yomari*
Pseudocereals (Beverages)	*Chyang, Khareng, Raksi, Sigolya, Tongba, Thon*
Pulses and legumes	*Adauri, Bara, Furaula, Kinema, Kwati, Maseura, Satu*
Rice-pulse	*Bagiya, Dal-puri, Lakhamari*
Vegetables	*Achar, Gundruk, Kalfpapro, Kumbharauri, Sinki, Titaudo*
Fruits	*Achar, Chuk, Khalpi, Mada, Nimki, Titaura*
Oilseeds	*Chiurigheu, Mustard oil, Philinge-achar, Til ko laddu*
Milk	*Churpi, Dahi, Gheu, Gundpak, Mohi, Nauni-gheu, Pustakari*
Meat	*Choyala, Kachila, Sargyangma, Sukuti, Womyuk*
Fish	*Fish cake, Sidra, Sukuti-maccha*
Sugar	*Chaaku, Sakkhar*
Miscellaneous	*Khamirmana, Manapu, Murcha, Tama (Mesu), Tadi*

Some efforts by the government have also been made to provide information about traditional food items and underutilized indigenous grains to improve food habits through yearly food fairs at various locations within the country. On the other hand, traditional foods can also be a source of income if used wisely among the tourists visiting the various sites. As food and tourism are two sides of a coin, there is tremendous scope for the development of tourism with traditional foods and vice versa.

1.5 Conclusion

The consumption of traditional foods has decreased immensely during the past few years, probably due to the poor perception of quality, urbanization, and acculturation, where western influences have overhauled the food culture. It is an understatement to say that Nepal is a treasure trove for diverse traditional food items. Regrettably, the pace of the development and preservation of NTFBs is lacking in many ways. There is a need for documentation and promotion of traditional foods and to improvise the production technology without obstructing the historical culture. This will promote the acceptability and longevity of traditional foods that are in essence the epitome of Nepali history, culture, and diversity.

CHAPTER 2

Traditional fermented food of Nepal and their nutritional and nutraceutical potential

Dambar Bahadur Khadka[1] **and Jiwan Prava Lama**[2]
[1]Central Campus of Technology, Tribhuvan University, Dharan, Nepal
[2]Nepal Agribusiness Innovation Centre, Kathmandu, Nepal

Contents

Nutritional and Health Aspects of Food in South Asian Countries
DOI: https://doi.org/10.1016/B978-0-12-820011-7.00022-8

2.1 Background

Food is essential for social and cultural heritage. It plays a multifunctional connecting role between society and sustainable food systems (Cavicchi and Stancova, 2016). Traditional foods and practices are a valuable aspect of society's culture and technology and reflect accumulated knowledge, skills, and technology of local people extracted from their direct interaction with local environment (Oniango et al., 2006). It is very important in times of crisis to preserve foods, for biodiversity, nutritional diversity, and in attaining food security (FAO, 2013). Nepal is a country rich in cultural, ethnic groups, and geographical diversity that provide an opportunity for various food production, preparation, and consumption of traditional foods. However, protein–energy malnutrition and micronutrient deficiency are widely distributed across the country. In spite of some improvement in Nepal, still stunting, wasting, and underweight prevail in under-five children, which are respectively 36%, 10%, and 27%. Around 17% women are thin, and 22.5% are overweight and obese. Undernutrition is higher in far west hill and mountain regions than in the *Terai* region. Micronutrient deficiencies such as iron deficiency are high among women (41%) and in children (53%) and are distributed unevenly in the country with higher prevalence in *Terai* regions (Ministry of Health Nepal, 2017). At the same time, noncommunicable disease prevalence is increasing in the country. About 52.2% of households are still food insecure and 10% are severely food insecure, and the condition is more aggravated in the mountain region and far-western hills (Acharya et al., 2018).

The agriculture practices are more seasonal and primitive in Nepal and lead to an occasional shortage of food, primarily nutritionally sensitive food. Traditional foods either fermented or nonfermented can be the basis for preservation and for food and nutrition security, besides their cultural and ethnical identity and role. Traditional foods can be useful for fulfilling the seasonal shortage of food and nutrients and enhance livelihood. Traditional fermented food can be an important nutrient supplement or source of functional components for the people and also enhanced diversity in periods of seasonal shortfall. However, most traditional knowledge and technology are passed as trade secrets of families of certain communities and are protected from tradition. Complete scientific information on the preparation method and mode of consumption and their nutritional value and nutraceutical potential are still lacking. Therefore this chapter mainly focuses to explore the available information of various traditional fermented foods and their nutritional values along with the possibilities of their exploitation as a nutraceutical and functional potential.

2.2 Geography and the natural landscape

Nepal is a Himalayan country, located between latitude 26°22′ to 30°27′ north and longitude 80°4′ to 88°12′ east with a total area of 147,181 square kilometers. It occupies 0.3% and 0.03% land of Asia and the world, respectively (CBS, 2015). Geographically, the country has tremendous diversity and is closely related to its two giant neighbors India and China. Nepal has a total population of 26.5 million with an annual growth rate of 1.35% (CBS, 2015). Nepal lies in the temperate zone with an added advantage of having altitudes of 70–8848 m. Nepal is divided into three regions (northern mountain, mid hill, and southern *Terai*) comprising 7%, 46%, and 47% of the population and 35%, 42%, and 23% of the total land area, and it has seven provinces (CBS, 2016). The climatic condition ranges from tropical to arctic depending upon the altitude. The *Terai* region lies in the tropical southern part of the country and has a hot and humid climate. The mid hills and mountain region is pleasant almost all year around. The northern mountain region around with an altitude above 3353 m has an alpine climate with considerably lower temperature and thin air in winter. Nepal has four climatic seasons: spring (March–May), summer (June–August), autumn (September–November), and winter (December–February) (CBS, 2016).

The agricultural sectors contribute nearly 35% of Nepal's gross domestic products supporting the livelihood of more than 75% of the population (CBS, 2011). The diversified agroclimatic conditions provide a huge opportunity to grow, cultivate, process, and consume diverse agricultural and livestock products. Southern *Terai* is more fertile and has arable land compared to the mid-hill area, whereas mountains are nearly infertile in nature (MoAD, 2016). The main cereals cultivated in Nepal are paddy, maize, wheat, buckwheat, barley, and millet. The production of paddy, maize, and wheat is mainly concentrated in the *Terai* regions, while the production of buckwheat, millet, and barley is more concentrated in hills and some of the mountainous regions. The diverse climate of the country also supports the cultivation and production of a variety of fruits and vegetables. The major livestock of hills and *Terai* is cow, buffalo, goat, poultry, pig, duck, and sheep, while yak is domesticated only in mountain regions (MoAD, 2016).

2.3 History of fermentation and fermented food

Fermented foods have been used since humans arrived on earth after the existence of microbes and plants (Steinkraus, 1994). Historically, with the dawn of civilization, humans lived as hunter-gatherers, started agriculture, and learned ways of processing food. Fermentation after drying is the oldest food preservation method. It is believed that the first fermentation might have been developed accidentally when the storage of surplus food in ancient times was in practice and became popular with the dawn of civilization when they were accepted organoleptically. The science behind the fermentation was unknown even after the initiation of fermentation for 200 years and only flourished after 1700 CE along with the discovery of the microscope and Pasteur's discovery of fermentation (Mehta et al., 2012).

The art of fermentation seems to have originated in the Indian subcontinent in the settlement that predates the great Indus valley civilization. There are indications of highly developed systems of agriculture and animal husbandry during the Harappan spread or prevedic times. Artifacts from Egypt and the Middle East suggest that fermentation was known from ancient times in those regions. Fermented bread and beer were known in ancient Egypt and Babylonia in early 4000 and 3000 BCE (Farnworth, 2008; Hutkins, 2006). China was thought to initiate fermentation of vegetables and use of molds to make food around 300 BCE (Farnworth, 2008). Alcoholic fermentation involved in the making of wine and brewing is considered to have been developed during the period of 2000–4000 BCE by the Egyptians and Sumerians. It is documented that fermented drinks were being produced over 7000 years ago in Babylon (now Iraq), 5000 years ago in Egypt, 4000 years ago in Mexico, and 3500 years ago in Sudan (Dirar, 1993).

The culture of the South Asian countries has relatively few artifacts regarding the beginning of fermentation and fermented food. *Rig-Veda* (about 1500 BCE) has mentioned the "*Somras*," fermented juice and wine. In Hindu mythology, the use of *soma/somras*, as well as *sura*, by various groups in the society for anesthetic and calming effects has been mentioned around 2000 BCE (Farnworth, 2008; Prajapati and Nair, 2008). In Nepal, human existence had been reported before 9000 BCE. According to Nepalese history, animal husbandry and agriculture have been mentioned since ancient times by the Gopala dynasty (a cattle herder and buffalo herder from Ahira's dynasty) before *kirant* (from 1800 BCE to 300 CE) from Tibeto-Burman and Indo-aryan (*Licchavi*) ruled in Nepal (Bhattarai, 2008; Shrestha, 2002). The origin of fermented food in Nepal has been lost in antiquity. It perhaps originated in ancient times or has been introduced by different rulers who migrated from Indo regions and Tibeto-Burman regions along with their culture across the country (Tamang, 2010).

2.4 Ethnicity, origin, and distribution of ethnic groups

The ethnicity of Nepal can be grouped into three broad groups based on their ancestral origin, Indo-origin, and Tibeto origin and their pool of indigenous groups (Shrestha, 2002). Indo-Nepali groups mostly inhabit the fertile lower hills, rivers valley,

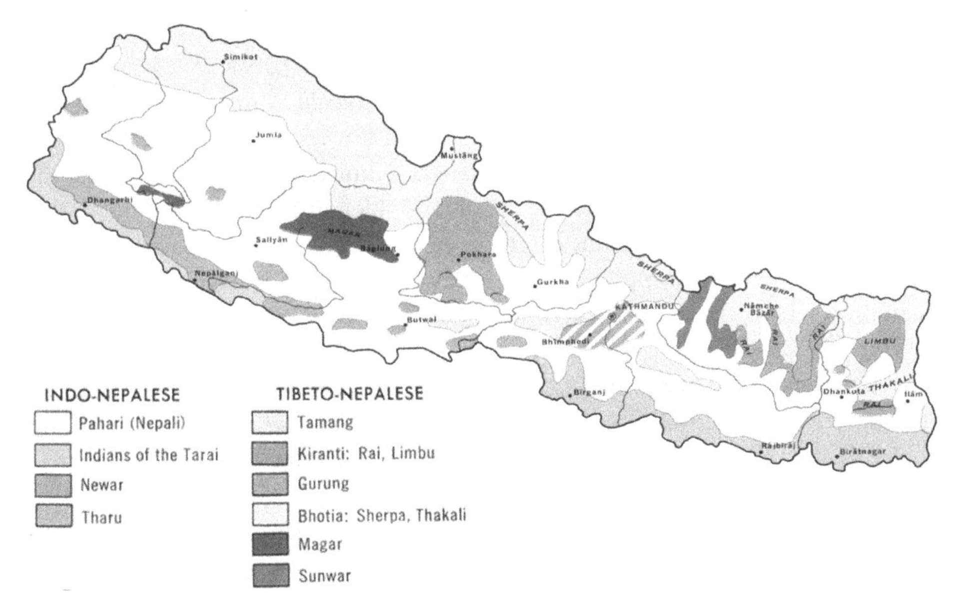

Figure 2.1 Ethnic groups and their distribution in Nepal.

and *Terai* plain. The Indo-Nepali groups include two distinct groups. The hill Indian origin group known as hill dwellers (*Pahari*) includes high caste Hindus, mostly of Brahmins and Kshatriya status. They have spread throughout Nepal. They usually constitute a significant portion of the local community. The second group of Indo-Nepal primarily includes the *Terai* habitants generally identified as *Madhesi*; they came to Nepal from northern India as shown in Fig. 2.1 (Bhattarai, 2008).

Tibeto-Nepali, coming from Tibet (*Bhot*) mostly occupy the higher hills (Fig. 2.1). The Tibeto-Nepali are generally found in higher altitudes, and they are mainly *Sherpas* (*Bhote*), *Gurung*, *Rai*, *Limbu*, *Thakali*, and *Tamang* tribes (Bhattarai, 2008; Shrestha, 2002). *Bhote* tribes are mainly found in the Trans-Himalayan zone. *Sherpa* tribes occupy northeast mainly around Everest (*khumbu*) regions and mainly practice Buddhism. Moving westward along the hills, there is a higher concentration of *Tamang* population, *Gurung* in west-central hills, while the *Magar* are found in the hills and further west. The *Thakali* are well known for Himalayan trade having settled along the upper reaches of *Kali Gandaki* river basin, which was a major trade route between Tibet and India in the past before 1950 (Bhattarai, 2008; Shrestha, 2002).

2.5 Food culture and traditions

Nepal is a multilanguage and multicultural country with various ethnic groups living together across the country. Altogether 125 castes/ethnic groups are residing in the country, and about 123 languages are being spoken. The 10 major caste and ethnic groups reported are *Chhetri*, *Brahman*, *Magar*, *Tharu*, *Tamang*, *Newar*, *Muslman*, *Kami*, *Yadav*, and *Rai*. Ten different religious groups *Hindu*, *Buddhist*, *Islam*, *Kiranti*, *Christian*, *Prakriti*, *Bon*, *Jain*, *Bahai*, and *Sikha* reside in Nepal (CBS, 2014).

Food culture and tradition often relate to ethnicity, religion, and tradition. Nepalese food culture reflects the diffusion and blending of the Hindu and the Tibetan cuisines, with modifications based on ethnic preferences and social philosophy over a period of time (Tamang, 2010). Himalayan ethnic foods have evolved because of traditional wisdom and experiences of generations over periods of time based on agroclimatic condition, available edible sources, ethnical preferences, and social and cultural acceptances (Tamang, 2010). *Bhat* (boiled rice) with *daal* (pulses soup), *tarkari* (vegetables curry), *dahi* (milk curd)/*mohi* (buttermilk), and *achar* (pickle) is the main meal of Nepalese. When there is a scarcity of rice in hilly areas, *dhinro* (bolied maize) with *mohi* is often consumed. Besides in the form of *tarkari*, various traditional foods, both fermented and nonfermented, are being consumed. Nepal is rich in traditional food culture and cuisines. More than 105 traditional foods are consumed in Nepal and about 24 different fermented foods are prepared and consumed since time immemorial (Subba, 2012). Based on seasonal and local substrate availability, different food groups—cereals (41), followed by legume and pulses (9), vegetable-based (12), milk-based (12), meat-based (5), fish-based (3), sugar-based (2) and others (7)—are used to prepare, store, and consume various dishes (Subba, 2012). Some fermented foods are unique to festivals such as *selroti* and are prepared and consumed mainly in religious and cultural festivals such as *Deepawali* or *Tihar* (Katawal, 2012). *Dahi* is often used in making *tika* and *achhata* for worshiping goddesses and applying on forehead for different ritual activities in *Hindu* culture. In *Newari* festivals, *Raksi* is important for guest hospitality and also in various ritual activities. *Jand* and alcoholic products are especially famous among *Matwalis* (*Rai* and *Limbu*) tradition and culture (Tamang, 2010). Some traditional foods are typically related to ethnic groups, and some are intercultural and interregional adaptations. Their different modes of consumption are presented in Table 2.1.

2.6 Traditional fermented food and types

Due to various ethnic tribes, cultural habitat, and availability of local substrates in Nepal, different fermented foods are prepared and consumed. Traditional fermented foods can be basically divided based upon the major substrate used for fermentation such as cereal-based fermented foods (*selroti*, *jand*, *tongba*, *nigar*), legume-based fermented foods (*kinema*, *masyaura*), fruits and vegetable-based fermented foods (*gundruk*, *sinki*, *khalpi*, *mesu*), milk-based fermented foods (*dahi*, *mohi*, *gheu*, *solar*, *somar*), and meat- and fish-based fermented foods (*sidra*, *sukaako machha*, *sukuti*, *masular*). Fermented foods can

Table 2.1 Traditional fermented food, their ethnic and regional origin and mode of consumption.

Basic foods groups	Fermented food	Preservation technique	Ethnical origin	Regional origin	Consumption pattern	References
Cereals	*Selroti*	Fermentation and frying	Intercultural	Interregional	Sweet confectionary, Snacks	Dahal et al. (2005), Subba (2012)
Pseudocereals	*Jand*	Fermentation	Intercultural	Eastern mountain	Beverage	Dahal et al. (2005), Subba (2012)
	Raksi	Fermentation and distillation	Intercultural	Interregional	Beverage	
	Nigar	Fermentation	Intercultural	Interregional	Beverage	
Legumes	*Masyaura*	Drying	Intercultural	Interregional	Curry, side dish	Dahal et al. (2005), Subba (2012)
	Kinema	Fermentation	*Limbu*	Eastern hill and mountain	Curry	
Vegetable	*Gundruk*	Fermentation and drying	Intercultural	Interregional	Side dish/appetizer	Dahal et al. (2005), Subba (2012)
	Sinki	Fermentation and drying	Intercultural	Interregional	Side dish/appetizer	
	Khalpi	Fermentation	Intercultural	Interregional	Appetizer	
	Mesu	Fermentation	*Limbu*	Eastern mountain	Side dish/appetizer	
Milk	*Dahi*	Fermentation	Intercultural	Interregional	Side dish, beverages	Dahal et al. (2005), Subba (2012)
	Mohi	Fermentation	Intercultural	Interregional	Beverages	
	Gheu	Dehydration	Intercultural	Highland Himalaya	Frying medium, as such for energy	
	Somar	Fermentation	*Bhotia, Sherpa*	Highland Himalaya	Soup	Rai et al. (2016)
	Chhurpi	Fermentation, and drying	Intercultural	Interregional	Curry, soup	
Fish	*Sidra*	Salting and drying	Intercultural	Interregional	Snacks	Subba (2012)
	Sukuti	Drying and smoking	Intercultural	Interregional	Snacks	Rai et al. (2016)
	Sukkako maachha	Drying	Intercultural	Interregional	Snacks	
	Masular	Drying	*Tharu*	East and west Tarai	Side dish/curry soup	Gartaula et al. (2014)

also be classified based on the fermentative organism involved and type of fermentation as alcoholic and nonalcoholic fermented food. *Jand*, *tongba*, and *nigar* belong to alcoholic fermented food. Vegetable-based fermented foods such as *gundruk*, *sinki*, *khalpi*, and *mesu* as well as milk-based *dahi*, *mohi*, *gheu*, etc. can be placed in the group of lactic acid fermented food. *Kinema* can be categorized as alkaline fermented food, while *masyaura* and *selroti* can be considered as mixed spontaneous fermented food.

2.7 Cereal, legume-based fermented food products

2.7.1 Selroti

Selroti is a ring-shaped fried bread/doughnut prepared by mixing rice flour paste [rice: water 1:1 (w/v)], banana (one small piece/kg paste), honey (5%), ghee (5%), and some spices. Sometimes banana and honey are replaced with sodium bicarbonate (0.25%) and sugar (10%). The well-mixed batter is allowed to ferment for either 4 h (during summer) or 24 h (during winter). The kneaded batter is filled in a small funnel and deposited as continuous rings into the hot oil. These rings are fried until brown and served while hot (Yonzan and Tamang, 2009).

2.7.2 Kinema

Kinema is a nonsalted and solid-state alkaline fermented soybean food product of the eastern hills of Nepal (Rai, 2012; Tamang, 2010). It is mainly consumed by non-Brahmin Nepalese inhabiting Nepal, Darjeeling and Sikkim of India, and in some parts of Bhutan. It has a pungent smell of ammonia, slimy texture, and short shelf life. It resembles the *Bacillus* fermented Japanese *natto*, Korean *chungkukjang*, *thuanao* of northern Thailand, *pepock* of northern Myanmar, and *seing* of Cambodia (Tamang, 2010). The preparation method of *Kinema* is lost in antiquity. In the traditional method, soybeans (*Glycine max* L.) are cleaned, washed, and soaked in water overnight at ambient temperature (10°C–25°C), and excess water is drained off. Soaked beans are cooked in an open cooker until they can be crushed easily between the fingertips. Then, the water is removed and crushed lightly by a wooden pestle to de-hull the seed. A small amount of firewood ash is often added. The soybean grits containing torn hulls are then wrapped with fresh fern (*Athyrium* sp.) or *Leucosceptrum canum* smith leaves, covered by a sackcloth and kept in a bamboo basket above an earthen oven in the kitchen to ferment for 1–3 days (maximum 1 week in winter) till formation of the typical flavor is dominated by ammonia. *Kinema* after fermentation has stringy threads when touched with fingers; the longer the threads, the better the quality of *kinema* (Sarkar et al., 1994). Fresh *kinema* is fried in edible oil along with salt, spices, and tomatoes and eaten as a side dish with rice. The predominant microflora of the *kinema* are

Bacillus subtilis and *Enterococcus faecium* bacteria and *Candida parapsilosis* and *Geotrichum candidum* as yeast (Sarkar et al., 1994).

2.7.3 Masyaura

Masyaura or maseura is an ethnic, fermented black gram or green gram product prepared by Nepalese living in the Himalayas. It is a cone-shaped hollow, brittle, and friable product mostly consumed by Newari communities of Nepal (Chetri and Tamang, 2008). *Masyaura* is a product similar to North Indian *wari* and South Indian *sandige*. They are brittle and spongy textured dried balls, 2–5 cm in diameter (Dahal et al., 2005). *Masyaura* is especially prepared from split black gram (*Phaseolus mungo*) and colocasia (*Colocasia esculenta*) or radish and ash gourd depending upon the availability of raw materials (Dahal et al., 2005). The dried balls are stored at ambient conditions. It is mixed with curry to make soup and served with rice as a side dish. Dried *masyaura* contains a final moisture content of 8%–10%. It is a cheap and rich source of protein (18%–20% on fresh weight), carbohydrates (67%–70% on fresh weight), and minerals. It is also known as meat for vegetarians (Dahal et al., 2005; Dahal et al., 2003). The major microflora identified are lactic acid bacteria (*Lactobacillus fermentum*, *Lactobacillus salivarius*, *Pediococcus pentosaceus*, and *Enterococcus durans*), spore former (*B. subtilis*, *Bacillus mycoides*, *Bacillus pumilus*, and *Bacillus laterosporus*), and yeast (*Saccharomyces cerevisiae*, *Pichia burtonii*, and *Candia castelli*) (Chetri and Tamang, 2008). During preparation of *masyaura*, seeds of black gram are cleaned, washed, and soaked overnight. Soaked seeds are dehulled by pressing through hands; hulls are removed and ground into a thick paste using mortar and pestle. Water is carefully added while grinding until the paste becomes sticky. Washed, peeled, and shredded colocasia tuber is mixed and hand-molded into small ball or cones. The mixture is placed on a bamboo mat and fermented in an open kitchen for 2–3 days and sun-dried for 3–5 days depending on weather conditions (Chetri and Tamang, 2008).

2.8 Nutritive value of cereal and legume-based nonalcoholic fermented products

Most of the cereals and legume-based fermented products are good sources of calories and proteins as shown in Table 2.2. Legume-based fermented products are easily digestible and enriched with vitamins, minerals, and amino acids. *Kinema* is rich in linoleic acid produced by microbial lipase during fermentation (Sarkar et al., 1996) and reported to contain all the essential amino acids (Sarkar et al., 1997). It has a higher content of riboflavin and niacin (Sarkar et al., 1998). *Masyaura* has high soluble proteins (74.8%–82.1% of total protein), amino nitrogen (1.0–2.02 mg/100 g, db), nonprotein nitrogen (0.83%–1.61%, db), and vitamin B-complex (vitamin B_1 from 116 to 246 mg/100 g, db and vitamin B_2 from 88 to 141 mg/100 g, db), and decreases

Table 2.2 Cereal- and legume-based fermented product and their nutritional composition (per 100 g dry basis).

Product	Substrate	Microflora	References
Selroti	Rice, wheat flour, and spices	Lactic acid bacteria (LAB): *Leuconostoc mesenteroides, Enterococcus faecium, Pediococcus pentosaceus, Lactobacillus curvatus* Yeast: *Saccharomyces cerevisiae, Saccharomyces kluyveri, Debaryomyces hansenii, Pichia burtonii, and Zygosaccharomyces*	Katawal (2012), Yonzon and Tamang (2010)

Moisture (%)	Protein (%)	Fat (%)	CHO (%)	Fiber (%)	Ash (%)	Energy (kcal)	Ca (mg)	P (mg)	Mg (mg)	Na (mg)	K (mg)
11.4	4.7	26.5	68.4	0.12	0.3	532	6.4	12.7	24.9	17.4	46.7

Product	Substrate	Microflora	References
Kinema	Soybean	Bacteria: *Bacillus subtilis, Enterococcus faecium* Yeast: *Candida parapsilosis, Geotrichum candidum*	Sarkar et al. (1994)

Moisture (%)	Protein (%)	Fat (%)	CHO (%)	Ash (%)	Energy (kcal)	pH	Acidity as lactic acid (%)
63.0	48.7	16.1	29.6	5.6	478	8.10	0.10

Product	Substrate	Microflora	References
Masyoura	Black gram, Colocasia tubers	Lactic acid bacteria (LAB): *L. fermentum, L. salivarius, Pediococcus pentosaceus, Enterococcus durans* Bacillus: *Bacillus subtilis, Bacillus mycoides, Bacillus pumilis*, and *Bacillus laterosporus* Yeast: *Saccharomyces cerevisiae, Pichia burtonii*, and *Candia castelli*	Chetri and Tamang (2008), Dahal et al. (2003), Lama (1988)

Moisture (%)	Protein (%)	Soluble protein as % of total protein	CHO (%)	Crude fiber (%)	Ash (%)	Vitamin B_1 (μg)	Vitamin B_2 (μg)
8–10	18–20	74.2–84	67–70	5.12	4.8	116–246	88–141

in pH (6.1−5.4), starch (57.7%−54.1%, db), free sugar (9.45%−4.61%, db), and reducing sugar (2.0%−0.75%, db) contents as compared with the raw ingredients (Dahal et al., 2003).

2.9 Cereal-based alcoholic fermented beverages

2.9.1 Jand

Jand (also spelled as *jandh/jaanr/jnar/jnard)* is a generic term that refers to a sweet-sour cereal beer made by solid substrate fermentation of cereals such as finger millets (*Eleusine coracana*), rice (*Oryzae sativa*), wheat (*Triticum* spp.), and maize (*Zea mays*) using *murcha* (Rai, 2006). It is an indigenous nondistilled alcoholic beverage of Nepal. Finger millet is a preferred substrate for *jand*, as it is believed to provide superior quality (Rai, 2012). It has found a very prominent place in *Limbu* and *Rai* culture in particular and other ethnic groups in general (Rai, 2006). *Murcha, an* amylolactic starter, contains saccharifying mold, lactic acid bacteria, and fermenting yeast (Rai, 2012). The basic steps of *jand* making include cooking of cereals, cooling to room temperature, mixing with *murcha* powder and leaving for a day or two to develop biomass, and fermenting in a tight close-necked earthen pot. The duration of fermentation is a week to several months.

Jand is consumed in different ways. It can be served after mixing with the requisite amount of water squeezed as strained *jand* and is also consumed as *tongba* or *tungba* by adding luke-warm water to loosely stuffed fermented millet in a cylindrical vessel. *Nigar* is more similar to cereal wine (Japanese *Sake*), while *jand* that contains live yeast and suspended particles has been categorized as cereal beer. If *jand* is pot distilled, it becomes *raksi*, a nonaged traditional spirit of varying alcohol content (15%−50%) (Rai, 2012).

2.10 Nutritive value of cereal-based alcoholic beverages

Cereal-based alcoholic products such as *jand*, *nigar*, and *raksi* have calorific values due to alcohol content (Table 2.3). Vitamin-like cyanocobalamine, which is not present in the finger millet, has reported to be synthesized by fermenting microorganisms (Basappa, 2002). Compared with unfermented mash, fermented finger millet has been reported to have an increment in protein content by twofold (7.62%−15.7% db) and ash content by 1.8-fold (2.76−4.62) along with a significant increase in phosphate, sodium, potassium, and zinc but no significant change in iron (Karki, 2013). The essential amino acids such as valine, threonine, leucine, and isoleucine are in higher concentrations in *koddoko jand* or *chyang* (Basappa et al., 1997). Because of high calorific values, both *bhaate Jand* and *koddoko jand* are consumed to regain strength by ailing persons and pregnant women (Tamang and Thapa, 2006; Thapa and Tamang, 2004).

Table 2.3 Cereal-based fermented alcoholic product and their nutritional composition (per 100 g dry basis).

Product	Substrate	Microflora	pH	Acidity[a]	Alcohol (%)	References
Bhaate Jand	Rice, wheat	Mold: *Mucor circinelloides, Rhizopus chinensis* Yeast: *Saccharomyces fibuligera, Pichia anomala, Saccharomyces cerevisiae, Candida glabrata* Lactic acid bacteria (LAB): *Pediococcus pentosaceus, Lactobacillus bifermentans*	4.04	0.24	5.9	Tamang et al. (2012), Tamang and Thapa (2006)

Product	Moisture (%)	Protein (%)	Fat (%)	CHO (%)	Crude fiber (%)	Ash (%)	Energy (kcal)	Ca (mg)	Fe (mg)	Mg (mg)
Bhaate Jand	83.4	9.5	2.0	86.9	1.5	1.7	405	12.8	7.7	50

Product	Substrate	Microflora	pH	Acidity[a]	Alcohol (%)	References
Koddoko Jand	Finger millet	Mold: *Mucor circinelloides, Rhizopus chinensis* Yeast: *Saccharomyces fibuligera, Pichia anomala, Saccharomyces cerevisiae, Candida glabrata* Lactic acid bacteria (LAB): *Pediococcus pentosaceus, Lactobacillus bifermentans*	4.04	0.27	4.8	Tamang et al. (2012), Tamang and Thapa (2006)

Product	Moisture (%)	Protein (%)	Fat (%)	CHO (%)	Crude fiber (%)	Ash (%)	Energy (kcal)	Ca (mg)	Fe (mg)	Mg (mg)
Koddoko Jand	69.7	9.3	–	83.7	4.7	5.1	394	281	24	118

[a]As % lactic acid.

2.11 Fruits and vegetable-based fermented food products

A number of fermented fruits and vegetable products have been prepared and consumed in different communities and regions of Nepal. *Gundruk*, *sinki*, and *sinnamani* are the fermented products obtained particularly from leafy vegetables and radish stem, with some variation in the substrate used and method of preparation. The words *gundruk* and *sinki* are derived from *Newari* words (Dahal et al., 2005; Kharel et al., 2007; Tamang, 2010).

2.11.1 Gundruk

Gundruk is prepared by spontaneous lactic acid fermentation of leafy vegetables and is commonly consumed by all the Nepalese and Gorkha tribes of northeastern states of India (Tamang, 2010). It is commonly prepared from mustard (*Brassica juncea*), radish (*Raphanus sativus*), *rayo sag* (*Brasicca rapa*), and cabbage (*Brassica oleracea*) and some other locally grown vegetable leaves (Tamang and Tamang, 2010; Tamang et al., 2009). *Gundruk* is usually prepared from December to February when the weather is less humid.

During the preparation, the leaves are withered in the sun for 1–2 days. The withered leaves, after a mild crushing, are hand pressed in a perforated tin or earthen jar with a heavy article such as a large stone to remove surplus water. They are then left to ferment in a warm and dry place for 15–22 days. In the village setup, a hole of diameter and depth of about 1 m is dug in the ground and dried by fire. A 30 cm layer of banana or bamboo leaves are placed in the bottom; the dried crushed leaves of the vegetables to be fermented are placed above this layer and covered with a layer of banana or bamboo leaves. A heavy stone is kept to compress the substrate, which is allowed to ferment in situ until a fermentation odor develops (15–22 days). The fermented *gundruk* is then taken out and sun-dried (Dahal et al., 2005). The dominant floras identified in *gundruk* fermentation were *Lactobacillus plantarum*, *Pediococcus pentosaceous*, and *Lactobacillus cellubiosus*. Lactic acid and acetic acid were the major organic acids in *gundruk* and *sinki* (Karki, 1986).

2.11.2 Sinki and Sinnamani

Sinki and *sinnamani* are prepared from the whole radish stem. *Sinnamani* is similar to *sinki*, but drying after fermentation is usually not done in the case of *sinnamani*. *Sinnamani* is used as a pickle in the fresh and soft stage, and it is sourer than *sinki* (Dahal et al., 2005). The method of preparation of *sinki* is also similar to that of *gundruk*, except that the substrate is radish root (*R. sativus*) and the fermentation takes 30–40 days. *Sinki* fermentation is initiated by heterofermentative *L. fermentum* followed by another heterofermentative *Lactobacillus brevis* and succeeded by homofermentative *L. plantarum* (Tamang and Sarkar, 1993). The preparation and shelf life of *sinki* are similar to those of *gundruk*, and *sinki* is mainly consumed as an appetizer or pickle with the main dish (Karki, 1986).

2.11.3 Khalpi

Khalpi is a well-known lactic acid fermented pickle of Nepal, prepared in almost every home. *Khalpi* is prepared with ripe cucumber, spices, and salt. The cucumber is washed, sliced lengthwise, and the inner soft portion is removed, and it is cut into pieces (5−8 cm), mixed with rapeseed powder, red chili powder, turmeric powder, and salt, and heated with mustard oil. The mixture is transferred to an earthen or glass pot, covered with cloth or lid and allowed to ferment for 3 days (Dahal et al., 2005). In *Khalpi* fermentation, initially, *Leuconostoc fallax*, *L. brevis*, and *Pediococcus pentosaceus* are active and later dominated by *L. plantarum* (Tamang and Tamang, 2010).

2.11.4 Taama/Mesu

Mesu (*Me* means young bamboo shoot and *su* means sour in *Limbu* language) is a pickle, similar to *naw-mai-dong* of Thailand. It is prepared from the tender edible bamboo shoot of common variety of bamboo such as *choya bans* (*Dendrocalamus hamiltonii* also known locally as *tama bans*), *mal bans* (*Bambusa nutans*), *bhalu bans* (*Dendrocalamus sikkimensis*), *dhungre bans* (*Dendrocalamus gigantea*), and *Karati bans* (*Bambusa tulda Roxb.*) depending on their availability and seasons (Kharel et al., 2007; Tamang, 2010; Tamang and Sarkar, 1996).

The shoots (*taama*) are finely chopped (1−2 cm) and transferred into bamboo vessels or a glass bottle, tightly packed, and capped to provide an airtight environment. The material is allowed to ferment at ambient temperature (20°C−25°C) for 7−8 days. Lactic acid bacteria seem to be the dominant organism in *Mesu* fermentation (Tamang and Sarkar, 1996). *Mesu* fermentation is initiated by *Pediococcus pentosaceus* followed by *L. brevis* and dominated by *L. plantarum* presented naturally in fresh shoots (Tamang and Sarkar, 1996). *Mesu* is usually prepared from June to September. It has a sour taste and strong ammonia odor. The curry called *allu-taama-bodi* (potato-*mesu*-white beans) is one of the more popular items in the *Newari* community of Nepal (Dahal et al., 2005). A very common pickle by mixing *mesu* with salt and green chilies is also prepared. It is also used in the preparation of meat curry after frying (Tamang and Sarkar, 1996).

2.12 Nutritive value of vegetable-based fermented product

The nutritive value of *gundruk*, *sinki*, *khalpi*, and *mesu* is presented in Table 2.4. *Gundruk* is a good source of B-vitamins and minerals along with essential amino acids (Karki, 1986; Karki et al., 2016). The level of palmitic acid, oleic acid, and linoleic

Table 2.4 Vegetable-based fermented product and their nutritional composition (per 100 g dry basis).

Product	Substrate	Microflora	pH	Acidity[a]	References
Gundruk	Leafy vegetables	*Lactobacillus plantarum* *Pediococcus pentosaceous, Lactobacillus cellubiosus*	4.40	0.8–0.9	Karki (1986), Karki et al. (2016)

Protein (%)	Fat (%)	CHO (%)	Energy (kcal)	Ca (mg)	Na (mg)	K (mg)
35.9	2.1	48.9	321	92.2	6.7	678

Product	Substrate	Microflora	pH	Acidity[a]	References
Sinki fresh	Radish tap root	*Lactobacillus plantarum, Lactobacillus brevis, Lactobacillus fermentum*	3.30	1.2	Tamang and Sarkar (1993)

Moisture (%)	Protein (%)	Fat (%)	Ash (%)	–	–
93.5	14.6	2.5	11.3	–	–

Product	Substrate	Microflora	pH	Acidity[a]	References
Sinki dried	Radish trap root	*Lactobacillus fermentum, Lactobacillus plantarum, Lactobacillus brevis*	4.40	0.72	Tamang and Sarkar (1993)

Moisture (%)	Protein (%)	Fat (%)	Ash (%)	Ca (mg)	K (mg)	Fe (mg)
21.3	14.6	2.5	11.5	121	443	18.0

Product	Substrate	Microflora	pH	Acidity[a]	References
Khalpi	Cucumber	*Lactobacillus plantarum, Lactobacillus brevis, Leuconostoc fallax*	3.9	0.95	Tamang and Tamang (2010), Tamang (2010)

Moisture (%)	Protein (%)	Fat (%)	CHO (%)	Energy (kcal)	Ash (%)	Ca (mg)	Na (mg)	K (mg)
91.4	12.3	2.6	70.9	356	14.2	6.4	2.3	125

Product	Substrate	Microflora	References
Mesu	Tender and young bamboo shoots	*Lactobacillus plantarum, Lactobacillus brevis, Lactobacillus curvatus, Leuconostoc citreum, Pediococcus pentosaceus*	Tamang and Sarkar (1996), Tamang et al. (2012)

Moisture (%)	Protein (%)	Fat (%)	CHO (%)	Energy (kcal)	Ca (mg)	Na (mg)	K (mg)
89.0	27.0	2.6	55.6	352.4	7.9	2.8	282

[a]As % lactic acid.

acid is much higher in mustard leaf *gundruk* as compared with the unfermented vegetables (Karki et al., 1983b; Karki et al., 2016). In mustard leaf *gundruk*, free amino acids such as glutamic acid, alanine, lysine, and threonine increased with a decrease in asparagine, glutamine, histidine, and arginine (Karki et al., 1983a; Karki et al., 2016). The level of iron and calcium is high, but carotenoids are reduced (>90%) probably due to sun drying (Dietz, 1984). *Gundruk* contains cyanate and isothiocyanate as the main flavor compounds followed by alcohols, esters, and phenylacetaldehyde (Karki et al., 1983c). *Gundruk* is considered as a good appetizer (Tamang and Tamang, 2010).

The *sinki* collected from different regions has been reported to vary in its proximate composition (Tamang and Tamang, 2010). The protein, fat, carbohydrate, and the calorific value of *sinki* are almost the same as its substrate (radish). Dried *sinki* is a rich source of organic acid, and minerals such as calcium, iron, and potassium (Table 2.4). The mean protein, fat, and ash content of dried *sinki* has been reported to be 14.6%, 2.5%, and 11.5%, respectively (Tamang and Tamang, 2010).

2.13 Milk-based fermented food products

Milk is a highly nutritious and versatile food for infants to old age people. Nepalese people enjoy drinking milk in its natural form or use it to make a wide range of fermented and nonfermented products (Kharel et al., 2007). The major fermented milk products, such as *dahi*, *mohi*, *gheu*, and *chhurpi*, are famous in all regions of Nepal.

2.13.1 Dahi

Dahi is the main naturally fermented traditional milk product of Nepal, Darjeeling hills, and *Sikkim*. It is also used for the preparation of several other milk products such as *mohi* (butter milk), *nauni ghee* (butter like), *gheu* (ghee), soft *churpi*, and hard *chhurpi* (Rai et al., 2016). Different types of *dahi* are prepared in Nepal. A special *dahi* mainly prepared in the Bhaktapur and Kathmandu valley called as *juju-dhau* is very famous because of its texture, taste, and flavor (Dahal et al., 2005).

Traditionally, *dahi* is prepared from cow or buffalo milk by adding starter culture from previously made *dahi* locally known as *jordan* for fermentation. Milk is boiled and cooled to room temperature. *Jordan* is added and fermented in specially designed cylindrical wooden vessels (locally known as *Theki*) or in earthen pots (mainly in local shops) for 1–2 days (Kharel et al., 2007). *Dahi* is consumed directly as a beverage in Nepal, Darjeeling and Sikkim, and Bhutan. It is also consumed by mixing with *chiura* (beaten rice) or rice (Rai et al., 2016).

2.13.2 Mohi, Nauni-gheu, and Gheu

Nauni-gheu is a butter-like product achieved by traditional, manual churning of the *Dahi*. It contains 77%–78% fat, which is slightly less than butter (80%–82%). In the villages, it is customary to consume *nauni-gheu* with rice, which is considered as the staple food of most Nepalese. Churning is carried out in *Theki* manually with the help of a wooden churner locally known as *Madani*. The separated *nauni-gheu* is melted and boiled in an open pan until water evaporates. When it is cooled, a clear upper layer (known as *gheu*) separates from *bilauni* (precipitated material collected at the bottom of the pan). *Gheu* is filtered and stored for future use (Kharel et al., 2007). The liquid portion called *mohi* (resembles buttermilk) contains almost all proteins, lactose, and vitamins found in milk and appreciable amounts of fat (residual) and hence is widely consumed as a nutritious beverage.

If *mohi* is too sour, it is commonly used to prepare a spicy soup called *sollar*. *Sollar* is prepared by adding sour *mohi* to already fried spices (fenugreek, chopped onion, cumin seed, and turmeric powder) having a golden brown color. *Solar* is consumed by all, although it is believed to be more beneficial for people suffering from cold, fever, and sore throat (Kharel et al., 2007). *Gheu* is consumed with rice, mixed with *daal* (lentil soup) and used in traditional sweets or as frying medium in the preparation of a number of cereal snacks and in cooking. *Mohi* is often consumed as a cool beverage during summer or to overcome tiredness (Rai et al., 2016).

2.13.3 Chhurpi and Somar

Chhurpi is a *chhana* (curd)-based milk product indigenous to Nepal, Sikkim, and Bhutan (Rai et al., 2016). Traditionally, soft *chhurpi* is obtained when *mohi* (butter milk) is boiled for about 15 min and curd is collected by separation using a muslin cloth, which is hung tightly by a string to drain out remaining whey. If it is kept in a tight container for 10–15 days, the product is known as *somar* (Rai et al., 2016). If soft *chhurpi* is overpressed by stone for 2 days and sun-dried, it can be converted into hard *chhurpi* (Rai et al., 2016). This hard variety of *chhurpi* prepared from yak milk is also known as *dudh Chhurpi*.

However, the *chhurpi* making process varies from region to region. *Chhurpi* is also prepared from cream-separated skim milk. The milk either raw or boiled is kept on a wooden vat at room temperature for 1 day, and the cream is separated. The cream-separated milk (skim milk) is then boiled for 30 min to make the curd. Curdling of skim milk by using alum or citrus fruit juices (citric acid) is also widely practiced in Nepal (Kharel et al., 2007). The remaining process is similar to the traditional method of making soft and hard *chhurpi* (Kharel et al., 2007; Rai et al., 2016).

2.14 Nutritive value of milk-based fermented food

The nutritional composition of *dahi, mohi, gheu,* and soft and hard *chhurpi* is presented in Table 2.5. Milk-based fermented food products have the high calorie content. They are good sources of milk proteins except for *Gheu. Gheu* has the highest calorie content because of very high fat content. Among minerals, calcium is present in higher concentrations. The nutritive value of products solely depends on the type of milk used for preparation. The protein and fat content in *chhurpi* made from yak milk has been reported to be higher than those made from cow's milk (Dewan, 2002; Tamang, 2010).

2.15 Fermented fish products

People from Nepal prepare and consume different types of traditionally prepared smoked dried fermented salted fish products. Dried (*sidra*), dried salted (*sukuti*), dried smoked (*sukako maachha*), and *masular* (sun-dried mix of *sidra* and bottle guard leaf) are widely prepared and consumed in Nepal and some parts of Northeast India (Gartaula et al., 2014; Thapa, 2016). The microorganism reported in *sidra, sukako maccha,* and *sukuti* are almost the same and are mainly lactic acid bacteria (*Lactococcus lactis* subsp. *cremoris, L. Lactis* subspp. *lactis, L. plantarum, Leuconostoc mesenteroides, Enterococcus faeciem, Enterococcus faecalis, P. pentosaceous,* and *Weissella confusa*) and yeast (*Candida chiropetror-um, Candida bombicola,* and *Saccharomycopsis* spp.) (Thapa, 2016).

2.15.1 Sidra

Sidra is an ethnic sun-dried product commonly consumed in Nepal, Northeast India, and Bhutan. Small types of fish (*Puntis sarana Hamilton*) are generally used in *sidra* making. Collected fish are washed, dried in sun for 4–7 days, and stored at room temperature for 3–4 months. It is generally consumed by making chutney or pickling.

2.15.2 Sukako Maachha

Sukako Maachha is a dried, salted, and smoked fish product. Hill river fish such as *dothay asala* (*Schizothorax richardsoni Gray*) and *chuchay asala* (*Schizothorax progastus McClelland*) are generally collected in bamboo baskets from rivers or streams, washed and mixed with salt and turmeric powder, hooked in a bamboo-made string, and hung over an earthen oven in the kitchen. It can be kept for 4–6 months and usually eaten as a curry with or without soup (Thapa, 2016).

2.15.3 Sukuti

Sukuti is another popular traditional fermented fish cuisine of Nepal, Bhutan, Darjeeling hills, and Sikkim. Fish (*Harpodon* nehereus *Hamilton*) are collected, washed,

Table 2.5 Milk-based fermented product, and their nutritional composition (per 100 g dry basis).

Product	Substrate	Microflora	pH	Acidity[a]	References
Dahi	Cow's milk, Buffalo milk, Yak milk	LAB: *L. bifermentans*, *L. alimentarius*, *L. paracasei* subspp. *pseudoplantarum*, *Lactococcus lactis* subspp. *Lactis*, *Lactococcus lactis* subspp *cremoris* Yeast: *Saccharomycopsis* and *Candida*	4.2	0.73	Dewan and Tamang (2007), Tamang (2010)

Moisture (%)	Protein (%)	Fat (%)	Ash (%)	CHO (%)	Energy (kcal)	
84.8	22.5	24.5	4.7	48.2	503	–

Product	Substrate	Microflora	pH	Acidity[a]	References
Mohi	Cow's milk or yak milk	*LAB: L. alimentarius*, *Lactococcus lactis* subspp. *lactis*, and *Lactococcus lactis* subspp. *cremoris* Yeast: *Saccharomycopsis* and *Candida*	3.9	0.73	Dewan (2002), Dewan and Tamang (2007), Tamang (2010)

Moisture (%)	Protein (%)	Fat (%)	Ash (%)	CHO (%)	Energy (kcal)	
92.6	44.7	12.4	2.7	40.2	451	–

Product	Substrate	Microflora	pH	Acidity[a]	References
Gheu	Cow or yak milk	Lactic acid bacteria (LAB): *Lactococcus lactis* subsp. *lactis*, *Lactococcus lactis* subsp. *cremoris*	5.9	0.28	Dewan (2002), Tamang (2010)

Moisture (%)	Protein (%)	Fat (%)	CHO (%)	Energy (kcal)	Ca (mg)	Fe (mg)	Mg (mg)	Mn (mg)	Zn (mg)
12.6	1.6	96.1	1.2	876	81.2	1.0	32.4	1.8	43.9

Product	Substrate	Microflora	pH	Acidity[a]	References
Somar	Cow or yak milk	Lactic acid bacteria (LAB): *L. paracasei* subsp. *Pseudoplantarum*, *Lactococcus lactis* subspp. *cremoris*	6.0	0.04	Dewan (2002), Tamang (2010)

Moisture (%)	Protein (%)	Fat (%)	CHO (%)	Energy (kcal)	Ca (mg)	Fe (mg)	Mg (mg)	Mn (mg)	Zn (mg)
36.5	35	15.4	46.9	466	31.2	0.4	13.7	0.5	5.2

Product	Substrate		Microflora				pH	Acidity[a]		References	
Chhurpi hard/ Dudh chhurpi	Yak milk or cow's milk		Lactic acid bacteria (LAB): *L. farciminis*, *L. paracasei*, *Weissella confusa*, and *L. bifermentans*				6.0	0.29		Dewan (2002), Tamang (2010)	
	Moisture (%)	**Protein (%)**	**Fat (%)**	**Ash (%)**	**CHO (%)**	**Energy (kcal)**	**Ca (mg)**	**Fe (mg)**	**Mg (mg)**	**Mn (mg)**	**Zn (mg)**
	16.8	57.2	6.1	5.2	31.6	409	19.8	0.5	6.3	0.4	10.0

Product	Substrate		Microflora			pH	Acidity[a]		References	
Chhurpi soft	Cow's milk or yak milk		Lactic acid bacteria (LAB): *L. plantarum*, *L. curvatus*, *L. paracasei* subsp. *Pseudoplantarum*, *L. kefir*, *L. fermentum*, *L. alimentarius*, *L. hilgardii*, *Enterococcus faecium*, and *Leuconostoc mesenteroides*			4.3	0.61		Dewan (2002), Tamang (2010)	
	Moisture (%)	**Protein (%)**	**Fat (%)**	**CHO (%)**	**Ash (%)**	**Ca (mg)**	**Fe (mg)**	**Mg (mg)**	**Mn (mg)**	**Zn (mg)**
	73.8	65.3	11.8	16.3	6.6	44.1	1.2	16.7	0.6	25.1

[a]As percent lactic acid.

rubbed with salt, and sun-dried for 7–8 days and stored for 3–4 months. It is commonly consumed as pickle, curry, and soup, and is commonly sold in the marketplaces (Thapa, 2016).

2.15.4 Masular

Masular (*Masu* means fish and *Lar* means syrup or soup in *Tharu* language) is a dried food prepared from *sidra* and young tender bottle-gourd leaves (*Lagenaria siceraria Standl.*), mashing them together in *okhalli/dhikki* and finally providing the shape similar to pancake followed by sun drying. It is the traditional food of the *Tharu* communities of the *Terai* regions of Nepal. The preparation is limited to the household level; the final product has characteristics of dry fish. It is mainly prepared and consumed in the *Deepawali* festival by *Tharus* living in *Terai* areas, but can also be prepared in any season over the years. It is mainly consumed by making paste or syrup after cooking with tomatoes and other spices and salt (Gartaula et al., 2014).

2.16 Nutritive value of fermented fish products

All the fish products are sun-dried and hence have a low moisture content. They are slightly acidic as pH ranges from 6.4 to 6.5. Fermented fish products *sidra*, *sukako machha*, and *masular* are fair sources of calories and good sources of proteins (Thapa and Pal, 2007). Because of low moisture content and acidic nature, they can be stored for a longer time and are important for protein supplementation of local diets during off-seasons. They are also good sources of calcium and phosphorous (Tamang, 2010). The fermented fish products and their nutritive values are presented in Table 2.6.

2.17 Nutraceutical potential and health benefit of traditional fermented food

Fermented foods are transformed food products produced by the action of microbial growth and enzymatic conversions of major and minor food components. Traditional fermented foods contain both functional and nonfunctional microorganisms (Tamang et al., 2016c). The functional microorganisms that are present in traditionally fermented foods are responsible for the enrichment of nutraceutical values and health beneficial functional properties and reduction of antinutritional factors and allergens (Marco et al., 2017; Pervez et al., 2006). A summary of possible nutraceuticals and the health benefits of traditionally fermented food is compiled in Table 2.7, and a brief discussion follows.

2.17.1 Probiotics properties

Lactobacillus strains belong to the *L. acidophilus* group. *L. paracasei*, *L. plantarum*, *L. reuteri*, and *L. salivarius*, which represent the respective phylogenetic group, are known to

Table 2.6 Fermented fish products and their nutritional composition (per 100 g dry basis).

Product	Substrate	Microflora	pH	References
Sukako Machha	Dothay Asala Chuchay Asala (hill river fish)	Lactic acid bacteria (LAB): *Lactococcus lactics* subspp. *cremoris*, *Lactococcus lactis* subspp. *lactis*, *Lactococcus plantarum*, *Leuconostoc mesenteroides*, *Enterococcus faecium*, *Enterococcus faecalis*, *Pediococcus pentosaceus* Yeast: *Candida chiropetrorum*, *Candida bombicola*, *Saccharomyces* spp.	6.4	Thapa (2016), Thapa and Pal (2007)

Product	Moisture (%)	Protein (%)	Fat (%)	CHO (%)	Ash (%)	Energy (kcal)	Ca (mg)	Fe (mg)	Mg (mg)	Mn (mg)	Zn (mg)
Sukako Machha	10.4	35.0	12.0	36.8	16.2	395.2	38.7	0.8	5.0	1.0	5.2

Product	Substrate	Microflora	pH	References
Sidra	*Puntius sarana* (small fishes of freshwater and lake)	Lactic acid bacteria (LAB): *Lactococcus lactics* subspp. *cremoris*, *Lactococcus lactis* subspp. *lactis*, *Lactococcus plantarum*, *Leuconostoc mesenteroides*, *Enterococcus faecium*, *Enterococcus faecalis*, *Pediococcus pentosaceus* Yeast: *Candida chiropetrorum*, *Candida bombicola*, *Saccaharomyces* spp.	6.5	Thapa (2016), Thapa and Pal (2007)

Product	Moisture (%)	Protein (%)	Fat (%)	CHO (%)	Ash (%)	Energy (kcal)	Ca (mg)	Fe (mg)	Mg (mg)	Mn (mg)	Zn (mg)
Sidra	15.3	25.5	12.5	36.8	16.6	395	25.8	0.9	1.6	0.8	2.4

Product	Substrate	Microflora	pH	References
Masular	*Puntius sarana* (*Sidra*) + Bottle gourd leaves	Not available	–	Gartaula et al. (2014)

Product	Moisture (%)	Protein (%)	Fat (%)	Crude fiber (%)	Ash (%)	pH
Masular	10.1	41.5	13.97	4.77	20.11	–
						–

Table 2.7 Nutraceutical potential and health benefits of fermented food products.

Food	Nutraceuticals and functional components	Possible health benefits	References
Selroti	Bacteriocins, soluble nitrogen, and trichloroacetic acid (TCA) soluble nitrogen	Antimicrobial activity, enhancement in protein digestibility.	Anal (2019), Yonzon and Tamang (2010)
Kinema	Polyphenolic compounds, Isoflavon Glycon, Group B Saponin and derivatives	Antioxidant, estrogenic, antiosteoporotic, and anticarcinogenic activity	Moktan et al. (2008), Omizu et al. (2011), Samruan et al. (2012), Tamang et al. (2016b)
Masyaura	Omega fatty acids, soluble nitrogen (bioactive peptides)	Antioxidant activity	Dahal et al. (2005)
Kooddoko Jand	Soluble protein, protein hydrolyzed, fiber	Helps in digestion and absorption, consumed to regain strength by an ailing person and pregnant women, antioxidant activity	Karki (2013), Thapa and Tamang (2004)
Bhaate Jand	Maltooligosaccharides, pyranose derivatives, polyphenolics	Inhibits the intestinal pathogens antioxidants, antimutagenics, free radical scavenging and immune-stimulatory activities consumed to regain strength by an ailing person and pregnant women	Das and Deka (2012), Ghosh et al. (2015), Phutthaphadoong et al. (2010), Ray et al. (2016)
Gundruk	Organic acids, probiotics, fiber, bacteriocins	Increases digestion and absorption good appetizer, antimicrobial, beneficial in diarrhea and constipation	Gautam and Sharma (2015), Karki (1986), Karki et al. (1983a,b), Tamang et al. (2009)
Khalpi Mesu Sinki	Organic acids, probiotics, fiber, bacteriocins	Increases digestion and absorption good appetizer, antimicrobial, beneficial in diarrhea and constipation	Tamang et al. (2009)
Dahi	Probiotics, antimicrobials, functional enzymes, bioactive peptides	Effective against infectious diseases including viral, bacterial, or antibiotic-associated diarrhea, relief of chronic bowel inflammatory diseases, immunomodulation, lowering of serum cholesterol, decreased the risk of colon cancer, improves lactose digestion, reduces allergies, and has an effect on intestinal microbiota	Saad et al. (2013) Balamurugan et al. (2014), Khatri and Khadka (2018)
Gheu	Conjugated linolenic acid (CLA), phospholipids, Shingolipid	Antioxidant, anticarcinogenic, antidiabetic, antiobesity, antiatherogenic, osteosynthetic, and immunomodulatory effects	Kwak et al. (2013)

contain probiotic strains. Probiotics are the live organisms having the ability to resist gastric pH and exposure to bile and are able to grow and colonize in the gastric tract, conferring a health benefit to host (Hill et al., 2014; Saad et al., 2013). These probiotic organisms have wide applications in the treatment of infectious diseases including viral, bacterial, or antibiotic-associated diarrhea, relief of chronic bowel inflammatory diseases, immunomodulation, lowering of serum cholesterol, decreased risk of colon cancer, improved lactose digestion, and reduced allergies and adverse effect on intestinal microbiota (Saad et al., 2013). Some strains (out of 94 strain isolated) of lactic acid bacteria from fermented vegetables of Himalayan regions have shown to have the adhesion potential in gut epithelial cells indicating chances of being probiotic in nature (Tamang et al., 2009). *Lactobacillus sphicheri* G_2, a *gundruk* isolated strain has shown to have probiotic properties (Gautam and Sharma, 2015). Similarly, some strains of lactic acid bacteria (*Lactobacillus*, *Lactococcus*, and *Leuconostoc*) from homemade milk curd (Balamurugan et al., 2014) and some strains of *Lactobacillus* from traditionally prepared *dahi* have been reported to possess probiotic potential (Khatri and Khadka, 2018).

2.17.2 Antimicrobial properties

Many lactic acid bacteria present in fermented milk and vegetable products can produce antimicrobial components such as bacteriocin and nisin. Several strains of lactic acid bacteria isolated from fermented vegetables (*gundruck*, *khalpi*, *mesu*) have shown the ability to have antimicrobial properties (Tamang et al., 2009). *L. lactis* isolated from *dahi* has shown to produce nisin Z that inhibits *Listeria monocytogenes*, *Escherichia coli*, *Salmonella*, and *Bacillus* (Mitra et al., 2010). Isolated lactic acid bacteria from *Selroti* are reported to possess antimicrobial activity (Yonzon and Tamang, 2010). The antimicrobial properties and their compounds can have important applications for biopreservation and maintaining food safety (Gaggia et al., 2011). They can also be important for maintaining gut health and acute diarrhea (Balamurugan et al., 2014) and for immunomodulatory effects (Granier et al., 2013). Lactic acid fermented vegetables such as *gundruk* and *sinki* are believed to be consumed by local people as remedies against diarrhea and stomach disorder (Tamang and Tamang, 2010).

2.17.3 Antioxidant properties

The antioxidant activity of *Bacillus* fermented soybean-based Asian foods, for example, Japanese *natto* (Ping and Shih, 2012), Korean *chunkokjang* and *doenjang* (Shin and Jeong, 2015), Chinese *douchi* (Shon et al., 2011), and Thai *Thuanao* (Samruan et al., 2012), are well documented. Nepalese *kinema* largely resembles these food products. Extracts of *kinema* have a higher antioxidant activity than soybean extracts (Moktan et al., 2008). In soybean fermentation, an increase in polyphenolic compounds with increased antioxidant properties has been reported (Hong et al., 2012). Glycosidic isoflavones are hydrolyzed in soya bean fermentation to aglycon and isoflavin that increases antioxidant activity along with estrogenic, antiosteoporotic, and anticarcinogenic activity (Samruan et al., 2012; Tamang et al., 2016b). In soybean fermented products such as *kinema*, Group B saponin (DDMP-2,3-dihydro-2,5-dihydroxy-6-metyl-4*H*-pyran-4-one) and its derivatives that have a preventive role against hypercholesterolemia, colon cancer, and lipid peroxidation were reported to be increased (Omizu et al., 2011; Tamang et al., 2016a). An increase in antioxidant activity along with soluble protein and volatile acid has also been reported in finger millet fermented *jand* (Karki, 2013). *Koodoko jand* are rich in crude fiber (Thapa and Tamang, 2004) and soluble proteins (Karki, 2013) that are beneficial for food digestion and absorption. Fermented rice bran has been reported to have anticancer properties against various types of cancers including colon, stomach, and bladder cancer (Phutthaphadoong et al., 2010). The fermented rice beer contains maltooligosaccharides (maltotetrose, maltotriose, and maltose), which inhibits the intestinal pathogens and is very nutritious for infants and the elderly. Beside these, it also contains a number of pyranose derivatives (1,2,3,4-tetra-*O*-acetyl-4-*O*-formyl-D-glucopyranose, B-D-galactopyranose pentacetate) and polyphenolics and flavanol compounds that provide elevated antioxidants, antimutagenics, free radical scavenging activities, and immune-stimulatory activities (Das and Deka, 2012; Ghosh et al., 2015; Ray et al., 2016).

2.17.4 Bioactive peptides

Bioactive peptides produced in fermented products have been reported to have various health effects such as antioxidants, antihypertensive, ACE inhibition activity, immunomodulatory effect, and antimutagenic and anticarcinogenic (Martinenz-Villaluenga et al., 2017; Qian et al., 2011). Bioactive peptides are formed by proteolysis organisms by acting on the substrate proteins (Tamang et al., 2016b). *Dahi* has been reported to contain bioactive peptides and shown to have antihypertensive properties (Ashar and Chand, 2004). Studies on bioactive peptides in other Nepalese fermented foods are rarely available. However, the increase in soluble nitrogen level in *selroti* (Anal, 2019; Yonzon and Tamang, 2010), *kinema* (Sarkar et al., 1997), *masyaura* (Dahal et al., 2003), and *jand* (Karki, 2013) may reflect sign of profound proteolysis, indicating some possibilities of bioactive peptides formation in those food during fermentation and further storage.

2.17.5 Conjugated linoleic acid

Fermentation can change free fatty acids into conjugated linoleic acid (CLA) that has a number of health benefits (Paszczyk et al., 2016). *Ghee* or *Gheu* is a concentrated source of fat and is a good source of CLA, phospholipids, and sphingolipids. These components have been reported to have various health benefits including antioxidant, anticarcinogenic, antidiabetic, antiobesity, antiatherogenic, osteosynthetic, and immunomodulatory effects (Kwak et al., 2013).

2.18 Conclusion

Traditionally fermented food has been consumed since historical times, and they are physically, socially, and culturally accepted food in most of the communities in Nepal. Fermentation alone or in combination with other methods such as drying and frying are basic methods of food preservation in many households or communities, as well as sources of income generation and livelihood of people. Fermentation also brings a reduction in antinutrient factors; improves utilization of the nutrients, and can be a vital supplement of diverse nutrients that would not be present otherwise in the natural substrate. Traditionally, fermented foods can be a nutritionally important part of a regular diet and fulfill the non-seasonal food shortages. Similarly, fermentation also enhances the nutraceutical and health beneficial properties. Fermented foods possess a number of beneficial compounds depending upon the functional organisms and possible transformation of substrate components to health-related nutraceuticals, ranging from good appetizers to antioxidants, antiatherogenic, antiinflammatory, cholesterol-lowering to anticarcinogenicity. Hence, traditional fermented foods are not only nutritionally important but also have exploitation potential for health benefits. However, future studies with clinical trials and animal models are required to substantiate the claims of functional foods and the functionality of fermentative organisms to safeguard their holistic use and applications.

References

Acharya, A.K., Paudel, M.P., Wasti, P.C., Sharma, R.D., Dhital, R.D., 2018. Status Report on Food and Nutrition Security in Nepal. Ministry of Agriculture, Land Management and Cooperatives, Nepal.

Anal, A.K., 2019. Quality ingredients and safety concerns for traditional fermented foods and beverages from Asia: a review. Fermentation 5 (1), 8.

Ashar, M.N., Chand, R., 2004. Fermented milk containing ACE-Inhibitory peptide reduces blood pressure in middle aged hypertensive subjects. Milchwissenschaf 59 (7), 363–366.

Balamurugan, R., Chandragunasekran, A.S., Chellappan, G., Rajaram, K., Ramamoorthi, G., Ramakrishna, B.S., 2014. Probiotic potential of lactic acid bacteria present in home made curd in southern India. Indian J. Med. Res. 140 (3), 345–355.

Basappa, S.C., 2002. Investigations on chhang from finger millet (*Eleusine coracana* Gaertn.) and its commercial perspects. Indian Food Ind. 21 (1), 46–51.

Basappa, S.C., Somashekar, D., Renu Agrawal, K., Suma Nharati, K., 1997. Nutritional composition of fermented ragi (Chhang) by Phab and defined starter culture compared to unfermented ragi (*Eleucine coracan* G.). Int. J. Food Sci. Nutr. 48, 313–319.

Bhattarai, K.P., 2008. In: Charles, F.G. (Ed.), Nepal, edn. Chelsea House Publisher, New York.

Cavicchi, A., Stancova, C.A., 2016. Food and Gastronomy as Elements of Regional Innovation Strategies. European Commission, Joint Research Centre, Institute for Prospective Technological Studies, SpainEUR 27757 EN. Available from: https://doi.org/10.2791/284013.

CBS, 2011. Nepal Living Standard Survey NLSS III Report. Central Bureau of Statistics, National Planning Secretariat. Government of Nepal.

CBS, 2014. Population Atlas of Nepal 2014. Central Bureau of Statistics, National Planning Secretariat. Government of Nepal.

CBS, 2015. Nepal in Figures. Central Bureau of Statistics, National Planning Commission Secretariat. Government of Nepal.

CBS, 2016. Nepal in Brief. Statistical Pocket Book Nepal-2016. National Planning Commission Secretariat, Central Bureau of Statistics, Government of Nepal, Kathmandu, Nepal.

Chetri, R., Tamang, J.P., 2008. Microbiological evaluation of Maseura, an ethnic fermented legume based condiment of Sikkim. J. Hill Res. 2 (1), 1–7.

Dahal, N.R., Rao, E.R., Swamylingapa, B., 2003. Biochemical and nutritional evaluation of MAsyaura—a legume based traditional savoury of Nepal. J. Food Sci. Technol. 40 (1), 17–22.

Dahal, N.R., Karki, T.B., Swamylingapa, B., Li, Q., Gu, G., 2005. Traditional food and beverages of Nepal—a review. Food Rev. Int. 21 (1), 1–25.

Das, A.J., Deka, S.C., 2012. Fermented food and beverages of the North-East Asia. Int. Food Res. J. 19 (2), 377–392.

Dewan, S., 2002. Microbiological Evaluation of Indigenous Fermented Milk Products of the Sikkim Himalayas. Ph.D. thesis, Food microbiology Laboratory. Sikkim Government College (under North Bengal University), Gangtok, India.

Dewan, S., Tamang, J.P., 2007. Dominant lactic acid bacteria and their technological properties isolated from the Himalayan ethnic fermented milk products. Anton. van. Leeuw. 92, 343–352.

Dietz, H.M., 1984. Fermented dried vegetable and their role in nutrition in Nepal. Proc. Inst. Food Sci. Technol. 17, 208–213.

Dirar, H.A., 1993. The Indigenous Fermented Foods of the Sudan: A Study in African Food and Nutrition. CAB International, Wallingford, Oxon.

FAO, 2013. Indigenous methods of preparation: what is their impact on food security and nutrition? Global Forum of Food Security and Nutrition, summary of discussion no. 89.

Farnworth, E.R. (Ed.), 2008. Handbook of Fermented Functional Foods. second ed CRC Press, Taylor and Francis Group, London, Newyork.

Gaggia, F., Diana, D., Baffoni, L., Biavati, B., 2011. The role of protective and probiotic culture in food and feed and their impact in food safety. Trends Food Sci. Technol. 22, 558–566.

Gartaula, G., Dhami, B., Dhungana, P.K., Vaidya, B.N., 2014. Masular—a traditional fish product of Tharu community of Nepal. Indian J. Tradit. Knowl. 13 (3), 490–495.

Gautam, N., Sharma, N., 2015. Evaluation of probiotic potential of new bacterial strain *Lactobacillus spicheri* isolated from Gundruk. Proc. Nat. Acad. Sci.ences 979–986. India.

Ghosh, K., Ray, M., Adak, A., Dey, P., Halder, S.K., Das, A., et al., 2015. Microbial, saccharifyingand antioxidant properties of an Indian risce based fermented beverage. Food. Chem. 168, 196–202.

Granier, A., Goulet, O., Hourou, C., 2013. Fermentation product: immunological effect on human andanimal model. Pediatr. Res. 74 (2), 238–244.

Hill, C., Guarner, F., Gibson, G.R., Merenstein, D.J., Pot, B., Morelli, L., et al., 2014. Expert consensus document. The International Scientific Association for Probiotics and Prebiotics consensus statement on the scope and appropriate use of the term probiotic. Nat. Rev. Gastroenterol. Hepatol. 11 (8), 506–514.

Hong, G.-E., Mandal, P.K., Lim, K.-W., Lee, C.-H., 2012. Fermentation increase Isoflavone aglycon content in black soybean pulp. Asian J. Anim. Vet. Adv. 7, 502–511.

Hutkins, R.W. (Ed.), 2006. Microbiology and Technology of Fermented Food. first ed. IFT Press; Blackwell Pub., Iowa, USA.

Karki, T.B., 1986. Some Nepalese fermented food and beverages. Traditional Food: Some Product and Technologies. Central Food Technological Research Institute, Mysore, India, pp. 84–96.

Karki, D.B., 2013. Improvement on traditional millet fermentation process and its brewing quality assessment. Central Department of Food Technology. Tribhuvan University, Dharan, pp. 1–256.

Karki, T.B., Itoh, H., Hayashi, K., Kozaki, M., 1983a. Chemical changes during gundruk fermentation part II-1 aminoacids. Lebens Wiss. Technol. 16, 180–183.

Karki, T.B., Itoh, H., Kiuchi, K., Ebine, H., Kozaki, M., 1983b. Lipid in gundruk and takana fermented vegetables. Lebens. Wiss. Technol. 16, 167–171.

Karki, T.B., Itoh, H., Kozaki, M., 1983c. Chemical changes occuring during gundruk fermentation Part II Falavor components. Lebens. Wiss. Technol. 16, 203–208.

Karki, T.B., Ojha, P., Panta, O.P., 2016. Ethnic fermented foods of Nepal. In: Tamang, J.P. (Ed.), Ethnic Fermented Foods and Alcoholic Beverages of Asia. Springer, India. Available from: https://link.springer.com/chapter/10.1007/978-81-322-2800-4_4.

Katawal, S.B., 2012. Technological and Nutritional Evaluation of Sel-Roti. Central Department of Food Technology. Tribhuvan University, Dharan, pp. 1–296.

Kharel, G.P., Rai, B.K., Acharya, P.P., 2007. Handbook of Traditional Food of Nepal. Highland Publication (P). Ltd., Bhotahity, Kathmandu. Available from: https://vdocuments.net/indigenous-foods.html.

Khatri, H.P., Khadka, D.B., 2018. Probiotic potentiality of lactic acid bacteria isolated from traditional fermented product Dahi. In: Proceedings of the Eighth National Conference on Food Science and Technology, Kathmandu, Nepal.

Kwak, H.S., Ganesan, P., Mijan, M.A., 2013. Butter, ghee and cream product. In: Park, Y.W., Haenlein, G.F.W. (Eds.), Milk and Dairy Product in Human Nutrition: Production, Composition and Health. John Willey & Sons Ltd, pp. 390–411. Available from: https://onlinelibrary.wiley.com/doi/book/10.1002/9781118534168.

Lama, J.P., 1988. Preparation and quality evaluation of Maseura-based on locally available raw materials. *Food Technology, Central Campus of Technology, B.Tech. (Food) thesis*. Tribhuvan University, Dharan.

Marco, M.L., Heeney, D., Binda, S., Cifeli, C.J., Gotter, P.D., Folingne, B., et al., 2017. Health benefits of fermented food: microbiota and beyond. Curr. Opin. Biotechnol. 44, 94–102.

Martinenz-Villaluenga, C., Penas, E., Frias, J., 2017. Bioactive peptide in fermented food: production and evidence for health effects. Fermented Food in Health and Disease Prevention. Elsvier Inc., pp. 23–47.

Mehta, B.M., Kamal-Eldin, A., Iwanski, R.Z., 2012. Fermentation effect on food properties. In: Sikorski, Z.E. (Ed.), Chemical and Functional Properties of Food Components *Series*. CRC Press, Taylor & Francies Group, Boca Raton, FL.

Ministry of Health Nepal, New ERA and ICF, 2017. Nepal Demographic Health Survey. Ministry of Health, Nepal, Kathmandu, p. 2016.

Mitra, S., Chakrbarty, P.K., Biswas, S.R., 2010. Potential production and preservation of dahi by *Lactococcus lactis* W8, a nisin producing strain. LWT Food Sci. Technol. 43 (2), 337–342.

MoAD, 2016. Statistics Information on Nepalese Agriculture 2015/16, Monitoring, Evaluation and Statistic Division—Agri statistic section. Ministry of Agricultural Development, Government of Nepal.

Moktan, B., Saha, J., Sarkar, P.K., 2008. Antioxidant activities of soybean as affected by *Bacillus*-fermentation to kinema. Food Res. Int. 41 (6), 586–593.

Omizu, Y., Tsukamoto, C., Chhetri, R., Tamang, J.P., 2011. Determination of saponin content in raw soybean and fermented soybean food of India. J. Sci. Ind.Res. 70, 533–538.

Oniango, R., Allotey, J., Malaba, 2006. Contribution of Indigenous knowledges and practices in food technology to the attainment of food security in Africa. J. Food. Sci. 69 (3), 87–91.

Paszczyk, B., Brandt, W., Luczynska, J., 2016. Content of conjugated linoleic acid (CLA) and trans-isomers of C18:1 and C18:2 acids in fresh and stored fermented milk produced with selected starter culture. Czech J. Food Sci. 34 (5), 391–396.

Pervez, S., Malik, K.A., Ah khang, S., Kim, H.Y., 2006. Probiotic and their fermented food products are beneficial for health. J. Appl. Microbiol. 100 (6), 1171–1185.

Phutthaphadoong, S., Yamada, Y., Hirata, A., Tomita, H., Hara, A., Limtrakul, P., et al., 2010. Chemopreventive effect of fermented brown rice and rice bran (FBRA) on the inflammation-related colorectal carcinogenesis in ApcMin/+ mice. Oncol. Rep. 23 (1), 53–59.

Ping, S.P., Shih, S.C., 2012. Effect of isoflavone aglycon content and antioxidation activity in Natto by various culture of *Bacillus subtilis* during fermentation period. J. Nutr. Food Sci. 2 (7).

Prajapati, J.B., Nair, B.M., 2008. The history of fermented food. In: Farnworth, E.R. (Ed.), Handbook of Fermented Functional Food, second ed. CRC Press, Taylor & Francies, London, New York.

Qian, R., Xing, M., CuI, L., Deng, Y., Huang, M., Zhang, S., 2011. Antioxidant, antihypertensive, and immunomodulatory activities of peptide fraction from fermented skim milk, with *Lactobacillus delbruecki* spp. *bulgaricus*. J. Dairy Res. 78 (1), 72–79.

Rai, B.K., 2006. Preparation of starter culture using Yeast and mold isolated from local *murcha*. Central Department of Food Technology. Tribhuvan University, Dharan.

Rai, B.K., 2012. Essential of Industrial Microbiology. Lulu Publishing, USA, pp. 362–382. Available from: http://www.lulu.com/spotlight/basanta.

Rai, R., Shangpliang, H.N.J., Tamang, J.P., 2016. Naturally fermented milk product of the Eastern Himalayas. J. Ethn. Food 3, 270–275.

Ray, M., Ghosh, K., Singh, S., Mondal, K.C., 2016. Folk to functional: an explorative overview of rice based fermented food and beverage in India. J. Ethn. Foods 3 (1), 5–18.

Saad, N., Delattre, C., Urdaci, M., Schmitter, J.M., Bressolier, P., 2013. An overview of the last advances in probiotic and prebiotic field. LWT Food Sci. Technol. 50 (1), 1–16.

Samruan, W., Oonsivilai, A., Oonsivilai, R., 2012. Soybean and fermented soybean extract antioxidant activity. Int. Sch. Sci. Res. Innov. 6 (12), 1134–1137.

Sarkar, P.K., Tamang, J.P., Cook, P.E., Owens, J.D., 1994. Kinema—a traditional soybean fermented food: proximate composition and microflora. Food Microbiol. 11, 47–55.

Sarkar, P., Jones, L., Gore, W., Graven, G., 1996. Changes in soybean lipid profiles during kinema production. J. Sci. Food Agric. 71, 321–328.

Sarkar, P.K., Jones, L., Graven, G., Somerest, S.M., Palmer, C., 1997. Amino acid profiles of kinema, a soybean fermented food. Food. Chem. 59 (1), 69–75.

Sarkar, P.K., Morrison, E., Ujhang, T., Somerest, S.M., Craven, G., 1998. B-group vitamin and minerals content of soybeans during kinema production. J. Sci. Agric. 78 (4), 498–502.

Shin, D., Jeong, D., 2015. Traditional fermented soybean product: Jang. J. Ethn. Food 2, 2–7.

Shon, M.Y., Lee, J., Choi, J.H., Choi, M.S., 2011. Antioxidant and free radical scavenging activity of methanol extract of Chunkukjang. J. Food Compos. Anal. 20, 113–118.

Shrestha, N.R., 2002. *Nepal and Bangladesh, A Global Studies Handbook*. ABC-Clio., Santa Barbara, CA.

Steinkraus, K.H., 1994. Nutritional significance of fermented foods. Food Res. Int. 27 (3), 259–267.

Subba, D., 2012. Present status and prospects of Nepalese indigenous foods. Proceedings of the National Conference on Food Science and Technology (Food Conference-2012). Nepal Food Scientists and Technologists Association, Kathmandu, Nepal.

Tamang, J.P., 2010. *Himalayan Fermented Foods Microbiology, Nutrition and Ethnic Values*. CRC Press, Tylor & Francis Group, London.

Tamang, J.P., Sarkar, P.K., 1993. Sinki: a traditional lactic acid fermented radish tap root product. J. Gen. Appl. Microbiol. 39 (4), 395–408.

Tamang, J.P., Sarkar, P.K., 1996. Microbiology of mesu, a traditional fermented bamboo shoot product. Int. J. Food Microbiol. 29, 49–58.

Tamang, J.P., Thapa, S., 2006. Fermentation dynamics during production of bhaati jaanr, a traditional fermented rice beverage of the Eastern Himalayas. Food Biotechnol. 20 (3), 251–261.

Tamang, B., Tamang, J.P., 2010. In situ Fermentation dynamics during production of gundruk and khalpi, ethnic fermented vegetable products of Himalayas. Indian J. Microbiol. 50 (Suppl. 1), S93–S98.

Tamang, J.P., Tamang, B., Schilinger, U., Guigas, C., Holazapfel, W.H., 2009. Functional properties of lactic acid bacteria isolated from ethnic fermented vegetables of the Himalayas. Int. J. Food Microbiol. 135 (1), 28-23.

Tamang, J.P., Tamang, N., Thapa, S., Dewan, S., Tamang, B., Yonzan, H., et al., 2012. Microorganism and nutritional value of ethnic fermented foods and the alcoholic beverages of North East India. Indian J. Tradit. Knowl. 11 (1), 7–25.

Tamang, J.P., Shin, D.H., Jung, S.J., Chae, S.W., 2016a. Functional properties of microorganism in fermented foods. Front. Microbiol. 7, 578.

Tamang, J.P., Watanable, K., Holzapfel, W.H., 2016b. Diversity of microorganism in global fermented food and beverages. Front. Microbiol. 7, 1–28.

Thapa, N., 2016. Ethnic fermented and preserved fish products of India and Nepal. J. Ethn. Food 3 (1), 69–77.

Thapa, S., Tamang, J.P., 2004. Product characterization of kodo ko jaanr: fermented finger millet beverage of Himalayas. Food Microbiol. 21, 617–622.

Thapa, N., Pal, J., 2007. Proximate composition of traditionally processed fish products of the Eastern Himalayas. J. Hill Res. 20 (2), 75–77.

Yonzan, H., Tamang, J.P., 2009. Traditional processing of Selroti – a cereal based ethnic fermented food of Nepalis. Indian J. Tradit. Knowl. 8 (1), 110–114.

Yonzon, H., Tamang, J.P., 2010. Microbiology and nutritional value of selroti, an ethnic fermented cereals food of the Himalayas. Food Biotechnol. 24 (3).

Further reading

Sanlier, N., Gokcen, B.B., Sezgin, A.C., 2017. Health benefits of fermented foods. Crit. Rev. Food. Sci. Nutr. 1–22.

SteinKraus, K.H., 1995. Handbook of Indigenous Fermented Food. Marcell Dekker Inc., New York.

CHAPTER 3

Health and nutritional aspect of underutilized high-value food grain of high hills and mountains of Nepal

Uma Koirala
Gender Studies Program, Tribhuvan University, Kathmandu, Nepal

Contents

3.1 Introduction

Among the numerous plant species found in nature, approximately 120 are cultivated for human consumption as food (Adhikari et al., 2017). Worldwide-abundant edible plant species are neglected and/or underutilized; however, they are a potential source of nutrients for human beings, for example, energy, fiber, protein, fat, vitamins, and many other vital micronutrients essential for quality human life. These food grains are called as forgotten or underutilized foods, which are domesticated plant species that have been used for human or animal food, fiber, fodder, oil or medicinal properties, but have decreased in importance over time in terms of global production and consumption systems. In the modern context, only three grain crops—rice, wheat, and maize—are abundantly used grains and are responsible for supplying more than half of the dietary energy supply for the human body (FAO, 2009). However, through the lens of sustainability and food and

Nutritional and Health Aspects of Food in South Asian Countries
DOI: https://doi.org/10.1016/B978-0-12-820011-7.00023-X

nutrition security of people of Nepal, these three crops are not adequate and are hard to procure for many people of hilly areas too. Among 17 of United Nation's Sustainable Development Goals (SDG), Goal 2, "*end hunger, achieve food security and improved nutrition and promote sustainable agriculture*" is directly related to the fundamental rights of human beings that are ensured by all nations. This is also closely related to Goal 3, which is "*ensure healthy lives and promote wellbeing for all at all ages.*" Thus to achieve SDG nos. 2 and 3, it is necessary to promote the consumption of those underutilized food crops that are local, sustainable, and nutrient-dense and are beneficial for human life of all ages. The genetic resources of these underutilized crops are vital for sustaining agriculture and adapting to climate change because many of these species are well adapted to stressful environmental conditions especially of high hills and mountainous areas (Padulosi et al., 2012).

Nepal is famously categorized into three ecological regions: mountains, hills, and the *Terai*. Climate, landscape, geography, resources, and socioeconomic development are distinctly varied among these three ecological regions. The mountain region accounts for 35% (51,817 square kilometers) of the total land area and ranges in altitude from 4877 to 8848 m above sea level, where 7% of the total population of Nepal reside (Government of Nepal, 2012). Occupying nearly 42% of the total land area, the hill region ranges from 610 to 4876 m above sea level, is thickly populated where about 43% of the total population of the nation resides. Due to hill and high hill topography, the terrain is rugged, uneven, and hard for farming and easy access to other developmental means; however, it is also known as a very fertile part consisting of areas such as *Kathmandu, Dhading,* and *Pokhara.* The *Terai* region is plain and covers 23% (34,019 square kilometers) of the total land area. It has highly fertile land where nearly 50% of the population lives (ibid).

The national household food security percentage of Nepal is only 48.2, and in rural areas it is about 38.8. The severely food-insecure households are about 10% (NDHS, 2016). The mountain region of Nepal suffers with high food insecurity, where only 38.4% of households are considered as food secure compared to *Terai* where similar data is around 51%. In total, the severely food-insecure households in mountain regions are about 13.8% compared to 9.2% of the *Terai* region. Province-wise, the Karnali Province has the lowest level of food security where only 22.5% of households are food secure and severely food-insecure households are about 17.5% (ibid).

Except for the high hill region, other regions (hill and *Terai*) are surplus in major cereals. Among 16 high hill districts such as *Taplejung, Sankhuwasabha, Solukhumbu, Dolkha, Sindhupalchowk, Rasuwa, Manang, Mustang, Dolpa, Mugu, Humla, Jumla, Kalikot, Bajura, Bajhang,* and *Darchula*, 12 districts, except *Sankhuwasabha, Solukhumbu, Dolkha, and Sindhupalchowk*, have a food deficit situation. Nepal is in a food surplus situation at the national level. It is positively indicated that food security can be achieved by balancing the cereal distribution system within the country. However, this is not indicative of nutrition security in the nation. There is a need for production and utilization of various traditional/local grains including diversified foods including pulses, vegetables, fruits, eggs, milk, fish, and meat in cereal-based diets for nutrition security. So, certainly, there is a need for the promotion of underutilized food grains in the country for sustainable nutrition security (NDHS, 2016).

3.2 Historical overview

In the past, the Nepalese household food plate consisted of many different edible food grains and plant species in the high hill region. However, due to continuous changes in technology and commercialization of local food systems, food habits, policy priorities, and exposure to various media along with the movement of people, traditional crops are largely neglected and/or underutilized today (Adhikari et al., 2017). In this region, millets, sorghum, buckwheat, barley, and beans are some of the grains mostly considered as underutilized, and these were habitually used by community from large areas of high hills and mountains. However, these grains continue to be cultivated and consumed by minor localities because of habituation and health benefits. After decades of negligence, many researchers and nutritionists are promoting these underutilized grains as good food for health and nutrition security in place of rice, which has now become a staple for most people. Mostly, tourism sectors are promoting these foods as local and nutritious in their cuisine that provides an opportunity for income generation and expresses a typical identity through food.

Nepalese farmers have historically grown several species of food crops including many varieties of millet, barley, and buckwheat. These food crops were primarily consumed by the growers, and remaining was sold in the local market for income generation. Even today, these food crops are major sources of nutrition for many communities in Nepal. Yet, people are shifting toward rice as their main staple food instead of high-value food grains such as barley, buckwheat, or other millets.

3.3 Cultural value

Food has always been an expression of love, affection, happiness, and sorrow. It is also a means of welcoming guests and respecting them. Traditional food systems are now being recognized as a cultural identity of the Nepalese. It is a powerful medium of conservation of the local ecosystem and traditional local food. Local people's skills and knowledge have transferred over time, and new generations are eagerly modernizing these skills acknowledging the culture and tradition of the society/place/ethnicity. For example, buckwheat noodles are excellent food for young as well as aged persons in the mountainous areas of the Hindukush region including Nepal. Similarly, *dhindo*,[1] *roti*, *pakoud*, and cakes made by buckwheat and millet flour are in demand even in good modern restaurants in the name of traditional cuisine. *Satu*[2] prepared by barley

[1] Soft porridge made by flour cooked in hot water.

[2] *Satu* is prepared by roasting and grinding barley and adding sugar, cardamom, and cinnamon powder.

flour is considered as a sacred food and especially offered to God *Bishnu* (during the festival of Sakranti) and Siva (on the day of *Akcchyaya Tritiya*, a religious auspicious day) with juices. Barley and buckwheat are taken as holy food by pure vegetarians, priests, and common people even during fasting, and this reflects the sentiment of connectivity with health, land, tradition, and acknowledgment of their own produce. Culturally, millet is considered as inferior food grain and hardly used by traditional higher caste people: *Brahmin* and *Chhetri*. However, now there is no such taboo for millet, and they are equally being used by all.

3.4 Value addition on nutrition security

With respect to food and nutrition security, Pearl S. Buck (2018) stated that "A hungry man cannot see right or wrong. He just sees food."[3] Previously, our focus was only on food rather than its quality or diversification to address overall food and nutrition security. Asia and Pacific Region have 79 million children, or one child in every four below the age of five, suffering from stunting and 34 million children are wasted, while 12 million suffer from severe acute malnutrition with drastically increased risk of death (FAO, 2018). More than half of the world's malnourished children live in Asia and the Pacific. It is also home to the fastest growing prevalence of childhood obesity in the world. This paradox is attributed to the nutrition transition with children increasingly exposed to cheap and convenient unhealthy processed foods rich in salt, sugar, and fat but poor in essential nutrients. This double burden of malnutrition sees undernourished and overweight children living in the same communities and households, and it can even occur in the same child (FAO, 2018).

Nepal Living Standard Survey (2011) found that 38% Nepalese live with less than the minimum daily requirement of calories required for a healthy life. However, a significant disparity prevails between ecological zones, development regions, and rural–urban divisions. Compared to 24% of *Terai*, the population living with insufficient calorie intake is higher, that is, 36% and 38% in hilly and mountainous areas respectively. Disparity is evident in the extent of incidences of low-calorie intake among various landscapes and provinces[4] ranging from 24% in Province 1%–36% in Karnali Province. By provinces, the two western provinces—Karnali and Province 7—are more calorie-deficient compared to the other four provinces, 1, 2, 3, and *Gandaki*. Thus hilly and mountainous areas of the western parts of Nepal are worst hit by food insecurity and insufficient calorie intake.

[3] Quotation drawn from the site https://www.pinterest.com/pin/365213851007853526/visual-search/?x=16&y=16&w=530&h=530.

[4] The Constitution of Nepal (2015) has declared the provision of seven provinces in Nepal.

Nepal is struggling to reduce a very high rate of child malnutrition (36% and 27% of children under five are stunted and underweight, respectively—NDHS, 2016) since decades. About 17% of Nepali women belonging to the reproductive age group have chronic energy deficiency with a body mass index[5] of less than 18.5, and 41% of them are anemic. Similarly, women and children also suffer from vitamin and mineral deficiencies that can be emphasized by the fact that vitamin A deficiency is the cause of deaths of approximately 6900 children in Nepal each year. Nearly 21% of children are born with low birth weight reflecting gestational malnutrition (ibid). Diabetes and cardiovascular disease prevalence are serious and show an increasing trend. Iodine deficiency in pregnancy causes more than 200,000 babies a year in Nepal to be born mentally impaired and intelligence quotients that are 10–15 points lower than those who are not deficient.

The proportion of food-insecure households in the mountain areas of Nepal is significantly higher than in the plains and in comparison to the national level. In mountain areas, 59.5% households are food insecure and in hills 52.8%. Similarly, the consequences of food insecurity in the form of child stunting, wasting, and underweight are also very high: in mountains—52.9%, 10.9%, and 35.9%; and in hills—41.1%, 10.6%, and 26.6%, respectively (Rasul et al., 2019). The growing trend of consuming refined white rice replacing high-value grains is affecting the health of people of these regions, especially children and women. The result of the household survey 2016/17 (Government of Nepal, 2018) has indicated that Nepalese consume 3.5 kg of millet, 0.1 kg of buckwheat, and 0.1 kg of barley per year in comparison to 86.8 kg of rice. These data draw serious attention for making every effort to encourage the production and consumption of high-value grains in a systematic way to reduce undernutrition in these high hills and mountain regions. Below is a brief discussion regarding some of the underutilized high-value food grains of Nepal, which are significant for their nutrition and health.

3.5 Millet (*Pennisetum glaucum*)

Millets are small-seeded grains, originated in Africa and grown extensively in Africa, Asia, India, and Near East as a staple grain. There is evidence of the cultivation of millet in the Korean Peninsula around 3500–2000 BCE a very ancient religious book *Yajurveda* has mentioned about millets and indicates that production and consumption of this grain was an indigenous practice especially in the Asian region (around 4500 BCE). Before the Green Revolution, millets made up around 40% of all cultivated grains (contributing more than wheat and rice). However, since the revolution, the production of rice has doubly increased and wheat production has tripled so

[5] Body mass index (BMI): BMI=weight(kg)/height $(m)^2$.

millets were less valued for production. There are many types of millets produced in the globe; however, here, only popular varieties of millets that are cultivated in relation to hills and mountain regions of Nepal are discussed.

3.6 Finger millet (*Eleusine coracana*)

Finger millet (*Ragi*) is the fourth most important crop of Nepal after rice, maize, and wheat in area and production. It occupies an average of 7.9% (268,050 ha) of the total area covered by cereal crops and accounts for 3.3% (308,488 mt) of total cereal production (MoAD, 2015). It has been cultivated from Kachorwa (Terai, 60 m) of *Bara* district (Amgai et al., 2004) to Burnouse of Humla district (High Hill, 3500 m) in Nepal with cultivation records in all 77 districts. The major production districts of millet are *Khotang*, *Sindhupalchok*, *Baglung*, *Syangja*, *Kaski*, *Gorkha*, and *Sindhuli*. It is an important crop in terms of food and nutrition security of Nepal, especially for both mid-hill and mountain areas. Nepal produced a total of 306,704 tons of millet in the year 2017, of which 77% was from hill districts and 20% from mountain districts (Factfish, 2018).

In the mid-hill agroecosystem, the crop is important for different traditional food uses and is strongly associated with a maize-based cropping system. Finger millet is important for human food and animal feed and is included in various cropping patterns. In addition, the crop is widely tailored to marginal lands in high hill with cold stress and also well adapted to lands where low fertile and dry soils are the general characteristic stresses. Its cultivation has been found with low infestation of crop pests and diseases. So, this millet grain can be stored for years without any losses by pests and insects; that is why it is a suitable and preferred food grain in famine/drought-prone areas. It is especially valued for filling specific niches or needs because it often succeeds in stressful situations where other crops generally fail to grow.

After rice, finger millet is another crop that produces grain for human consumption and straw for cattle fodder. Several food preparations are made from finger millet. The most commonly eaten varieties are a semiliquid cooked item *khole*,[6] a thick porridge locally known as *dhindo* and *roti*.[7] Other improved but modern look-alike food items can be made with millet flour such as pancakes, cake, cookies, noodles, and super flour (MoAD, 2013). Finger millet is also popular for making fermented beverages—beer and local alcohol among certain communities of the country. As much as one-fourth of the total production of finger millet in Nepal goes into fermented alcoholic beverages *raksi*.[8] Finger millet is one of the most important food crops of the

[6] Finger millet flour cooked in water adding salt or sugar.
[7] Thick or thin bread cooked in flat iron pan.
[8] Alcoholic drink locally made by millet.

economically suppressed but physically hard-working people. It is appreciated by the people because it is digested slowly (apparently due to its rather high fiber content) and thereby furnishes energy for hard work throughout the day after being eaten as a single morning meal (Seetharam et al., 1986). The harvest residue of finger millet particularly green, as well as dry straw, is extensively used for animal feeding.

Finger millet is tasty, mildly sweet with a nut-like flavor, highly nutritious, nonglutinous, and is good for health. Finger millet is an excellent source of fiber, calcium, iron, manganese, and methionine—an amino acid lacking in the diets of hundreds of millions of the poor who live on starchy foods such as cassava, plantain, polished rice, and maize meal (FAO, Statistics, 2005 Data). Finger millet provides 320 kcal, 7.0 g protein, 11.2 g of fiber, 364 mg of calcium, and 4.2 mg of iron per 100 g. It also provides other vitamins and minerals (Longvah et al., 2017). Different from myth, millet is not an acid-forming food and therefore is soothing and easy to digest. In fact, it is considered to be one of the least allergenic and most digestible grains available, and it is considered as hot grain that helps to keep the body warm in cold weather. Consuming millet helps to keep skin healthy, reduces wrinkles, discoloration, and pigmentation, keeps bones healthy, helps in weight management (Railey, 2019a,b), and is a heart-healthy choice, which acts as a cofactor for more than 300 enzymes. The seeds are also rich in phytochemicals, including phytates, which is believed to lower cholesterol and is associated with reduced cancer risk (ibid).

Due to so-called modernization and attraction toward refined processed foods, millets are looked down upon as "coarse grains," though their ancestors lived on them. Food habit is changing and many valuable traditional grains such as finger millet, which are far better than refined grains are utilized less. As a result, millet production has been reducing over the years (315,067 mt. tons in 2012 to 306,704 mt. tons in 2017) (Fact fish, 2018).

3.7 Chino (*Panicum miliaceum*)

In high hills and mountainous areas of Nepal, *Chino* (*Proso* Millet) is considered as a second-most important crop of the millet group from the food security point of view. However, it ranks third after pearl millet and foxtail millet in total global millet production (about 5×10^6 tons of grain per year). Literature shows that this grain was grown first as a domestic crop in Northern China at least 10,000 years ago (Liu et al., 2016). Later, around 3000 years ago, it was introduced as a cereal in Europe. Now, it is cultivated as a staple grain in several locations such as the high belt of Afghanistan, Bhutan, China, India, Nepal, and Pakistan as well as in Central Asia. It is comfortable for farmers to not wait longer for harvesting because of its short cycle (60–90 days) of growing and maturation. It grows well in many varieties of soil and climatic conditions and can be cultivated in altitudes up to 3500 m (Baltensperger,

2002). The crop has a climate-resilient capacity and could survive in low water and nutrient requirements, allowing it to be cultivated at a wide range of altitudes, even on marginal land where other cereals can hardly survive (Lagler et al., 2005).

Chino grain is being utilized for many local food varieties such as *bhat* (boiled), *kheer* (sweet pudding cooked in milk), *dhindo* (porridge), roti (pancake and flatbread), and *raksi* (locally produced alcohol). In Nepal, *proso* millet is grown in 1900 ha with a productivity of 0.81 t/ha (DoA, 2017). Major districts producing *proso* millet are Mugu, Dolpa, Humla, Jumla, Kalikot, Bajura, and Jajarkot (Ghimire et al., 2017). It is considered as a healthy and nutritious food because of its nutritional composition with 11% protein (significant amounts of essential amino acids, particularly those containing sulfur, methionine, and cysteine), 4.22% fat, 72.9% carbohydrate, 1% fiber, and 3.25% minerals such as iron, calcium, and phosphorus (Ministry of Agriculture Development, 2013). Being gluten-free and easily digestible, it is considered as a perfect food for gluten-intolerant people. *Chino* millets are rich in micronutrients such as niacin, B-complex vitamins, vitamin B_6, and folic acid (Hulse et al., 1980; Pathak, 2013). This grain contains a good amount of lecithin, which provides brilliant support to the health and normal functioning of the nervous system by helping to reestablish nerve cell functions, regenerate myelin fiber, and intensify brain cell metabolism. Although nearly unknown for urban habitat, now it is considered as the crop of the future in the context of climate change with great potential to cope with food insecurity in remote areas of the country.

3.8 Kaguno (*Panicum italicum*)

Kaguno falls under the millet family and is popularly known as Foxtail Millet. It is a gluten-free grain and the second-most commonly grown species. It is one of the oldest cultivated millet of Nepal generally grown in high hill areas. Characteristically, it has a low water requirement, although it does not resist drought conditions well due to a shallow root system. *Kaguno* is preferred by hill and high hill people due to its short growing season, higher yield potential, disease resistance, and attractive panicles that could be considered as an important genetic resource to develop climate-resilient varieties to cope with the adverse effects of climate change (Ghimire et al., 2018). Its maturation time is almost 65–70 days. This millet can be planted when it is too late to plant most other crops. It is a gluten-free grain, and the structure is very similar to rice paddy. In Nepal, it is used as a food grain and is cultivated in high hills and mid hills mainly in the districts of the *Karnali* Province and *Kaski and Lamjung of Gandaki* provinces. There is a practice of cultivating *Kaguno* as a monocrop in *Ghanpokhara* whereas *Karnali* province farmers cultivate it as a mixed crop together with finger millet. Currently, the trend of cultivation and production of *Kaguno* is decreasing all over

Nepal. Farmers find the process of weeding and postharvest handling to be more tedious. Shortage of labor has demotivated farmers to grow this grain.

Kaguno is very easy to consume any time of the day either as a snack or staple food. Young/immature panicles can be roasted and consumed. Indigenous people carry it as travel food while going for wild honey hunting, which is one of the unique features of Nepal, especially among the *Gurung* community (Gurung, 2016). Popular dishes of *Kaguno* are *bhaat*, *kheer* (porridge cooked in milk), *selroti* (deep-fried bun-like product made by mixing *kaguno* flour with ghee and sugar), and *raksi* (local liquor, made by mixing with finger millet).

Kaguno is highly nutritious and superior to rice and wheat grain. This grain has a low glycemic index with high fiber content with hypoglycemic and hypocholesterolemic action that is extremely beneficial for preventing cardiovascular diseases and diabetes. Despite its importance for local food security and nutrition, little research has been done in foxtail millet making it a neglected and underutilized species from a research and development perspective (Hariprasanna, 2016). As per the food composition table (MoAD, 2012), *Kaguno* has 12.3% protein, 60.9% carbohydrate, 4.3% fat, and 3.3% minerals. It is also a rich source of micronutrients.

3.9 Buckwheat (*Fagopyrum esculentum*)

In the series of important staple food grains of Nepal, buckwheat comes sixth after rice, wheat, maize, finger millet, and barley. It is cultivated widely on marginal land of 61 out of 77 districts of Nepal ranging from 60 to 4500 m altitude such as *Rukum, Rolpa, Jajarkot, Dolpa, Humla, Jumla, Dolakha, Solukhumbu, Mustang, Kalikot, Kavre, and Okhaldhunga* districts. *Karnali* zone is popularly known for abundant cultivation of this grain. Basically, it is a summer crop of hills (high altitude >1700 m), autumn and spring crop in mid-hills (600–1700 m), and winter crop in *Terai* (Luitel et al., 2017). In recent times, it has been grown extensively in some *Terai* districts such as *Chitwan, Jhapa*, and *Nawalparasi* for commercial purposes especially for green vegetables that have very high demand due to flavonoid (rutin) content. It can resist the poor, infertile, and acidic soil, as well as nutrients, moisture, and heat stress with wider adaptability so its cultivation is easy for farmers. These rare characteristics of buckwheat show great potential as a future crop for food security among food-deficit areas of Nepal. Buckwheat is cultivated in 10,510 ha area with a production of 10,355 tons/year and a yield of 0.983 tons/ha (ibid).

Popularly known as a poor man's crop, buckwheat is taken as an alternative cereal grain for the habitat of high hills ensuring food security year-round. Due to the short duration of cropping and easy adaptation to various climatic situations, buckwheat is considered as an imperative food grain. There are many varieties of buckwheat found in Nepal such as *Barule, Bharule, Chuchche, Chode, Kalo, Seto, Tilkhude, Tite, Tote*

Phaper, *Batule*, *Bharule*, *Mithe*, *Murali*, and *Tilkhunde*. Sweet buckwheat varieties are generally grown in mid-hill and *Terai*, but Tartary buckwheat varieties are grown in higher altitudes. Buckwheat is a drought-tolerant crop and requires approximately 100 mm rain for its whole cropping life. Although buckwheat is a short duration crop, its flowering period is more than 30 days, which is very useful for bee-keepers to collect good quality honey. The productivity buckwheat varies from district to district and also depends upon the type of local variety (Luitel et al., 2017).

Buckwheat is a pseudocereal/minor food, or cash crop but it is one of the major staple food crops for the high mountainous region of Nepal. Buckwheat is a multipurpose crop and has been cultivated for its use as staple food, animal feed, vegetable, soup, beverage, and medicine. All parts of buckwheat plants are used in a variety of ways. The leaf contains rutin, which is an important pharmaceutical product used as tea brew and to treat hypertonia; flowers that bloom for about a month produce good quality nectar for honey; grain is the staple food; hulls of grain are used for making pillows; straw is good source feed for livestock; and green plants are used as green manure.

Many food items prepared from buckwheat are popular in Nepal such as *dhindo* (thick porridge), *roti* (bread), *momo* (dumpling), *lagar* (very thick bread), *dheshu* (bread thicker than *lagar*), fresh vegetables, dried vegetables, *chhyang or jaand* (local beer), *raksi* (alcohol), salad (leaves), pickle (fresh and dry leaves), soup, *ryale roti*, noodle, *sel roti*, *bhat* (rice), sausage, *dorpa dal*, tea, vinegar, jam, macaroni, biscuit, cakes, *mithai* (sweet), *haluwa*, *puri*, *puwa*, *bhuteko Phapar* (roasted grain), *satu*, *phuraula*, porridge, and *pakauda*. Nepalese from mountainous regions prefer *dhindo* than other items because of its specific sticky taste (Luitel et al., 2017).

Common buckwheat is mostly used as bread pancake, which is a delicious item for the tourists in the trekking root of Mustang. Thick porridge prepared by mixing the flour of bitter buckwheat with *Uwa* (Oat) or finger millet (in the ratio of 1: 3) is the common food of poor people in the hilly area. Buckwheat has a superior nutritional value because of balanced amino acids and high mineral content. Hundred grams of buckwheat provides 343 kcal along with 12.5% protein, 29% dietary fiber, and 4.7 mg iron. Similarly, it contains significant amounts of micronutrients, that is, riboflavin, vitamin B_6, magnesium, phosphorous, and potassium, which is essential for our bodily function (Alvarez-Jubete et al., 2010). It is an excellent source of lysine that is typically deficient in cereals. Due to its therapeutic value, buckwheat is now in demand, especially in urban areas. Rutin is an important bioactive component present in buckwheat that works as a strong antioxidant and can fight inflammation and protect the heart and brain. It also reduces bruising and vein issues (Ana Aleksic, 2018). Buckwheat diet is suitable for most of the noncommunicable diseases that have preventive action especially on leg edema, high blood pressure, high cholesterol, and cardiovascular disease.

Traditionally, buckwheat flour paste is applied as a curative treatment for wounds and burns, and its semicooked flour is used orally to cure cold, cough, jaundice, and fever. Similarly, fresh flour is used for dandruff treatment as well as for stopping hair fall, curing pimples, and skin scratches. Similarly, tender twigs and leaves of wild buckwheat are used in dysentery, pneumonia, and cholera. It is believed that soaked buckwheat flour is harmful to internal worms. Buckwheat grain flour is given regularly to goat and sheep in the hill and high hill areas. This grain is considered as a holy food, so Nepali Hindus prefer to eat food made from buckwheat during the fasting period or for religious activities (Ana Aleksic, 2018).

3.10 Barley (*Hordeum vulgare*)

Barley (*Jau* in Nepali language) is considered as an important crop culturally; however, its consumption as food grain is very low in Nepal. Barley is cultivated in approximately 26,000 ha (<1.5% of the total cultivated area for grain) of land, which is a very small area for food grain. Moreover, 40% of hill and 37% of mountainous area is under barley cultivation (Basnyat, 2015). It is cultivated starting from the low land of *Terai* at an altitude of around 4300 m (in *Dingboche* on the route to Everest). However, at higher altitudes, only barley grows successfully rather than buckwheat. It has an amazing quality of growing in high altitudes under extreme weather conditions. Barley tolerates poorer soils and lower temperatures better than wheat. In 2017, the barley yield for Nepal was 11,147 mt/ha. Although the yield of barley in Nepal fluctuated substantially in recent years, it increased through 1968–2017 ending at 11,147 mt/ha in 2017 (World Data Atlas, Grando and Macpherson, 2005).

The barley-growing season depends upon the geography of Nepal. Barley is grown as a winter crop in the hilly areas, whereas in the mountainous areas, barley is planted during spring. Barley that is grown as a winter crop matures earlier than wheat (at least a month), which allows plenty of time for planting a summer crop such as maize, rice, or buckwheat. In alpine climates, barley is grown as a spring crop that takes up to 10 months for maturation. Barley is valued not only as a grain, but its straw is preferred as a livestock feed, and the value of this straw is equal to that of the grain in areas where livestock feed is very limited. In the past, this crop had much economic value because it was traditionally traded with Tibet for salt.

Due to a massive impact of climate change and people's preferences, barley yields are declining gradually both in the hills and in the mountains. If we observe the consumption pattern, of total consumption, 70%, 16%, and 14% is consumed by mountainous, hilly, and *Terai* people, respectively. A naked type of barley, which is locally called *Uwe or Karu*, is cultivated extensively in mountainous areas and is valued as a highly nutritious food (Khadka).

Barley has nutritional benefits that provide both physical and spiritual sustenance to the people/especially of Nepal. It is considered as a rich source of vitamins B and micronutrients. It has plenty of fibers and therefore is very good for stomach muscle health and bowel movement, and it regulates blood glucose levels. There is also some evidence that consuming barley over a long period may help to decrease blood cholesterol.

Mostly people eat barley in the form of bread (*roti*), *satu* (prepared by roasting and grinding), and barley water during illness. In the Nepalese community, *satu* is offered especially to the God Vishnu and Shiva during the holy days of *Sakranti* and *Akcchaya Tritiya*. It is utilized as a livestock feed, for malt and for preparing foods. The roasted grains are coffee substitutes mostly used by hill and high hill people. This grain is beneficial not only for its nutritive value but also as a remedy for certain diseases. It is common knowledge that barley can be effective in the treatment of diabetes, stomach and colon issues, and kidney problems. It is also taken as a high-calorie food.

Nowadays, in many villages of the Himalayan region, instant noodles have replaced the eating of *Tsampa* (roasted barley) as a staple diet or snack especially among the younger generations. It is higher in rural areas than in cities mainly due to the ease of preparation and impression of having good food. However, for certain social occasions, such as gatherings for marriages and funerals, barley preparations are preferred. This grain is considered holy and is an essential offering to God during worship/*pooja*.

3.11 Future prospects

All high-valued grains mentioned previously that are widely cultivated in high hills and mountainous areas are valuable from the nutrition and food security context. Various studies have shown that low-quality diets are responsible for undernutrition, especially protein, calorie, and micronutrient deficiencies, which are high among mountain and high hill people. This situation could be improved through massive production and promotion of these high-value grains along with local but modified recipes. Similarly, these grains are climate-resilient and easy to store; however, more storage facilities and minimization in aflatoxin that is standardized by Food Standard[9] of Government of Nepal and Food Law could be a good action to improve the food security level of those areas of Nepal.

Moreover, more research on aflatoxin content in traditionally stored millets, buckwheat, and barley is needed for food safety and health for its wide promotion and use. Besides, nutritive value analysis is another important action highly recommended for better utilization of those grains by reducing local myths and negative fads. Identification and use of easy but smart postharvesting technology are also essential for better promotion of these grains. Similarly, improved storage facilities and safety measures against the climate as well as pest rodents and processing technology need to be addressed as an institutional priority for future prospects.

[9] Government of Nepal, Food Standard, Published in Nepal Gazette 2057.10.23.

3.12 Conclusion

Due to climate change and the need for sustainable development, traditional food grains such as millet, barley, and buckwheat are becoming an integral part of the food system of high hills and mountain areas. The cultivation and consumption of traditional food crops, however, are facing decreasing trends. Industrial farming patterns tremendously promote three grains—wheat, maize, and rice responsible for providing more than half of the global dietary energy supply, which is the cause for underutilization of many valuable grains despite their high nutritional and traditional value.

Low priority for local food grains, increased choices and easy access to ready-to-eat foods, and low awareness about nutritional needs and their sources have reduced the use of these valuable grains, and they are on the verge of disappearance. Farmers need to be motivated through policy and programming for cultivating and consuming these high-valued grains. Massive awareness campaigns with local and modern recipes originally made up of barley, buckwheat, and millets need to be initiated to protect and promote these underutilized food grains. These food grains not only supplement the necessary nutrients to improve the nutritional status of the people but can ensure household food security for more days. Moreover, one of the major attractions of tourism sectors is traditional food varieties with local grains and products, which has provided tremendous opportunities for encouraging more production and consumption. Hence, advanced technology for easy postharvest activities and advanced research for minimizing the attack of pests and aflatoxin contamination are also seen as future prospects of these food grains.

References

Alvarez-Jubete, L., Arendt, K., Gallagher, E., 2010. Nutritive value of pseudo-cereals and their increasing use as functional gluten- free ingredients. Trends Food Sci. Technol. 21, 106−113. Available from: https://doi.org/10.1016/j.tifs.2009.10.014.

Adhikari, L., Hussain, A., G. Rasul, 2017. Tapping the potential of neglected and underutilized food crops for sustainable nutrition security in the mountains of Pakistan and Nepal. In: Sustainability, ResearchGate, February 2017 (review article).

Ana Aleksic, M.Sc. (Pharmacy), Top 12 Rutin Benefits+Foods, Supplements & Side Effects Reviewed article, November 2, 2018. <https://selfhacked.com/blog/rutin/>.

Amgai, R.B., Joshi, B.K., Shrestha, P., Chaudhary, B., Adhikari, N.P., Baniya, B.K., 2004. Intra- and interpopulation variation in finger millet (*Eleusine coracana* (L.) Gaertn) landraces grown in Kachorwa, Bara, Nepal. In: Sthapit, B.R., Upadhyay, M.P., Shrestha, P.K., Jarvis, D.I. (Eds). On-farm Conservation of Agricultural Biodiversity in Nepal. Volume 1: Assessing the Amount and Distribution of Genetic Diversity On-farm. Proceedings of the Second National Workshop, Nagarkot, Nepal, pp. 84−95.

Baltensperger, D.D., 2002. Progress with Proso, Pearl and Other Millets. In: Janick, J., Whipkey, A. (Eds.), Trends in New Crops and New Uses. ASHS Press, Alexandria, VA.

Basnyat, B., M.D., B for Barley, Nepali Times Buzz2-8 January 2015.

Fact fish, 2018. Research made simple. Retrieved on February 19, 2019 from: <http://www.factfish.com/statistic-country/nepal/millet%2C%20production%20quantity>.

FAO, 2009. (Food and Agriculture Organization) and Traditional Knowledge: The Linkages with Sustainability. Food Security and Climate Change Impacts. Food and Agriculture Organization (FAO), Rome, Italy.

FAO, 2018. Asia and the Pacific Regional Overview of Food Security and Nutrition 2018 – Accelerating Progress Towards the SDGs. Bangkok. License: CC BY-NC-SA3.0 IGO.

Ghimire, K., Bhandari, B., Gurung, S.B., Narayan, B.D., Bimal, K.B., 2017. Diversity and Utilization Status of Millets Genetic Resources in Nepal.

Ghimire, K.H., Joshi, B.K., Gurung, R., et al., 2018. Geneict Resource Crop Evolution 65, 1147. Available from: https://doi.org/10.1007/s10722-017-0602-5.

Government of Nepal, 2012. Central Bureau of Statistics, National Planning Commission Secretariat. Available from: <http://www.CentralBureauofStatistics.Gov.NP>.

Government of Nepal, 2018. National Planning Commission, Central Bureau of Statistics (October) Annual Household Survey, October 17, 2016.

Grando, S., Macpherson, H.G. (Eds.), 2005. Food Barley: Importance, Uses and Local Knowledge. Proceedings of the International Workshop on Food Barley Improvement, 14–17 January 2002, Hammamet, Tunisia. ICARDA, Aleppo, Syria, x+156 pp. En.

Gurung, R., 2016. Kaguno (Foxtail Millet) Cultivation in Ghanpokhara, Lamjung. Retrieved on February 20, 2019, Originally published on October 13, 2015 from: <www.libird.org>.

Hariprasanna K., 2016. Foxtail Millet – Nutritional Importance and Cultivation Aspects, Indian Institute of Millets Research <https://www.researchgate.net/publication/303662897>.

Hulse, J.H., Laing, E.M., Pearson, O.E., 1980. Sorghum and the Millets: Their Composition and Nutritive Value. Academic Press, London, pp. 187–193.

Khadka, B.B., Coarse grains and pulses in Nepal, Role and Prospects, UN/ESCAP CGPRT Centre, Regional Co-ordination Centre for Research and Development of Coarse Grains, Roots and Tuber crops in the Humid Tropics of Asia and the Pacific.

Lagler, R., Gyulai, G., Humphreys, M., Szabo, Z., Horvath, L., Bittsanszky, A., et al., 2005. Morphological and molecular analysis of common millet (*P. miliaceum*) cultivars compared to a DNA sample from the 15th century (Hungary). Euphytica 146, 77–85.

Liu, M., Yue, X., Jihong, H., Zhang, S., Wang, Y., Lu, P., 2016. Genetic diversity and population structure of broomcorn millet (*Panicum miliaceum* L.) cultivars and landraces in China based on microsatellite markers. Int. J. Mol. Sci. 17, 370. Available from: https://doi.org/10.3390/ijms17030370.

Longvah, T., Ananthan, R., Bhaskarachary, K., Venkaiah, K., 2017. Indian Food Composition Tables. National Institute of Nutrition. ICMR, Hyderabad, India.

Luitel, D.R., Siwakoti, M., Jha, P.K., Jha, A.K., Krakauer, N., 2017. An Overview: Distribution, Production, and Diversity of Local Landraces of Buckwheat in Nepal, Hindawi, Advances in Agriculture, Volume 2017, Article ID 2738045, 6 pages. Available from: https://doi.org/10.1155/2017/2738045.

MOAD, 2012. Nepal Government, Ministry of Agriculture Development, Department of Food Technology and Quality Control, National Nutrition Program, Food Composition Table of Nepal.

MoAD, Department of Food Technology and Quality Control, 2013. Traditional and Underutilized Grains, Roots and Tubers Available in Remote and Hills Areas of Nepal: An Introduction (in Nepali). MoAD, DFTQC, Nepal.

MoAD, 2015. Statistical Information on Nepalese Agriculture, 2014/015. Ministry of Agricultural Development, Nepal.

NDHS, 2016. Nepal Demographic and Health Survey. Ministry of Health and Population Nepal; New ERA; USAID, Nepal.

Nepal Living Slandered Survey, 2010/2011. Central Bureau of Statistics, National Planning Commission Secretariat, Government of Nepal, November 2011.

14–16 June 2011 On-farm conservation of neglected and underutilized species: status, trends and novel approaches to cope with climate change. In: Padulosi, S., Bergamini, N., Lawrence, T. (Eds.), Proceedings of the International Conference, Friedrichsdrof, Frankfurt, Germany. Biodiversity International, Rome, Italy.

Pathak, H.C., 2013. Role of Millets in Nutritional Security of India. National Academy of Agricultural Sciences, New Delhi, pp. 1–16.

Railey, K., 2019. Whole Grains: Millet. Retrieve on February 19, 2019 from: <http://chetday.com/millet.html>.

Railey, K., 2019. Whole Grains: Millet, Marlian News. Retrieved on February 22, 2019 from: <https://www.merliannews.com/whole_grains_millet_by_karen_railey/>.

Rasul, G., Saboor, A., Tiwari, P.C., Hussain, A., Ghosh, N., Chettri, G.B., 2019. Food and nutrition security in the Hindu Kush Himalaya: unique challenges and niche opportunities. In: Wester, P., Mishra, A., Mukherji, A., Shrestha, A. (Eds.), The Hindu Kush Himalaya Assessment. Springer, Cham.

Further reading

Bhandari, P., 2018. Regional variation in food security in Nepal. Dhaulagiri J. Sociol. Anthropol. 12, 1–10. Available from: https://doi.org/10.3126/dsaj.v12i0.22174.

Bringing back millets- the super crop of our ancestors, Original post on April 15, 2017, <https://www.icrisat.org/a-short-history-of-millets-and-how-we-are-recognising-their-importance-in-the-modern-context/>.

Dong, Y.C., Zheng, D.S., 2006. Crops and Their Wild Relatives in China. China Agriculture Press, Beijing, China, pp. 331–359.

Ghimire, K.H., Khatri Chettri, H.B., Joshi, B.K., Bhatta, M.R., 2015. Plant Genetic Resources and Agriculture in Nepal. Country Report. The 3rd AFACI International Training Workshop on Germplasm Management System (GMS), 11–20 May 2015, RDA, Republic of Korea.

Habiyaremye, C., Matanguihan, J.B., D'Alpoim Guedes, J., Ganjyal, G.M., Whiteman, M.R., Kidwell, K.K., et al., 2017. Proso millet (*Panicum miliaceum* L.) and its potential for cultivation in the Pacific Northwest, U.S.: a review. Front. Plant Sci. 7. <https://www.frontiersin.org/article/10.3389/fpls.2016.01961>.

<https://www.ars.usda.gov/northeast-area/beltsville-md-bhnrc/beltsville-human-nutrition-research-center/nutrient-data-laboratory/docs/usda-national-nutrient-database-for-standard-reference/>. Retrieved on February 20, 2019.

Saud, N.B., 2010. Crops of Nepal and Their Sustainable Farming (in Nepali): Nepal ka bali naliratin kodigo kheti. Sajha Prakashan, Pulchok, Lalitpur, Nepal, pp. 223–227.

Status Report on Food and Nutrition Security in Nepal, 2013. Acharya, A.K., Paudel, M.P., Wasti, P.C., Sharma, R.D., Dhittal, S., Ministry of Agriculture, Land Pathak, H.C. (Eds.), Role of Millets in Nutritional Security of India, New Delhi. National Academy of Agricultural Sciences, pp. 1–16.

Wikipedia, 2019. Neglected and Underutilized Crop. Retrieved on February 25, 2019.

World Data Atlas Nepal Topics Agriculture Crops Production Yield. Significance of agriculture in improving malnutrition, Food and Nutrition Security in Nepal. <https://halokhabar.com/en/news-details/193/2018-11-24/>.

PART 5

Food, Nutrition, and Health in Bangladesh

CHAPTER 1

Introduction

S. M. Nazmul Alam
Department of Social Sciences, Faculty of Humanities, Curtin University, Perth, WA, Australia

Bangladesh, although a small country, is rich in ethnic and ecological diversity that influence its tradition, culture, and food types. The deltaic plains of Bangladesh have been famous for rice production from its alluvial agriculture landscapes that have prominently figured in the food habits of the Bangladeshi people. The arrays of water-bodies and the diverse fish therein offer many dishes to brand the nation with the epigram "Fish and rice make a Bengali" more meaningful. Being a country with a Muslim majority, Bangladeshi people usually adhere to the strict rules of the Islamic faith for all aspects of life, including food intakes and dining etiquette.

Wetland products, rice and fish, are traditional favorites with vegetables, *dal* (lentil soup), and occasionally meat also forming a part of the daily staple diet. The rural Bangladeshi people usually start their day with "Panta bhat" – semifermented plain boiled rice soaked overnight in water. This watery rice is then consumed with salt, onion slices, and green or fried chili to fill up the tummy. In urban areas, people generally have their breakfast with handmade *ruti* (bread) prepared from wheat flour, or *parata* with mixed fried vegetables, eggs, and tea. Some people take loaves of bread with banana and milk. There is no practice of taking cereals, but traditionally in winter, *muri* (puffed rice) or *cheera* (flattened rice) or *khoi* (popped rice) is preferred along with milk or yogurt and *gur* (molasses).

The coursewise lunch and dinner more or less comprise a similar set of items such as rice, curry, *vaji* (fried mixed vegetables or leaves), *bhorta* (mashed potato or vegetable or dry fish), and dal. Curry is a variety of dishes with fish, meat, and vegetables either alone or in combination with other vegetables cooked alongside with a blend of spices and herbs. *Bhorta* is made from smooth, fiery, and flavorful mashed veggies or fish either fresh or dry, made with mustard oil, onion, garlic, and red or green chilies to enhance smell and delicacy. *Alu bhorta* (mashed potato), *begoon bhorta* (mashed eggplants), and *shutki bhorta* (mashed dried fish) are the most common accompanying the meal in a rural diet. Innumerable varieties of freshwater fish (*rui, ilish, catfish, small shrimp, etc.*), assortments of fruits and vegetables (leafy green, beans, potato, tomato, pumpkin, *etc.*), and meat (beef, chicken, mutton, and duck) are always the distinctive features of a meal across Bangladesh. Bangladeshi recipes and dishes

Nutritional and Health Aspects of Food in South Asian Countries
DOI: https://doi.org/10.1016/B978-0-12-820011-7.00024-1

exhibit intense aromatic flavors derived from various spices and herbs such as garlic, ginger, lime, coriander, cumin, turmeric, and chili. In some dishes, cardamom and cinnamon are used for enhancing natural flavors in authentic Bangladeshi cooking.

The expression "Baro mashe tero parbon" translating into "Thirteen festivals in twelve months" indicates the occurrence of festivals throughout the year. Each of these festivals brings special food and making its cultural heritage richer. The *Pohela Baishakh* (first day of the Bengali New Year) is deemed to be noncelebratory without fried *ilish* (Hilsa fish) with *panta bhat.* The country's biggest harvesting celebration *Nabanno* usually marks the harvest of Aman paddy that turns in the preparation of different kinds of heritage "Pithas" (rice cakes) and sweets. Historical old Dhaka has an age-old tradition of hosting the "Iftar" market that brings unique and rare Iftar items during the month-long holy Ramadan. A grand Iftar delicacy in this market is known by the quirky name "Boro baper polay khay" meaning "Eaten by the son of wealthy man." It is made with a mixture of chickpeas, minced meat, potato, flattened rice, eggs, shredded chicken, spices, and butter. "Biriyani" or "Polao" served with meat curries, and desserts signify the religious celebration of a heavenly fervor. Chicken *roast*, mutton *rezala, borhani*, and desserts are featured in the wedding and social fiestas.

Snacks are ubiquitous in the daily lifestyle of Bangladesh with tea. A trendy snack is *shingara* with spiced vegetables, chickpeas, and potato wrapped in thin dough, and fried. *Dal puri* is another popular item where flattened flour dough is stuffed with mashed lentils and fried in hot oil. The favorite *fuchka* is a small crispy dough shell filled with thick *chatpati*, finished with grated eggs, and tasted with tamarind juice mix. *Moghlai parata, samosa, alu puri, piyaju, pakora, haleem, jhal muri*, and *kebab* are some much-loved items to add on the snack list.

Bangladesh is endowed with a subtropical monsoon climate that favors the production of a great variety of fruits. These are famous for their taste, flavor, and sweetness. Major fruits include mango, banana, papaya, jackfruit, pineapple, guava, lychee, pomelo, and lemon. The jackfruit is the national fruit for its large size and juiciness. Varieties of mangoes and lychees offer a unique taste and are a delicacy of the Rajshahi, Satkhira, Kustia, Jashore, and Dinajpur regions. Barisal, Patuakhali, and the southern districts are famous for Guava, Amra (*Spondias mombin*), and Chalta (*Dillenia indica*) production.

Homemade rice cakes popularly known as "Pitha" occupy an essential place in the Bangladesh tradition and culinary culture. Although pitha is a favorite for celebrating the winter, it is always prepared and cherished in any Bangladeshi dining table throughout the year. Most pithas are sweet, based on rice or wheat flour, and accompanied with sugar syrup, molasses or date juice, milk, coconut, and spicy gravy. Engraved with attractive designs, regional, and mouthwatering names of pithas have enriched the cultural heritage of Bangladesh. Bhapa pitha, puli pitha, chitoi pitha, and patishapta are some prominent pithas prepared round the year.

Bangladeshi cuisine has a rich tradition of *Misti* (sweets) and desserts. Sweets are mostly milk-based. Attractive sweet treats include *roshmalai* (miniature fried cottage cheese balls dipped in a creamy base), *Misti doi* (sweetened yogurt), *Chomchom* (a syrup-coated cake made from paneer), and *Jilepi* (dough fried in a coil shape dipped in sugar syrup). The art of Bangladeshi *Misti* has reached a stature of excellence bringing each region to have its own set of delicacies. From the *Porabari's Chomchom* of Tangail to the *Kachagolla* of Natore, and *Monda* of Muktagacha, *Roshmalai* of Cumilla, *Balish misti* from Kurigram, *Misti doi* (sweet yogurt) of Bogura, the massive list is bound to get the mouth of anyone watering. *Kheer*, *payesh*, and *jarda* are excellent rice-based desserts flavored with cardamom, saffron, sugar, milk, dry fruits, and nuts and typically served after a meal in festivals and special occasions.

Bangladeshis quench their thirst with a variety of juices, drinks, and traditional beverages. The familiar drink is green coconut water, while *cha* (tea) is the nation's standard beverage. Other trendy drinks include *bel-er shorbat* (wood apple juice), lemonade, sugarcane juice, date juice, yogurt-based *borhani* and *lassi*, and *faluda* (rose syrup with vermicelli and milk), which are equally enjoyed. An age-old *chelay mod* – traditional alcoholic beverage brewed from rice and wild herbs are the favorite drink among the *Adivasi* (tribal) people consumed during daily life and festivals.

Bangladesh by tradition is rich for its delicious foods, sweets, pithas, fruits, and savories. Certain food has become an essential element of a particular celebration and festival, while some special foods entice people in a colorful ceremony. Bangladeshis enjoy the tastes of these delicious traditional foods for ages, and generation after generation, attributing many of the properties of these foods for health and nutrition.

CHAPTER 2

Role of traditional foods of Bangladesh in reaching-out of nutrition

S. M. Nazmul Alam[1] and M. Niamul Naser[2]
[1]Department of Social Sciences, Faculty of Humanities, Curtin University, Perth, WA, Australia
[2]Department of Zoology, Faculty of Biological Sciences, University of Dhaka, Dhaka, Bangladesh

Contents

2.1 Introduction

Bangladesh, with rich cultivating land and vast water resources, has historically been an agrarian society and became eminent for producing sufficient foods to feed the people. There is a well-known saying *Gola bhora dhan, Goaal bhora goru, Pukur bhora machh* translating into "Homestead stores full of paddy, sheds packed of cows, and ponds brimming with fish," implying the abundance of foods in Bangladesh. The green and yellow paddy fields, rivers, and different kinds of wetlands in the deltaic plains of Bangladesh have influenced the food habits and cultural practices of the locals. Significant items in the traditional food basket in Bangladesh are rice, fish, pulses, wheat, vegetables, meats, sweets, and herbal drinks. Bangladeshis also enjoy

Nutritional and Health Aspects of Food in South Asian Countries
DOI: https://doi.org/10.1016/B978-0-12-820011-7.00025-3

various delicious savory snacks, fruits, desserts, and beverages. Some of them have a regional and custom presence.

People in Bangladesh make traditional cuisine with a blend of *vaji* (fried), *bhorta* (mashed), *torkari* (cooked), *charchari* (dry curry) and *dal* (lentil soup) from varieties of fish, vegetables, and meat available locally or seasonally. The common vegetables are potato, cauliflower, cabbage, tomato, beans, peas, carrot, radish, pumpkin, eggplants, bitter gourd, and others. The famous fish species include rui (*Labeo rohita*), catla (*Gibelion catla*), mola (*Amblypharyngodon mola*), tengra (*Mystus tengara*), kachki (*Corica soborna*), puti (*Puntius sophore*), taki (*Channa punctata*), bombay duck (*Harpadon nehereus*), and many more.

Shorshe ilish, Magur macher jhol, Kachki machher charchari, Rupchanda vaji, and *Muri ghonto* are among the most popular fish cuisine. Bangladeshi cuisine has been influenced by rulers from the past like the Mughal and the British who introduced rich food such as biriyani, polao, korma, chicken roast, mutton rezala, moghlai parata, kebab, tehari, and borhani. Common street foods such as shingara, samosa, dal puri, alu puri, jhal muri, alur chop, begooni, chola, haleem, and jilepi are all supremely delicious food. Seasonal fruit preparations such as *amra* (hog plum), green mango, guava, or pineapple chunk with traditional mustard sauce; *bel* (Bengal quince fruit), mango shakes are mouthwatering.

Traditional cakes called "Pitha" are diverse and are available under the names bhapa pitha, puli pitha, chitoi pitha, nakshi pitha, and patishapta that are prominently prepared around and enriched by the cultural heritage of Bangladesh. Some of the regional foods make the diversity of Bangladeshi cuisine even more extensive. Chattogram's mezbani, Sylhet's shatkora gosht, and Khulna's chui jhal are all favorite delicacies and utterly distinctive.

Paan (betel quid), an after-meal chewing treat, is a culture, custom, and ritual in Bangladeshi tradition. It is offered to the guests as an auspicious symbol of hospitality, and it retains ceremonial value particularly at weddings.

The diverse tribal communities in Bangladesh who preserve their culture and culinary habits have their exciting recipes using local ingredients and offbeat cooking methods. Rice, fish, fruit, vegetables, meat, pork, duck, and chicken are their favorite food and are consumed in raw, fermented, dried, or smoked forms. Bamboo chicken, bamboo shoots, *bini* rice, *nappi* (fermented fish paste), *shidal* (fermented fish sauce) *mochi* (smoked curry), and *chelay* (fermented beverage) are some of their favorite foods and local drinks.

From the historical perspective, Bangladeshi food whether it is plant or animal-based contributes to most of the total food mass and total dietary energy. Bangladeshi food culture has a rich literary tradition that provides essential nutrition when maintained and offers functional attributes for sustaining the physical well-being and keeping a healthy lifestyle.

2.2 Historical overview

Bangladeshi food has been influenced by historical rulers, empires, and religious regimes. From time immemorial, flood and wetland dominated subtropical landscapes provided fish and rice of various kinds. The highlands of northern Bangladesh are inhabited by Bengal goats, the Sylhet wetlands with water buffalos and ducks, and hill tracks with chicken. In following the historical line, the Mughals and the British rulers and also trade networks with the Arab world, Persia, Portugal, and Myanmar gradually introduced new food recipes to the culture. The Bangladeshi people progressively embraced and integrated a comprehensive cultural model comprising farming, ritual practices, seasonal variations, age-old skills, culinary techniques as well as ancestral customs and manners from the rulers (Uddin, 2018), and religious beliefs. After the 1550s, Bangladeshi food began absorbing elements of Mughal cuisine such as biriyani, moghlai parata, kebabs, and varied range of baked confectionaries such as *bakorkhani* and drinks such as *borhani*.

During the British regime (1757–1947), colonizers' preferences influenced to take items such as tea, cake, biscuit, meat curries, various kinds of dishes cooked with potato, and the varieties of bread into the local food culture (Huda, 2018). The Portuguese introduced cheese while other European traders introduced chilies, potatoes, tomatoes, and vinegar, which are all part of the staple diet. The influences from the Persian, Arabian, and Turkish cuisines are also quite apparent in Bangladeshi food. The betel leaf and betel nut are embedded in the Indian culture from its origin in Malaysia and the Indonesian archipelago during the early Gupta period (320 CE–550 CE) through which it was prevalent in the Bangladeshi culture (Ahuja and Ahuja, 2011). Despite geographic proximity, Bangladesh has some similarities with Indian, Sri Lankan, and Pakistani cuisines, but the cooking style varies distinctly in taste, texture, and flavor. All this variety from historical influences has helped to enrich the dish, bringing in a distinct and classical element of Bangladeshi cuisine.

2.3 The agricultural landscape

Geographically, Bangladesh is in the north-eastern part of South Asia between 20°34′ and 26°38′ north latitude and 88°01′ and 92°41′ east longitude (BBS, 2017). The total area of the country is 147,570 km^2 of which the agriculture area covers 91,942 km^2, forest area covers 14,264 km^2, and inland water area occupies 17,460 km^2 in 2016 (World Data Atlas, 2018). Bangladesh is predominantly an agrarian country due to the tropical weather and fertile plain land irrigated by a network of crisscrossed rivers, canals, tributaries, and floodplains. The country is divided into 30 distinct agroecological zones with 79% floodplain, 12.6% hilly areas, and 8.3% belong to terrace soil (Li and Siddique, 2018). The highly fertile and alluvial soil is, therefore, contributing to the agricultural sector (crops, livestock, forestry, and fisheries) abundantly to feed a growing population of 164.7 million in Bangladesh (World Bank, 2019; UNDP, 2019). The agricultural sector makes up about 17% of the country's gross domestic product and employs more than 45% of the total workforce (BBS, 2017) and making provision of accessible nutrition and healthy food to the people.

Rice is the primary crop using around 75% of the country's total cropped area representing over 58% of total crop production, achieving self-sufficiency in rice production during 2011–12 (Li and Siddique, 2018) and becoming the fourth largest rice-producing country in the world (FAOSTAT, 2017). The other cereal crops, wheat and maize, cultivation contributes 2.29% and 3.81% to the total crop production. More than a dozen pulse crop species grow in Bangladesh adding 1.23% to the entire crop production (BBS, 2017). The subtropical climate of Bangladesh makes it ideal for producing over 90 kinds of vegetables and over 60 kinds of fruits and providing essential human nutrition (BBS, 2017).

Cattle and buffalo milk, ruminant and poultry meat, and eggs, which are mostly raised by the rural household, are the leading animal-based food consumed, and they provide a ready source of income, power for cropping, source of fertilizer, and milk, meat, and eggs for human consumption. There are an estimated 393 million heads of livestock (cattle 14% and poultry 86%) in Bangladesh through which approximately 9.40 million tons of milk, 7.26 million tons of meat, and 15,520 million eggs were yielded in the year 2018 (DLS, 2019).

Bangladesh is blessed with the potential fisheries resources from its vast and well-diversified inland, and brackish and marine waters with nearly 260 freshwater fish and about 511 marine fish species with an annual production of 4.27 million metric tonnes (DOF, 2018). Bangladesh is credited as the world's third largest fish-producing country from inland water, and fifth in aquaculture produce (FAO, 2018). Globally, it is ranked fourth in rice production, sixth in tropical fruits, tenth in tea, and fifteenth in fresh vegetables (FAOSTAT, 2017). The top 10 foods produced during 2017 and the global ranking of Bangladeshi foods production are presented in Figs. 2.1 and 2.2.

2.4 Cultures and tradition

Bangladesh is a country of colorful festivals, customs, and traditions carried out with great passion and zeal throughout the seasons. Some colorful social and religious festivals are deeply rooted in our society, which is mainly based on ancient rituals, and the nature of the celebrations remains unchanged. Many of their preserved and nurtured traditions and cultures through the ages are predominantly centered on agricultural practices, food, and food products such as sweets, cakes, and drinks. Many special delicious meals have become iconic in these festivities. Celebrations from the indigenous and minority communities provide extra robustness to the national celebrations.

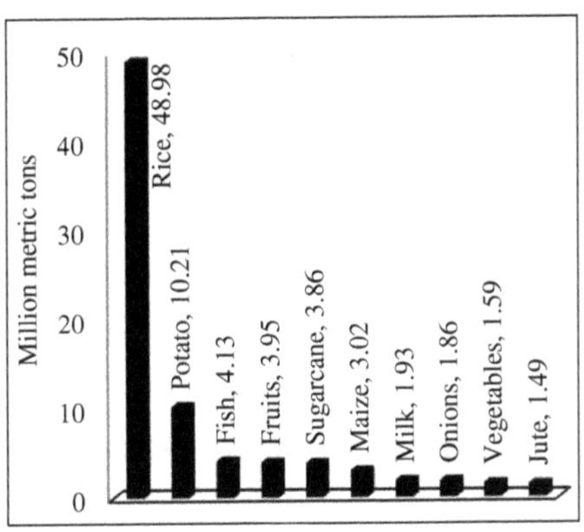

Figure 2.1 Top 10 food production of Bangladesh in 2017. *Authors calculation after FAO, 2018. Food and Agriculture Organization. The State of World Fisheries and Aquaculture 2018 – Meeting the Sustainable Development Goals. Rome. Licence: CC BY-NC-SA 3.0 IGO; FAOSTAT, 2017. Food and Agricultural Organization Statistical Databases. <http://www.fao.org/faostat/en/#home> (accessed 15.02.19.).*

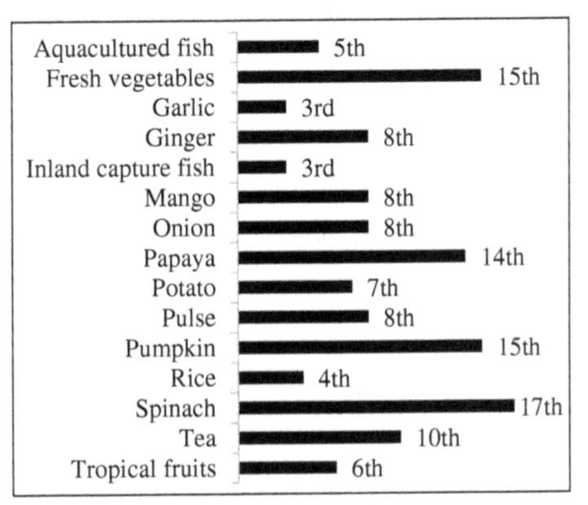

Figure 2.2 Global ranking of Bangladesh food production in 2017. *Authors calculation after FAO, 2018. Food and Agriculture Organization. The State of World Fisheries and Aquaculture 2018 – Meeting the Sustainable Development Goals. Rome. Licence: CC BY-NC-SA 3.0 IGO; FAOSTAT, 2017. Food and Agricultural Organization Statistical Databases. <http://www.fao.org/faostat/en/#home> (accessed 15.02.19.).*

People from all walks of life take part in these festivals with great enthusiasm, friendships, and cultural integrity.

2.4.1 Biju – the tribal traditions of essence and harmony

"Biju" is the largest and a unique tribal sociocultural festival that brings diverse ethnic communities in the celebration. The 3-day festival commencing on the 12 April and ending on the first day of the Bengali New Year becomes an explosion of colors, festive, and eating plenty of foods. The special attraction of the Biju festival is a traditional dish "Pajon" prepared with over 20 types of vegetables to treat the guests. *Tara*, a rare vegetable with unique flavor, grown during the festival period is the center of cooking this ethnic cuisine with some local vegetables (*bedagi, hathol dingyi, bigol biji*), different hill potatoes, bean seeds, peas, dried fish, bamboo shoots, jackfruits, and spices to make it tasty (Chakma, 2016). They also make their traditional pithas (cakes), sweets, and liquor (do-chawni, jagora, kanji) to celebrate the day.

2.4.2 Pohela Baishakh – a national celebration for the Bengali New Year

"Pohela Baishakh" – the Bengali tradition commencing on the first day of the Bengali New Year (conversely 14 April) is one of the most jubilant events for all the Bangladeshis regardless of social status, religious identity, and location that brings the entire country together in the celebration. The day also marks the beginning of business activities. Colorful parades, fairs, traditional music, and dance performances are a spectacular part of the festival. *Panta ilish* with different kinds of accompanying items has been the food of choice to mark the day in Bangladesh.

Traditional *panta bhat*, favorite summer's treat of the rural people, became popular among the urban people on the Pohela Baishakh festivity. The dish is usually topped with fresh green chili, salt, and onions and served with fried *ilish* (Hilsa fish) gaining the name *panta ilish*. In most instances *bhorta*, *vaji*, and *dal* are also supplemented in panta ilish and becoming a trend.

2.4.3 Roja (fasting) – the Ramadan

Ramadan is the Muslim tradition in the ninth month of the Islamic calendar. During the festive period, Muslims fast from Sehri (predawn) to Iftar (at sunset) for a month. During the fast, no food or drink is consumed throughout the day. The holy month of Ramadan allows Muslims an opportunity to practice self-discipline and resilience, and develop patience, modesty, and spirituality. Muslims break their fasting by taking traditional foods and beverages during Iftar.

Iftar is one of the religious observances of Ramadan, and people like to have Iftar at home with all family members. In Bangladesh, a wide variety of foods is prepared to break the fast at sunset. Some of the everyday Iftar items include *khejur* (dates), *shorbat* (fruit juice), jilepi, *piyaju* (made of lentils paste, chopped onions, green chilies fried on hot oil), *begooni* (made of thin slices of eggplant dipped in a light batter of gram flour), *chola* (cooked chickpeas), *muri* (puffed rice), potato chop, *haleem* (mutton stew with lentils, spices, and broken wheat, it is a slow-cooked delicacy), pitha, sweets, and different available fruits (Fig. 2.3).

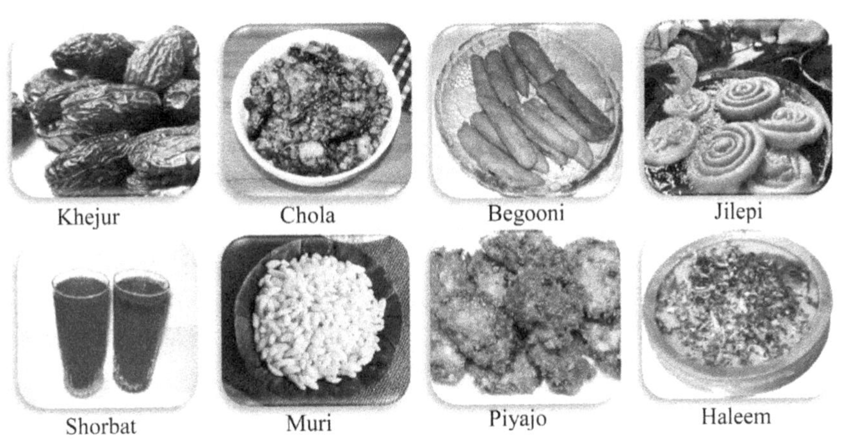

Figure 2.3 Bangladeshi traditional common Iftar items. *https://www.pinterest.com.au/.*

2.4.4 Food customs at religious festivals

The two major religious festivals celebrated by the Muslims every year in Bangladesh are Eid-ul-Fitr and Eid-ul-Azha. The days involve feasting on celebratory foods. The Eid-ul-Fitr marks the end of the month-long fasting in the Ramadan. People dress in their best clothes and after the prayer roam in the neighborhood, visit relatives to exchange the Eid greetings and taste special foods such as *semai* (vermicelli), chatpati, polao, biriyani, chicken roast, *jarda*, *payesh*, and traditional cold drinks. The well-off Muslims celebrate the Eid-ul-Azha with the sacrifice of cows or goats or sheep commemorating the great sacrifice of the Prophet Ibrahim (Abraham). According to Islamic law, the meat is distributed to the poor and the relatives, and the third portion is cooked at the home of the person who made the sacrifice. The cooked meat is the center of the feast with rice or polao and traditional desserts.

The Muslim devotees observe Shab-e-Barat, known as the night of fortune, with due religious fervor and solemnity spending the night at mosques and homes offering prayers and seeking blessings of the Almighty Allah (God). Many families prepare traditional foods such as handmade flat rice bread and *halua* (a kind of dessert usually made from semolina, carrot, chickpea, or papaya) and distributed among the poor, relatives, and neighbors. Milad (religious congregation) is another Muslim religious observance arranged on various occasions such as birthday, death anniversary, and survive from a shock or disease to seek something good or support from the mighty God. Relatives and neighbors are the attendees and are served with snacks such as jilepi, *shandesh*, samocha, or shingara and sometimes followed by lunch or dinner of a heavy meal.

Other religions in Bangladesh also have unique festivals or rituals with Christmas and Easter being the special ones for the Christian community, Buddha Purnima for the Buddhist community, and Durga puja for the Hindu community. The traditional and significant dish for the puja includes *khichuri*, *luchi*, *shukto*, *batasa*, *misti doi*, and *shandesh*.

2.4.5 Wedding ceremony

A Bangladeshi Muslim wedding is full of fun and laughter, can often be long, ritualistic, and elaborate with prewedding, wedding, and postwedding ceremonies observed under local traditions. The wedding function consists of four parts: bride's *Gaye holud* (turmeric the body), groom's *Gaye holud*, wedding ceremony (main occasion and feast arranged from bride side), and finishes with *Bou bhat* (wedding reception arranged by the groom's side). People spend to their utmost economic abilities to stage an elaborate and memorable wedding ceremony through organizing rich food, decorating the venues, and gifting.

It is a custom to send a pair of *rui* fish (*L. rohita*) to the bride's house by the groom's family on the morning of the *Gaye holud* function that symbolizes the eternity, good fortune and wisdom. The fish pair is dressed in funny and entertaining traditional attires to appear as the bride and the groom (Fig. 2.4A). The fish is then cooked and distributed among the relatives.

The wedding ceremony is hosted by the bride's family with much of the tradition around welcoming and treating the groom. Traditional dishes are greatly relished with polao or biriyani, chicken roast, mutton rezala, vegetable curry, salad, and drinks such as *borhani*. Traditional desserts such as *jarda* and *kheer* (cooked rice and milk and garnished with cashews and raisins) are served at the end of the wonderful meal. Finally, guests depart the wedding venue with *misti paan* or *paan masala* (mouth freshener) (Fig. 2.4C).

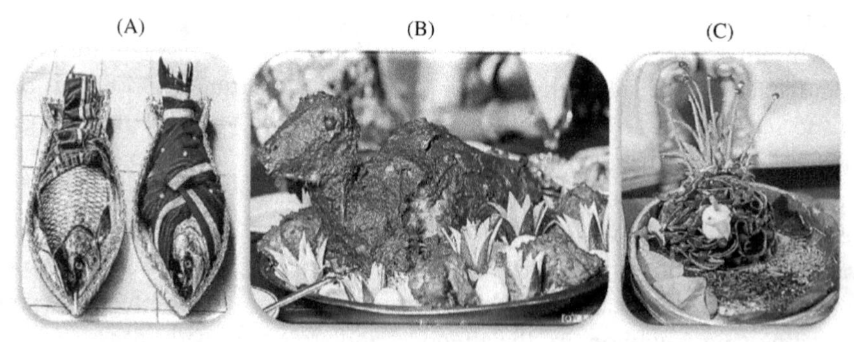

Figure 2.4 Ceremonials in the wedding observance.
(A) Fish duo with funny attires was sent to the bride's home on the day of the bride's *Gaye holud*.
(B) Shagorana – roasted whole goat with polao, chicken roast, and eggs in a decorated plate.
(C) Paan and paan masala in an ornamented basket sent out in both the *Gaye holud*. *Md. Sakib Ullah*.

After the lavish meal is served to the guests, the bride and the groom are seated together with their brothers, sisters, cousins, and friends for an even more extravagant feast *Shagorana* that comes with a whole roasted goat served alongside biriyani, chicken roast, kebabs, boiled eggs, and salads in a large plate with an elaborate decoration (Fig. 2.4B). It is all a bit of fun where the new brothers-in-law might try to stuff an entire egg in the groom's mouth. The groom starts slicing the roasted goat, and everyone jumps onto it. Following these rituals, the bride leaves her parents to begin a new life with her husband commonly fraught with tears. The uniqueness of a Bangladeshi wedding is mostly attributed to its culture and the ethnic tradition and heritage.

2.5 Regional dishes

Bangladesh is well known for its significant influence of some foods over others across its internal borders, which interestingly provides general differences by the administrative divisions. Each area has its methods of food preparation using locally available herbs, spices, vegetables, fruits, fish, and animals. Some foods are familiar in specific areas while some are the regional favorites while others are popular across the country and beyond (Fig. 2.5).

The capital Dhaka exhibits a great deal of Mughal influence in its cuisines as founded in 1608 as Jahangir Nagar, the capital of Mughal Bengal. The most notable of this is *kachhi biryani*. The layers of mutton, rice, and potatoes are infused with warm and delectable blends of aromatic spices to make it a mouthwatering

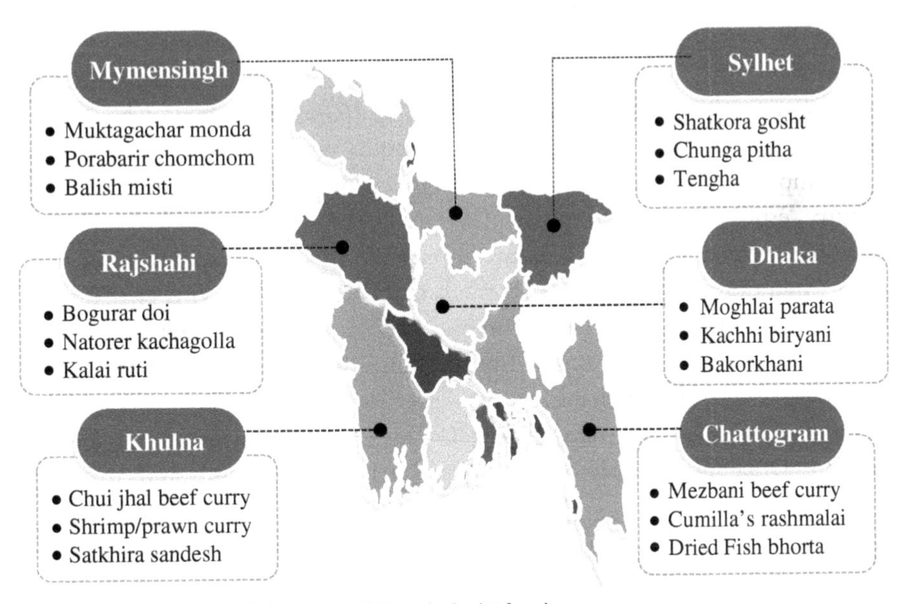

Figure 2.5 Mapping regional diversity of Bangladeshi foods.

experience. Bakorkhani, a thick and spiced or nonspiced baked flatbread gives old Dhaka a unique and distinct culinary identity. The old Dhaka is also famous for *moghlai parata*, *boti kebab*, *mutton chap*, *haleem*, *nehari*, *rezala*, *naan*, and desserts such as *jarda* and *phirni*, many of which have existed for over a century. Chowk Bazar of old Dhaka is famous for its large number of Iftar items including Mughal cuisine and other traditional items prepared during the holy Ramadan.

The port city of Chattogram is famous for *mezbani beef curry*. *Mezban* is the biggest celebratory and regional feast where people from all walks of life are invited to enjoy a meal with beef curry and white rice (Yesmin, 2016). The meat is braised with a secret combo of pepper, cumin, *garam masala*, and blend of other herbs to give the fulsome aroma of the meat. People arrange *mezban* on the occasions of death or death anniversary, birth and naming of a child, circumcision of a boy, and starting of a new business that has marked as the unique culture of Chattogram. Fresh fish *rupchanda* (pomfret) and dried fish of *churi* and *loitta* (bombay duck) are extremely popular in this region. Roshmalai of Cumilla, which is made of small soft beads of curdled meat sitting in thickened sweet and creamy milk, is extensively known throughout the region. Another favorite regional item is curd in Noakhali, as their variant is made of buffalo milk. The curd is recommended as being good for health, especially against cholesterol.

Sylhet, positioned in the north-eastern region of the country, is famous for its vast tea gardens. The best cuisine is *shatkora gosht* (*beef curry*), which is made of beef and a local lemon named shatkora available in the wild. Another traditional delicacy of Sylhet region is *chunga pitha*, a smoked cake of sticky rice cooked inside the cavity of the conventional *dolu* bamboo (*Schizostachyum dulloa*) over a fire. Later it is served with *doi* (yogurt). In *haor* (vast wetland) area, a high demanding semifermented *chepa shutki* is prepared from punti fish.

Chui jhal, a local name for stems of the plant (*Piper chaba*) is widely used for its stronger aroma in meat and fish dishes in the Khulna region. As this is the production area of shrimp and prawn, it is a popular choice of the local people to prepare a shrimp curry, especially for their guests (Yesmin, 2016).

In Rajshahi region, *kalai ruti*, handmade bread from *kalai* (black legume), is one of the famous traditional food items. It is thick flatbread blended with coarse flour and kalai powder and served with fresh onion and chili sauce. *Natorer kachagolla* is a unique sweet within the region. It is prepared by curdling the milk and separating the whey from it, added with sugar. Perhaps, no other heritage dessert item is as popular as the amazing and light sweetened curd that is *Bogura's misti doi*. Rajshahi's mangoes and lychees from Dinajpur are considered to be the best for its taste and aroma in the country.

The fame of some of the sweets that are prepared generation after generation bears the old glory of the Mymensingh region for more than a century. One of its famous sweets is the Muktagacha's *Monda*, a tradition of over 300 years old. It is a grainy sort of soft yogurt patty, where when biting into it, the individual granules of the cooked yogurt separate, filling the mouth with their sweet goodness. The Porabari's *Chomchom* of Tangail district is another famous sweet for its extreme sweetness, unique taste, crispness, and flavor, made up of flour, cream, sugar, lemon juice, and coated with coconut flakes. Another excellence of this region is *Balish* (pillow) misti of Netrokona district, which occasionally weighs up to 2 kg.

2.6 Seasonal foods

Bangladesh is known as *Chhoi ritur desh* meaning the land of six seasons: *Grissha* (summer), *Barsha* (rainy), *Sarat* (early autumn), *Hemonto* (autumn), *Sheet* (winter), and *Bashonto* (spring). Each 2-month season brings its essence of nature, distinct flavors, and festivals, which certainly showcase a variety of foods and dishes. However, the seasonal spirit and the reality encircle into three to four significant periods.

2.6.1 Summer season

Summer is the celebration of fruits. A favorable climate and tropical location contribute making Bangladesh a grower of over 60 varieties of fruits. Major summer fruits include *aam* (mango), *kathal* (jackfruit), *lichu* (lychee), *gaab* (sharonfruit), *bel* (wood apple), and *tormuj* (watermelon). Rajshahi, Dinajpur, Jashore, and Kustia regions are famous for growing celebratory mangoes, each having a fascinating name such as *amrapali, chausa, fazlee, gopalbhog himsagor,* and *lengra* contrasting in taste, changing sweetness, and even in flavor, essence, and texture. Jackfruit, the national fruit, is all inclusive for its sticky and delicious substance. The lychees of Rajshahi and Dinajpur are succulent and vivid, satisfying both eyes and the tongue. Banana, papaya, and lime are all season fruits available throughout the year and every corner of Bangladesh.

The most important cultural festival "Pohela Baishakh" takes place in this season with *panta bhat* as a delicacy meal. Some beverages such as sugarcane juice and *bel-er sharbat* (wood apple juice) are favorites to quench the thirst during hot days.

2.6.2 Rainy season

Heavy rainfall is a common characteristic of the monsoon season in Bangladesh. Notable festivals, fairs, and games are organized during the rainy season among where *nouka baichh* (boat race), *ha-du-du* (rural team game), and *pala gaan* (traditional song competition) are very popular in some rural areas in Bangladesh.

Rain is almost synonymous with eating *Khichuri* for Bangladeshi. There is hardly any Bangladeshi who does not crave for khichuri on a pouring rainy day. Khichuri is a traditional cuisine made with aromatic rice and *moong dal* (yellow beans) with herbs and spices and served with hilsa fish fry, bhortas, and other accompaniments. The flavorsome taste of different preparations of the hilsa is another specialty of the rainy season. Nutritious fruits such as pineapple, guava, and *dalim* (pomegranate) are grown plenty during this period.

2.6.3 Winter season

During the winter in Bangladesh, people taste some delicious food items such as pitha, *khejur er rosh* (date palm juice), and molasses (made from sugarcane or date palm juice) along with a variety of fresh vegetables and fruits. Pithas are made from freshly ground rice or wheat flour, molasses, coconut, oil, milk, and sweet or savory ingredients with distinctive sizes and shapes, salted or sugary, singed and bubbled, sun-dried or cooked. Bangladesh has hundreds of different types of pithas, tastes, and recipes varying from region to region.

The striking pithas are Chitoi pitha, Bhapa pitha, Patisapta, Bibikhana, Mera pitha, Pakan pitha, Puli pitha, different Nakshi pitha, and so on (Fig. 2.6). Chitoi pitha is a glue of rice flour prepared in clay pans. Patisapta is a mixed bag of hotcakes with *kheer* (awesome flavorful with milk thickened through constant bubbling) filling (Islam, 2012). Pithas are often eaten during breakfast or as a snack with tea. It is much related to several customs and festivals throughout the year, in particular, weddings and the *Nabanno* (new paddy harvesting). Nationwide pitha festival is organized during winter

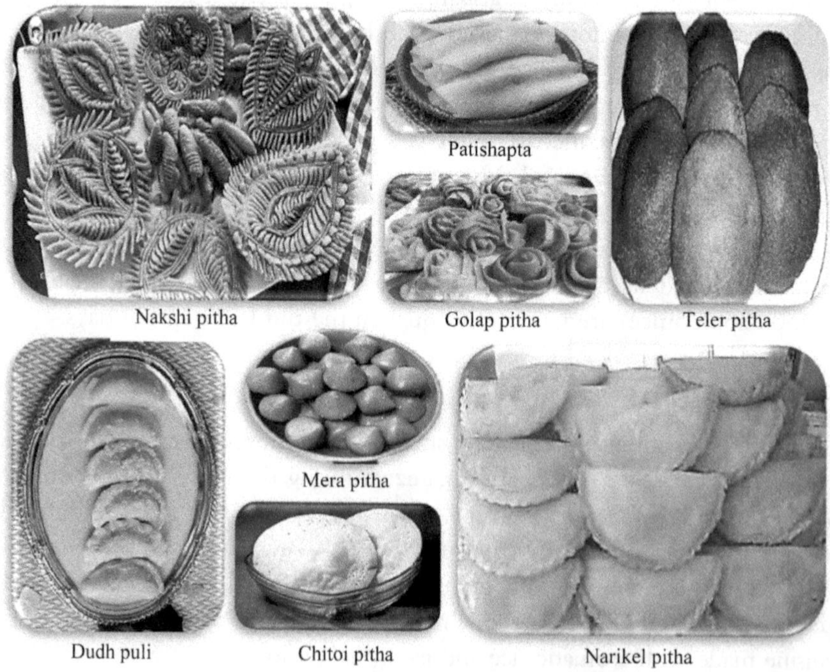

Figure 2.6 Traditional Bangladeshi pithas. *https://en.wikipedia.org/wiki/Pitha.*

to give pitha lovers to tantalize taste buds with varieties of pithas from the regions that prove to be a soulful union of heritage and tradition.

2.7 Nutrients and benefits of typical foods and food products

Bangladesh is famous for its distinctive culinary tradition and delicious food, snacks, and savories. The nutritional values and health benefits of traditional foods and food products vary according to the composition of the food. These food items account for almost 85% of the total calorie and protein intake. Rice and wheat alone contribute to 74% and 57% of the total per capita calorie and protein intake, respectively (BBS, 2017).

Rice, the center of a daily meal, is high in starchy carbohydrate, low in fat and cholesterol, and provides an excellent source of vitamin E, B vitamins (thiamine, niacin) and potassium (Paul, 2013). The health benefits of rice include supplying energy, fighting inflammation, supporting nervous system health, promoting heart health, preventing constipation, and supporting immune system health, and rice is a great source of selenium and a natural diuretic (Jessimy, 2019).

Panta bhat, on the other hand, has more micronutrients than cooked rice and provides immense health benefits (Table 2.1). The water intensifies nutritional elements of rice overnight, and in the morning, it offers a "cold drink" for a hot day and the field workforce. It increases the immune system of the human body and helps digestion, relieves constipation, maintains normal blood pressure, and reduces hypertension (Goswami et al., 2016). However, panta bhat causes a feeling of being drowsy as a side effect of fermentation.

In terms of nutrition, fish also occupies a significant position in the dietary habits of Bangladeshi people. Fish is widely known as healthy food, rich in protein and other nutrients accounting for approximately 60% of daily animal protein intake (DOF, 2018). The nutritional value of different fish species varies significantly per 100 g with iron ranging from 0.34 to 19 mg, calcium from 8.6 to 1900 mg, vitamin A from 0 to 2503 mg and vitamin B_{12} from 0.50 to 14 mg (Bogard et al., 2015).

Small indigenous fish and dried fish are common in the traditional Bangladeshi diet and are considered as nutrition powerhouse providing rich sources of many vitamins

Table 2.1 Micronutrients in cooked rice versus panta bhat (mg/100 g).

Type	Iron	Calcium	Sodium	Potassium
Cooked rice	3.4	21	475	77
Panta bhat	73.91	850	303	839

Source: Goswami, G., Baruah, H., Boro, R.C., Barooah, M. 2016. Fermentation reduces anti-nutritional content and increases mineral availability in Poita bhat. Asian J. Chem. 28, 1929–1932. Available from: http://dx.doi.org/10.14233/ajchem.2016.19820.

Table 2.2 Minerals and vitamin contents of small and big fish (per 100 g of edible parts).

Fish	Iron	Zinc	Calcium	Vitamin A	Vitamin B_{12}
	(mg)	(mg)	(mg)	(μg)	(μg)
Mola (*Amblypharyngodon mola*)	5.7	3.2	853	2503	7.98
Rui (*Labeo rohita*)	0.98	1.0	51	13	5.05

Source: Bogard, J.R., Thilsted, S.H., Marks, G.C., Wahab, M.A., Hossain, M.A.R., Jakobsen, J., et al., 2015. Nutrient composition of important fish species in Bangladesh and potential contribution to recommended nutrient intakes. J. Food Compos. Anal. 42, 120–133.

and minerals that are highly bioavailable. Small fish also enhances the absorption of micronutrients from other foods in the meal (Thilsted and Wahab, 2014). Small fish eaten whole with bones and organs have a high amount of calcium, iron, and vitamin A than bigger fish. Popular small fish such as mola (*Amblypharyngodon mola*) contains high amounts of calcium and vitamin A than rui (*L. rohita*), another favorite big fish (Table 2.2).

In contrast, *ilish* (Hilsa fish) is a massive fish in demand on various occasions like Pohela Baishakh and throughout the rainy and paddy harvesting season. This flavorful fish contributes about 12% of the total fish production in Bangladesh, and 65% of the world's hilsa is produced in Bangladesh. It received recognition of the "Global Identification" from the World Intellectual Property Organization for its geographical origin, qualities, and worldwide reputation. Hilsa fish is a fatty, oily fish filled with many nutrients. A 100-g serving of hilsa contains roughly 310 calories, 25 g of protein, and 22 g of fat (Fig. 2.7). It also supplies daily requirements of 27% of vitamin C, 2% of the iron, and an incredible 204% of calcium. It is rich in essential fatty acids (omega 3 fatty acids) and helps to develop a healthy brain and nervous system and lowers blood cholesterol level (Alam et al., 2012).

Fruits are low in calories and fats but contain reasonable amounts of vitamins and minerals (Anamika, 2017). All the green–yellow–orange vegetables are rich sources of calcium, magnesium, potassium, iron, β-carotene, vitamin A, vitamin B complex, vitamin C, and vitamin K in Bangladesh. Microbes transform the chemical constituents of raw substrates of plant and animal sources during fermentation, and enhance the nutritional value, improve the flavor and texture, produce antioxidant and antimicrobial compounds, and stimulate the probiotic functions (Farhad et al., 2010).

Cattle primarily used for agriculture and dairy farming are a prime source of a variety of dairy products in Bangladesh. Meat and poultry are excellent sources of protein and iron for the growth, development, and reproductive health of Bangladeshi women.

Throughout the ancient history of Bengal, garlic has been used for its health and medicinal properties. Its physiologically active organosulfur components (e.g., allicin, allylic sulfides) support the body's detox processes (Block, 1992). Garlic is low in

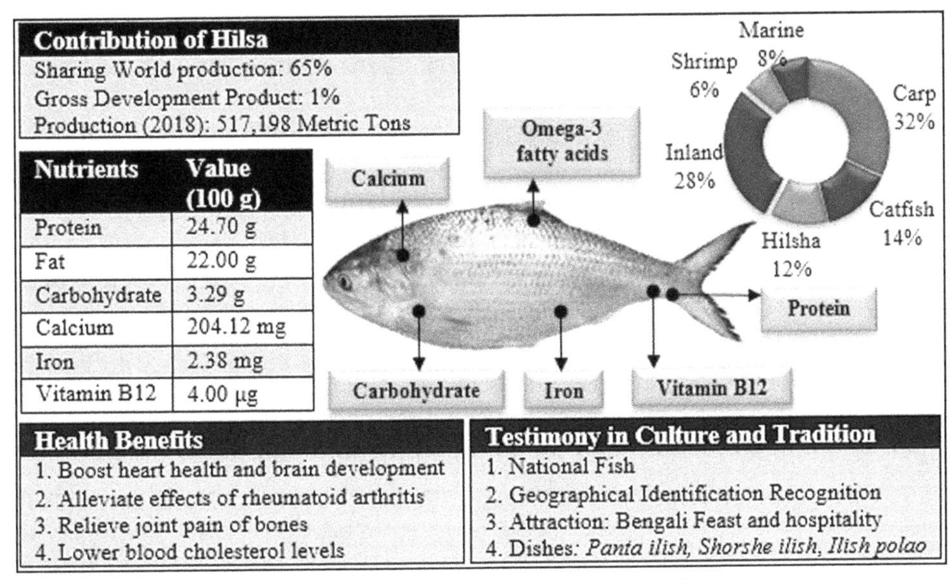

Figure 2.7 Salient features of the national fish—hilsa (*Tenualosa ilisha*).

calories and rich in vitamin C, vitamin B_6, selenium, and manganese. Garlic supplements help to prevent the severity of common illnesses such as the flu and common cold. In some instances garlic supplements are administered as regular medications for lowering blood pressure and reducing cholesterol levels (Silagy and Neil, 1994).

Ginger, on the other hand, has a very long history of use in various forms of traditional medicine. It is high in gingerol, a substance with potent antiinflammatory and antioxidant properties (Wang et al., 2014) that are effective in reducing symptoms of osteoarthritis (Altman and Marcussen, 2001). It has been used to help digestion, reduce nausea, and help fight the flu and common cold, to name but a few.

Bel (*Aggle marmelos* or wood apple) is a delicious and nutritious fruit, and *bel-er sharbat* (wood apple juice), a traditional drink, is a rich source of carbohydrate, carotene, calcium, iron, and vitamin B complex. Every 100 g of edible fresh *bel* juice contains 62.5 g water, 1.8 g protein, 31.8 g carbohydrate, 0.39 g fat, 87 kcal of energy, 55 mg carotene, 0.13 mg thiamine, 1.19 mg riboflavin, 1.1 mg niacin, 38 mg calcium, and 0.6 mg iron (Hossain et al., 2011). It helps in balancing the level of fluids in the body, aids in digestion, and fights constipation due to its antifungal and antibacterial properties (Nair, 2018).

Traditional foods eaten by the indigenous communities in Bangladesh have great qualities of nutrition and health benefits. Bamboo shoot-based food items contain 2.65% protein and possess moderate fiber, selenium, a potent antioxidant, and potassium, and improve appetite, digestion, weight loss, and curing cardiovascular diseases (Singhal et al., 2013). Rice beer, a traditional alcoholic beverage, is nutritionally rich and has high therapeutic values (Mousumi et al., 2016). Fermented fish products such as *shidal* contain 38.35% protein, 20.31% fat with antioxidant activity, and health beneficial bioactive compounds (Kakati and Goswami, 2013). There is a myth that "Pajon" is a symbol of unity as many vegetables are mixed up and are helpful for health and prevention of diseases. Ethnic communities believe that Pajon is their protector against any illnesses throughout the year (Chakma, 2016). Indigenous hill people feed on wild animal meat such as frogs, snakes, crabs, hedgehogs, python, scaly anteater, deer, and wild boar although most of them are threatened in the IUCN red list (IUCN Bangladesh, 2015).

Despite social, ceremonial, veterinary, and medicinal uses, the betel quid has adverse health effects and also considered a public nuisance when the users spit paan saliva onto public spaces. Excessive eating of betel leaf weakens the teeth, impairs health, and deadens the taste buds of the tongue (Ahuja and Ahuja, 2011). WHO (2004) found that chewing betel nut causes cancer of the mouth, esophagus, stomach, prostate, cervix, and lungs. Despite having many harmful effects on human health and in spite of promotional drives to curb the incidence of paan chewing, the passion for paan continues unabated across the planet.

2.8 Future outlooks

The favorite traditional food of Bangladesh is decreasing day by day due to the increased adoption of fast food along with other foreign cuisines. On the other hand, the increased population, rate of urbanization, and industrialization lead to a decrease in food production landscapes.

Changing agriculture production systems is influencing the traditional food culture of the country. Hybrid rice, caged chicken, and exotic fish such as tilapia, silver carp, bighead carp, and Thai sarputi are introduced replacing the long-practiced traditional foods. Exotic fruits, such as grapes, apple, and orange, and some vegetables are also making their space over conventional items. Nowadays, the distribution or exchange of home-grown agricultural products among the relatives and neighborhood are gradually disappearing from the social tradition due to the changing attitude of commercializing their produces.

Due to an increase in the spread of prepackaged snacks, traditional foods such as pitha are at risk of disappearing. It is becoming increasingly difficult to find raw ingredients such as date juice or molasses, and other primary ingredients risk being changed by genetic modification.

Changes in lifestyle and loss of the family tradition of eating together trigger the popularity and accessibility of fast foods and street foods among young adolescents. The shift from healthy, homemade food to more convenient fast foods combined with a sedentary lifestyle has resulted in obesity and related health complications.

There is a lack of policy to conserve the traditional food of Bangladesh. The trends of anthropological research of Bangladesh focus mostly on the ancient or recent civilizations but few on the food and agricultural practices of Bangladesh. The agriculture research and policy mainly involved in technological uplifting and introducing high yielding varieties to feed the demand overlooking the demise of traditional crops of the country have resulted in the loss of traditional food outcomes in communities. A survey conducted by Bangladesh Rice Research Institute in 2011 showed that there are 8000 varieties of rice in the country, but the figure was 18,000 in 1911 and 12,487 in 1984 (Zaman and Mohibub, 2017), while 64 species of freshwater fish are in threatened condition (IUCN Bangladesh, 2015). A separate governmental cell or department is in need for the conservation of traditional beliefs and foods of Bangladesh.

2.9 Conclusion

Being one of the few deltaic countries in the world, Bangladesh has a long history and tradition of culture and foods that are essential parts of the celebration. The rooted element of Bangladesh's culinary tradition is rice, prepared in many ways, often served with fish, or vegetables, or meat curry and accompanied by vaji or bhortas and dal. Rich foods such as polao, biriyani, mutton rezala, kebab, and desserts are occasionally arranged at home but more in functions and special events, particularly at weddings, birthdays, anniversaries, etc. Seasonal fruits and pithas have also enriched the Bangladeshi tradition alongside some distinctive cuisines from the diverse regions.

Bangladesh has an ancient history of distinctive cuisine made with the combination of the local ingredients, blended spices, taste, and serving styles such as dry, greasy with gravy, baked, or fried. Meals are occasionally accompanied with freshly squeezed fruit juices, especially mango, bel, lemon, coconut, and tea, of which Bangladesh produces numerous varieties. Besides various appetizers like *Achar* (pickles) made from green mango, *amra*, *boroi*, *tetul*, and chutney from tomato, *tetul*, and even from the leaf of drumsticks locally called Sajina (*Moringa oleifera*) are equally demanding during a meal. Many street foods have become a favorite among the urban population.

There is no such notable research on the traditional food of Bangladesh, especially on the aspects of nutrition and health benefits. Some food may not have any value as dietary supplements to health, although it is possible that little alternations to the existing recipes may enhance benefits to the locals.

Across Bangladesh, there are refreshingly unique ingredients and cooking styles that contribute to rich gastronomy. The deluge of delicacies, the geography, age-old tradition, festivities, and the everyday menu all combine to create an extraordinarily rich, diverse, tasty, and healthy Bangladeshi cuisine. Knowledge of preparing the traditional dishes needs to be transferred to the younger generation to uphold the long-established heritage of Bangladeshi foods.

There is a high risk for children to be affected by malnutrition and undernutrition with noncommunicable diseases (EAT-Lancet Commission, 2019). Raising food production is one of the solutions for reaching by 2050 the UN Sustainable Development Goals, and Paris Agreement will require substantial dietary shifts. It will be a challenge to see how traditional food can survive in the future or how it could help the population in uplifting nutrition security.

References

Ahuja, S.C., Ahuja, U., 2011. Betel leaf and betel nut in India: History and uses. Asian Agri-Hist. 15, 13–35.

Alam, A.K.M.N., Mohanty, B.P., Hoq, M.E., Thilshed, S., 2012. Nutritional values, consumption and utilization of Hilsa *Tenualosa ilisha* (Hamilton 1822). In: Proceeding of the Regional Workshop on Hilsha: Potential for Aquaculture, 16–17 September 2012, Dhaka, Bangladesh.

Altman, R.D., Marcussen, K.C., 2001. Effects of a ginger extract on knee pain in patients with osteoarthritis. Arthritis Rheum. 44, 2531–2538.

Anamika, M., 2017. Vegetables Nutrition Chart – How Vegetables Help Provide Nutrition? <https://www.stylecraze.com/articles/vegetables-nutrition-chart-how-vegetables-help-provide-nutrition/#gref> (accessed 10.03.17.).

BBS, 2017. Bangladesh Bureau of Statistics. Yearbook of Agricultural Statistics 2016. Statistics and Informatics Division. Ministry of Planning, Government of the People's Republic of Bangladesh, Dhaka, 591 pp.

Block, E., 1992. The organosulfur chemistry of the genus Allium-implications for organic sulfur chemistry. Angew. Chem. Int. Ed. Engl. 31, 1135–1178.

Bogard, J.R., Thilsted, S.H., Marks, G.C., Wahab, M.A., Hossain, M.A.R., Jakobsen, J., et al., 2015. Nutrient composition of important fish species in Bangladesh and potential contribution to recommended nutrient intakes. J. Food Compos. Anal. 42, 120–133.

Chakma, T., 2016. Pajon Aroma in the Hills for Biju. <https://www.thedailystar.net/frontpage/pachon-aroma-the-hills-biju-1208302> (accessed 25.02.19.).

DOF, 2018. Department of Fisheries. Yearbook of Fisheries Statistics of Bangladesh 2017-18, vol. 35. Fisheries Resources Survey System (FRSS), Bangladesh, p. 131.

DLS, 2019. Department of Livestock Services. Livestock Economy at a Glance. Bangladesh Government. Available from: http://www.dls.gov.bd/ (accessed 12.02.19.).

EAT-Lancet Commission, 2019. Healthy Diets from Sustainable Food Systems. Food Planet Health. Summary Report of the EAT-Lancet Commission. <https://eatforum.org/content/uploads/2019/01/EAT-Lancet_Commission_Summary_Report.pdf> (accessed 29.03.19.).

FAO, 2018. Food and Agriculture Organization. The State of World Fisheries and Aquaculture 2018 – Meeting the Sustainable Development Goals. Rome. Licence: CC BY-NC-SA 3.0 IGO.

FAOSTAT, 2017. Food and Agricultural Organization Statistical Databases. <http://www.fao.org/faostat/en/#home> (accessed 15.02.19.).

Farhad, M., Kailaspathy, K., Tamang, J.P., 2010. Health aspects of fermented foods. In: Tamang, J.P., Kailaspathy, K. (Eds.), Fermented Foods and Beverages of the World. CRC Press, Taylor & Francis group, New York, pp. 391–414.

Goswami, G., Baruah, H., Boro, R.C., Barooah, M., 2016. Fermentation reduces anti-nutritional content and increases mineral availability in Poita bhat. Asian J. Chem. 28, 1929–1932. Available from: https://doi.org/10.14233/ajchem.2016.19820.

Hossain, M.A., Bhuiyan, M.A.J., Islam, K.S., 2011. Improved Production Technology of Fruit Crops. Horticulture Research Centre, BARI, Gazipur. Bangladesh.

Huda, S., 2018. Gastronomy of Life: The Love for My Food. <https://www.thedailystar.net/supplements/now-lifestyle/the-love-my-food-1539103> (accessed 10.01.19.).

Islam, M.I., 2012. Traditional Food Culture & Food Security in Bangladesh. <https://www.academia.edu/32445513/Traditional_Food_Culture_and_Food_Security_in_Bangladesh> (accessed 18.01.19.).

IUCN Bangladesh, 2015. International Union for Conservation of Nature. Red List of Bangladesh. Volume 1: Summary. Bangladesh Country Office, Dhaka, Bangladesh, pp. xvi+122.

Jessimy, M., 2019. 11 Amazing Health Benefits of Rice. <https://www.naturalfoodseries.com/11-benefits-rice/> (accessed 05.03.19.).

Kakati, B.K., Goswami, U.C., 2013. Microorganisms and the nutritive value of traditional fermented fish products of Northeast India. Glob. J. Bio-Sci. Biotechnol. 2, 124–127.

Li, X., Siddique, K.H.M., 2018. Future Smart Food – Rediscovering Hidden Treasures of Neglected and Underutilized Species for Zero Hunger in Asia. Food and Agriculture Organization of the United Nations, Bangkok, Thailand, 242 pp.

Mousumi, R., Kuntal, G., Somnath, S., Keshab, C.M., 2016. Folk to functional: An explorative overview of rice-based fermented foods and beverages in India. J. Ethn. Foods 3, 5–18.

Nair, A., 2018. Wood Apple During Pregnancy – Health Benefits and Side Effects. <https://parenting.firstcry.com/articles/wood-apple-during-pregnancy-health-benefits-and-side-effects/> (accessed 12.03.19.).

Paul, A., 2013. Folk rice biodiversity: cultivation and culture. In: Proceedings of National Seminar on Recent Advances in Rice Genomics and Biotechnology. Department of Biotechnology, Visva-Bharati, Santiniketan, March 23–24, 2013. ISBN: 978-93-80663-98-2.

Singhal, P., Bal, L.M., Satya, S., Sudhakar, P., Naik, S.N., 2013. Bamboo shoots: A novel source of nutrition and medicine. Crit. Rev. Food. Sci. Nutr. 53, 517–534.

Silagy, C.A., Neil, H.A., 1994. A meta-analysis of the effect of garlic on blood pressure. J. Hypertens. 12, 463–468.

Thilsted, S.H., Wahab, M.A., 2014. Nourishing Bangladesh with Micronutrient-Rich Small Fish. CGIAR Research Program on Aquatic Agricultural Systems, Penang, Malaysia, Policy Brief: AAS-2014-08. <http://www.worldfishcenter.org/resource_centre/AAS-2014-08.pdf> (accessed 14.03.19.).

Uddin, M.F., 2018. Preserving the Cultural History of Bangladeshi Food. <https://www.nhbham.org/cultural-history-bangladeshi-food> (accessed 21.02.19.).

UNDP, 2019. United Nations Development Programme. Global Human Development Indicators. Available from: http://hdr.undp.org/en/countries/profiles/BGD (accessed 20.04.19.).

Wang, S., Zhang, C., Yang, G., Yang, H., 2014. Biological properties of 6-gingerol: a brief review. Nat. Prod. Commun. 9, 1027–1030.

World Bank, 2019. Bangladesh Population Data. World Bank. Available from: https://data.worldbank.org/country/Bangladesh (accessed 10.04.19.).

World Data Atlas, 2018. Country Profile: Bangladesh. https://knoema.com/atlas/Bangladesh (accessed 25.03.18.).

WHO, 2004. *World Health Organization*. Betel-Quid and Areca-Nut Chewing and Some Areca-Nut-Derived Nitrosamines, vol. 85. IARC Working Group on the evaluation of carcinogenic risks to humans, Lyon, France, 349 pp.

Yesmin, S., 2016. Bangladesh Cuisine Part I – Delectable and Diverse. <https://www.thedailystar.net/lifestyle/spotlight/bangladesh-cuisine-part-i-delectable-and-diverse-1325551> (accessed 08.02.19.).

Zaman, A.N.M., Mohibub, U., 2017. Indigenous Varieties of Rice Variety, Hybrid Varieties More Popular for High Yield. <http://www.daily-sun.com/printversion/details/219750/Indigenous-varieties-of-rice-vanishing> (accessed 03.03.19.).

CHAPTER 3

Nutritional and health issues in Bangladesh and solutions through traditional foods

S. M. Nazmul Alam[1] and M. Niamul Naser[2]
[1]Department of Social Sciences, Faculty of Humanities, Curtin University, Perth, WA, Australia
[2]Department of Zoology, Faculty of Biological Sciences, University of Dhaka, Dhaka, Bangladesh

Contents

3.1 Introduction

Bangladesh is a small country of 147,570 km^2 with an estimated population of 164.7 million (World Data Atlas, 2018; World Bank, 2019). Almost one in four Bangladeshis (24.3% of the population) lives in poverty, and 12.9% of the population live in extreme poverty line (BBS, 2017). This indicator perceptibly affects the nutritional sketch of Bangladesh. Although starvation and famine are related to the question of the general decline of food availability, they are also linked to the entitlements and deprivations (Sen, 1981). The people of deltaic Bangladesh are exposed to various types of climatic vulnerabilities such as flood (34.48%), drought (14.80%), waterlogging (13.88%), cyclone (21.31%), tornado (4.14%), storm/tidal surge (8.65%), river/coastal erosion (4.95%), landslides (0.08%), salinity (4.09%), hailstorms (11.88%),

Nutritional and Health Aspects of Food in South Asian Countries
DOI: https://doi.org/10.1016/B978-0-12-820011-7.00026-5

thunderstorm (14.94%), and others (7.90%) (BBS, 2016). These further affect the agriculture production, socioeconomic status, and household status of rural Bangladesh, which is detrimental to the nutritional security of poor households. Bangladesh has emerged from being a chronic food deficit country after the war in 1971 with a broken economy, dismantled infrastructure, and repatriation of the people in the country after the liberation. The population of the country has reached more than double in the last few decades, and food such as rice and fish production have been accelerating parallel to the population growth. Bangladesh has attained food self-sufficiency at the aggregate level in attaining calorie security. The per capita calorie intake was 2318 kcal/day in 2010, which is comfortably higher than the estimated minimum requirement of 2122 kcal/day (Osmani et al., 2016). However, the nutritional situation differed recently in Bangladesh depending upon factors such as policy, disaster, and poverty level.

3.2 Nutritional and health status in Bangladesh

Nutrition and food are among the basic needs of every human being. Agriculture remains a primary source of energy and nutrients for the Bangladeshi population. The nutritional status of Bangladesh can be visualized by the food and calorie intake data of the country. Rice, vegetables, and fish are the preferred items in the daily diets of the population. Dietary diversity has improved, along with a significant reduction of rice intake from 416.01 g in 2010 to 367.19 g in 2016 (Table 3.1). Rural people consumed more rice (386.09 g/day) than urban people (316.7 g/day) in 2016 (Table 3.2). Fish intake has increased from 49.41 g in 2010 to 62.58 g in 2016, which is above the desirable dietary intake pattern (60 g; BIRDEM, 2013). Although the consumption of pulses, meat, and eggs had increased in 2016, they are still far below the desirable

Table 3.1 Food (g/person/day) intake: 2016 and 2010 HIES in Bangladesh.

Foods	HIES[a] 2016	HIES 2010
Rice	367.19	416.01
Wheat	19.83	26.09
Pulse	15.6	14.3
Vegetables	167.3	166.08
Fish	62.58	49.41
Meat	25.42	19.07
Egg	13.58	7.25
Milk	27.31	33.72
Fruit	35.78	44.8

[a]Household Income and Expenditure Survey.
Source: BBS, 2017. Bangladesh Bureau of Statistics. Preliminary Report on Household Income and Expenditure Survey 2016. Ministry of Planning, Government of Bangladesh, 149 pp.

Table 3.2 Food (g/person/day) intake: rural versus urban people in 2016.

Foods	Rural	Urban
Rice	386.09	316.7
Wheat	17.44	26.22
Pulse	15.12	16.88
Vegetables	164.78	174.06
Fish	60.59	67.91
Meat	22.32	30.04
Egg	12.73	15.85
Milk	26.29	30.04
Fruit	32.24	45.23

Table 3.3 Calorie (kcal/capita/day) intake: rural versus urban people in 2016 and 2010.

Year	Rural	Urban	Total
2016	2240.2	2130.7	2210.4
2010	2344.6	2244.5	2318.3

Source: BBS, 2017. Bangladesh Bureau of Statistics. Preliminary Report on Household Income and Expenditure Survey 2016. Ministry of Planning, Government of Bangladesh, 149 pp.

dietary pattern. Consumption of milk has declined from 33.72 g in 2010 to 27.31 g in 2016 (Table 3.1). The intake of vegetables has increased since 2010 (166.08 g), although it is far away from the reaches of the FAO/WHO recommendations (400 g/day). The overall daily food intake by the rural people is lower than the food intake by the urban people (Table 3.2). The trends of food consumption score levels are widespread across the country.

The per capita calorie intake in 2016 was 2210.4 kcal/day, which was lower than 2010 per capita consumption (Table 3.3) and was comfortably higher than the estimated minimum requirement of 2122 kcal/day (BBS, 2017).

Similarly, the calorie intake level is higher in rural areas than in urban areas if the consumption is estimated separately. The per capita protein intake in 2016 was 63.80 g with the consumption being higher among the urban people (65.00 g/person/day) than the rural people (63.30 g/person/day) (BBS, 2017). It is evident that rural people consume less food than urban people due to the affordability and availability of the products.

The agricultural and food systems including livestock and fisheries are being strengthened to contribute adequately and efficiently toward meeting the dietary and nutritional needs of the population. The nutrition-related activities and policies of Bangladesh have focused on the increased production on meeting the nutrition required for the growing population of the country.

On the human development index for the year 2018, Bangladesh has been placed at the 136th position among 187 countries. Bangladesh scored 0.608 on the index with 72.8 years of life expectancy at birth, multidimensional poverty index of 0.194, and $3677 per capita gross national income (UNDP, 2019).

Bangladesh has a top-ranking position among the countries that provide free medical services to the people at the community level through various public health facilities. The primary healthcare is provided through an extensive network of health facilities extending down to the community level with upward referral linkage.

3.3 Malnutrition

Humans require energy, protein, vitamins, and minerals to reach their full physical, mental, and cognitive potential that results from consuming nutrient-rich food. Lack of awareness regarding the importance of nutrition and traditional food preparation and consumption patterns have led to decreased nutrient retention contributing to malnutrition. Children and women in Bangladesh suffer from high levels of malnutrition and micronutrient deficiencies such as low birth weight, undernutrition (underweight, stunting, and wasting), vitamin A deficiency, iodine-deficiency disorders, iron-deficiency anemia, and overweight being a significant emerging issue.

Tragically, the rates of malnutrition in Bangladesh are among the highest in the world. More than 54% of preschool-aged children, equivalent to more than 9.5 million children, are stunted, 56% are underweight, and more than 17% are wasted (FAO, 2019). All administrative divisions of Bangladesh were affected by child malnutrition. However, some differences in the prevalence of three anthropometric indicators exist. The prevalence of underweight ranged from 49.8% in Khulna to 64.0% in Sylhet, which also showed the highest incidence of stunting (61.4%) and wasting (20.9%). Despite the upper levels, rates of stunting have declined steadily over the past decade (Osmani et al., 2016; FAO, 2019).

Children of Bangladesh also suffer from high rates of micronutrient deficiencies, particularly vitamin A, iron, iodine, and zinc shortage in the body. Malnutrition among women is also extremely prevalent as more than 50% of women suffer from chronic energy deficiency. The prevalence of women with a body mass index (BMI) <18.5 kg/m^2 ranged from 47.6% in Khulna to 59.6% in Sylhet (Ahmed et al., 2012). Studies suggest that there has been little improvement in women's nutritional status over the past 20 years (FAO, 2019). Poor reproductive healthcare and anemia due to no-support given after baby-birth issues are related to the malnutrition in women in Bangladesh (Ahmed, 2000).

The Government of Bangladesh has made substantial investments to improve nutrition, including the establishment of the National Nutrition Program, which provides comprehensive nutrition-specific interventions to children and women at the community level. These include national-level infant and young child feeding counseling, food supplementation, vitamin A supplementation, and immunization programs, some of which have brought about dramatic changes in reducing vitamin A deficiencies, night blindness, and child morbidity and mortality (Yosef et al., 2015).

As an outcome of these interventions, Bangladesh has made significant progress in eliminating some forms of malnutrition including vitamin A and iodine deficiency. Bangladesh has made a considerable achievement in reducing child stunting and is commended as a success story in the global nutrition settings (Nisbett et al., 2017). The prevalence of stunting (low height-for-age) among children under five decreased from 55% in 1997 to 36% in 2014 (Osmani et al., 2016). Maternal undernutrition, as measured by "low" BMI, also declined significantly, from 52% in 1997 to 17% in 2014 (WFP, 2016). This trend has been conveyed as one of the most sustained diminutions in child undernutrition in the world (Headey et al., 2015).

The Bangladesh Government, in its 7th Five Year Plan (FY2016–20), set an ambitious target reducing 25% stunting of under 5-year children by 2020, that is, 3.8 million children, from the 5.5 million children estimated in 2014 (Fig. 3.1). As the rate of stunting-reduction has accelerated between 2012 and 2016, the World Health Assembly has targeted 3.6 million children by 2025. The current trend could support such a decrease of 4 million stunting of under 5-year children by 2025 (EC, 2017).

The underlying causes of malnutrition are multifaceted and go beyond the lack of availability and access to diverse, safe and nutritious food. Table 3.4 provides some of the drivers of malnutrition.

Malnutrition in early life has long-lasting and adverse effects on overall growth, which are influenced by cross-cutting and underlying socioeconomic, cultural, and political factors at the community and national levels.

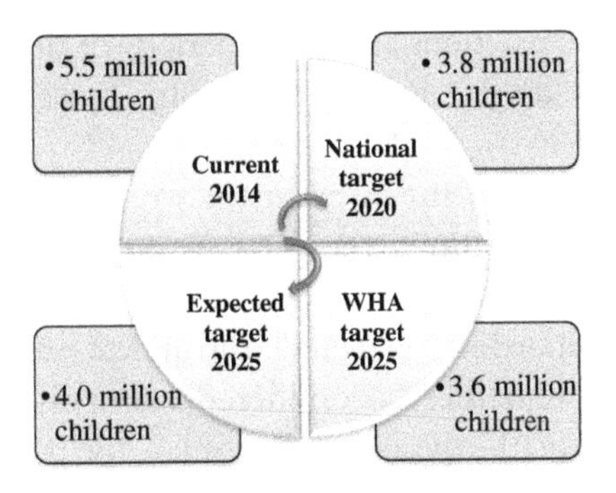

Figure 3.1 Current and projected plans for reducing stunting under 5-year old children. *EC, 2017. European Union. Country Profile on Nutrition, Bangladesh. European Commission, July 2017. https://ec.europa.eu/europeaid/sites/devco/files/2017_country_profile_on_nutrition_-_bangladesh.pdf (accessed 10.04.19.).*

Table 3.4 Root cause of malnutrition.

• Household food insecurity
• Inability to grow or purchase a nutritionally adequate amount and variety of foods
• Lack of dietary diversity
• Inappropriate knowledge of healthy diet and practices
• Inadequate maternal and childcare
• Lack of access to safe water and sanitation facilities
• Inadequate access to quality health services

Source: FTF, 2018. Feed the Future. Global Food Security Strategy: Bangladesh Country Plan 2018. <https://www.usaid.gov/documents/1867/global-food-security-strategy-gfss-bangladesh-country-plan> (accessed 04.04.19.).

3.4 Traditional beliefs and practices: food and health

Traditional beliefs refer to the knowledge that has been embedded in a society's cultural and spiritual belief system and has been passed on from generation to generation. Most communities are characterized by an intertwined set of specific beliefs and practices related to food and health including ways that food can be produced and prepared, which food could be prohibited, and better health can be maintained.

3.4.1 Food taboos versus food allergy

Dietary practices often take the form of rules stating which foods should not be eaten, that is, food proscriptions or taboos. In some cases the persistence of cultural beliefs and practices in the areas of food and health presents an obstacle to the improvement of food and nutrition outcomes.

There are a number of taboos found among rural and even urban people in Bangladesh. People avoid eating *shim* (green beans), *begoon* (brinjal), *chal kumra* (Hairy gourd), *boal fish* (freshwater shark, *Wallagonia attu*), and *gojar* fish (Great snakehead, *Channa marulius*), and *gura-chingri* (small freshwater shrimp) is forbidden for kids, old, and rural people for allergic reactions at certain periods of time. Every year during the rainy season, some people die by having pufferfish (*Tetraodon cutcutia* and *Tetraodon potoca*) curry due to its toxicity.

Several food taboos are prevalent in pregnant women who inadvertently deprive them of some vital nutrients. Among the rural women in Bangladesh, food such as ripe papaya, grape, and pineapple are avoided during pregnancy with the belief that such foods could cause abortion, placental disruption, difficult labor, and many others. The use of herbal remedies is considered culturally in Bangladesh, for promoting healthy deliveries of the gestational woman for a good intention but may medically cause anemia and hemorrhagic-related complications (Choudhury and Ahmed, 2011).

Food allergy represents a substantial health problem. Despite eating traditional food items, few foods have been identified as allergic to consumption. These are yams and vegetables such as leaf, stem, and root of *maan kochu bhorta* (Giant taro), *kochur mukhi* (Taro corms), and *maan kochu* (root of giant taro). Food allergies may increase stress and impact on both the quality and quantity of food choices resulting in inadequate intake of nutrients.

3.4.2 Traditional wisdom: *Khanar Bachan*

Culturally, many traditional beliefs exist in the country and in every household. Bangladesh has a long history of traditional food products related to agriculture or local products. The traditional knowledge goes back to the early civilization of Bengal. A poetess and legendary astrologer named Khana of ancient Bengal composed many small verses in the form of rhyme known as "Khanar Bachan" (Khana's verses) on agricultural and health-related topics between the 9th and 12th centuries CE. The existence of her sayings is observed reflecting in the then Bengali lifestyle, agriculture practices, health and nutrition, weather prediction, food habit and cooking, plantation, and animal husbandry (Nawaz, 1989).

Her verses were the basic guidelines for traditional agriculture practices, especially the time of sowing seeds, harvesting, and seasonal adaptation in Bangladesh. Her humongous influences are also used in modern agriculture advancement. Table 3.5 details some of the Khana's health and food-related remarkable quotes.

Table 3.5 Khana's Bachan on food and health.

Khana's Bachan	Interpretation
Kochi patha, buro mesh, Dodhir aag, gholer shesh	Ingest young goat, mature bull, and drink top creamy layer of yogurt, and bottom part of milk-shake
Tal, tetul, doi, Boiddo boley ooshud koi?	Toddy palm (*Borassus flabellifer*), tamarind, and yogurt can spoil the action of medicine in the body
Mangsey mansho bridhe, Ghreetey bridhe bol, Dudhey birjo bridhe, Shakey bridhe mol	Meat helps in developing body muscles while ghee (melting butter) increases energy, and milk improves sperms while leafy vegetable promotes feces
Tok, tita, chukka, jhal, Ei char purusher kal	Men do not like four things—higher bitterness, sourness, saltiness, and spicy-hot in food
Tel tamakey pittoo nashto, Jodi hoy ta baro maash	Oily food and smoking for years can result in health havoc
Jol khaey fol khaey, Jom boley aye aye	Eating fruit after having a glass of water is not suitable for health
Baro mashey baro fol, Na kheley jay rosatol	Twelve types of seasonal fruits during the 12 months and become healthy
Alo haowa bedhona, Rog e voge moriona	Do not obstruct light and air into the house to avoid suffering from the diseases

Source: Nawaz, A., 1989. *Khanar Bachan Krishi-O-Bangalee Sanskriti* (Khana's Quotes for Agricultural and Bengali Culture). Bangladesh Agricultural Research Council, Dhaka, Bangladesh, 320 pp. (in Bengali).

Table 3.6 Traditional beliefs and some common food items of health benefits.

Bengali term	English name	Traditional beliefs and uses
Lal shak	Red amaranth	For the anemic patient to recover hemoglobin level
Kolmi shak	Water spinach	To regain mineral and vitamin loss of the body
Kacha kola	Green banana	To recovery of taste from the loss of appetite and fever
Korola	Bitter gourd	Fresh juice for diabetic patient, and fry for an appetizer
Misti alu	Sweet potato	Source of carbohydrate for the patients after the fever
Shuji payesh	Rice pudding	Used as food supplements for the infant
Sajina torkari	Drumstick	Curry to overcome diseases such as chickenpox and others
Kakrol	Spiny gourd	Deep frying used as an appetizer and improves the taste
Kacha pepe	Green papaya	Cooked with a meat curry and help digestion
Kolar thor	Banana flower	Mashed that treats for infections, and premature aging.
Singh machh	Sting catfish	Mild curry/soup for recovering from illness
Magur machh	Catfish	Mild curry/soup for the sick patient
Rui machh	Rui fish	Fry used for celebration and offering to the bridal party
Ilish machh	Hilsa shad	Fried ilish served in traditional ceremonies
Shidol	Fish paste	Fermented fish paste used as a protein supplement
Chepa sutki	Punti fish	Paste for the protein supplement

Most Bangladeshi populations relate to agriculture directly or indirectly. Khana's verses pertinent to agriculture are verbal folk communication and the resource that poor farmers rely on for wisdom to apply in their daily life for ages. They are still being integrated into modern agriculture practices.

3.4.3 Common food items of traditional beliefs

In Bangladesh, some traditional food items are believed to achieve many of the nutritional and health benefits. Some selected plants and fish food used in traditional beliefs are listed in Table 3.6.

3.5 National guidelines for food intake

The nutrients including protein, energy, carbohydrates, fats and lipids, a range of vitamins, and a host of minerals and trace elements are essential to lead a healthy and energetic life. People can select nutritionally rich diets from a variety of available and affordable foods. A food-based dietary guideline is developed to improve the nutritional status of the Bangladeshi population and prevent nutrient deficiencies and diseases (Nahar et al., 2013). The guidelines are a set of advisory statements providing principles and criteria of good dietary practices to promote social well-being (Table 3.7).

Table 3.7 Food-based dietary guidelines in the Bangladesh context.

- Eat a well-balanced diet with a variety of foods at each meal
- Use in moderation foods high in fat and minimize fats and oils in food preparation
- Limit salt intake and condiments and use only iodized salt
- Take less sugar, sweets or sweetened drinks
- Drink plenty of water daily
- Consume safe and clean foods and beverages
- Maintain desired body weight through a balanced diet and regular physical activity
- Adopt and follow appropriate preparation and cooking practices with good eating habits
- Eat supplementary food and take extra care during pregnancy and lactation
- Practice exclusive breastfeeding for the first 6 months of life, introduce and continue complementary feeding along with breastfeeding up to 2 years

Source: Nahar, Q., Choudhury, S., Faruque, M.O., Sultana, S.S.S., Siddiquee, M.A., 2013. Dietary Guidelines for Bangladesh. FAO Research Grant from National Food Policy Capacity Strengthening Programme (NFPCSP) Phase II to Bangladesh Institute of Research and Rehabilitation in Diabetes, Endocrine and Metabolic Disorders (BIRDEM), Dhaka, Bangladesh, 53 pp.

3.5.1 Proportion of food in a healthy diet

The proportion of food items (in percent) for a healthy lunch is proposed by the food plate method (Nahar et al., 2013) that could be met through traditional food items in Bangladesh.

According to the benchmarks, 53% will be rice or wheat or any carbohydrate like mashed potato. Mixed vegetables are 15% while leafy vegetables are 15%. Many options are available in preparing this menu. Meat or fish could account for 6%, and plant protein lentil accounts for 4% of the prescribed diet. The remaining 7% is for fruits of seasonal origin.

3.5.2 Food guide pyramid

A complete dietary guideline for Bangladesh was developed by Nahar et al. (2013) with a food pyramid showing different types of foods to be taken. For Bangladeshis, the bottom of food pyramids exerts eating rice or wheat, fruits, and vegetables in the diets liberally. The middle zone of the pyramid is composed of fish, meat, and eggs, which are suggested for eating moderately. The top-notch of the pyramid is limited to sugar as well as fats and oils in the diet (Fig. 3.2).

3.5.3 Physical exercise

Physical exercise is not commonly practiced among the general population of Bangladesh. Socially, men go to work, and wives remain in households. There is a growing concern about overweight among the children and housewives in Bangladesh. Among the 17% of the overweight or obese adults in Bangladesh,

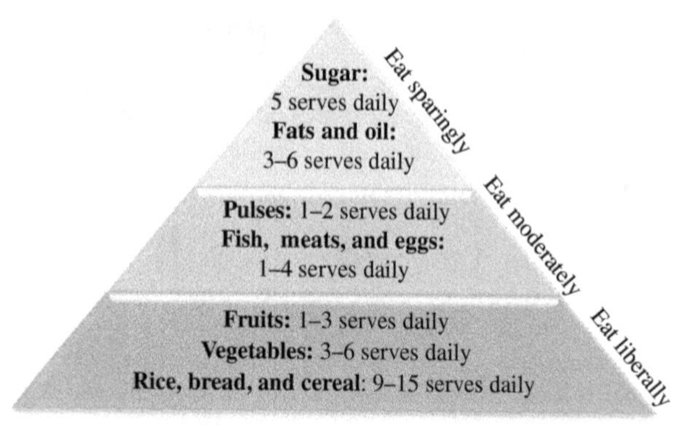

Figure 3.2 Food pyramid in a Bangladesh context.

Table 3.8 Guidelines for regular physical activity.

- Maintain ideal body weight by balancing food consumption through physical activity
- Take 30–45 min of daily physical activity such as walking, running, jogging, cycling, and household works
- Maintain body mass index (BMI: 18.5–23.0)
- Avoid the risk of obesity-related metabolic complications (waist circumference >90 cm for male and >80 cm for female)
- Maintain healthy waist-hip ratios (male 0.9: female 0.8)
- Engage in light activity such as household chores and walk after the meal

Source: Nahar, Q., Choudhury, S., Faruque, M.O., Sultana, S.S.S., Siddiquee, M.A., 2013. Dietary Guidelines for Bangladesh. FAO Research Grant from National Food Policy Capacity Strengthening Programme (NFPCSP) Phase II to Bangladesh Institute of Research and Rehabilitation in Diabetes, Endocrine and Metabolic Disorders (BIRDEM), Dhaka, Bangladesh, 53 pp.

4% were obese, and obesity rates in Bangladesh are increasing at a slower pace. Obesity rates in adults grew from 2% to 4%, and rates in children and adolescents remained at about 1.5% from 1980 to 2013 (Stewart and Persaud, 2014). The prevalence of overweight and obesity is found to be higher in girls than in boys among children and adolescents, and prevalence rates are higher in females than in males in the adults where it is also higher in urban people compared with rural people living in Bangladesh (Banik and Rahman, 2018). A guideline provided by Nahar et al. (2013) recommended engaging individuals with adequate levels of physical activity throughout their lives to achieve overall physical, mental, social, and spiritual health. Table 3.8 presents key messages from the guideline regarding physical activities.

Maintaining the desired body weight through regular physical exercise and a balanced food improves oxygen utilization, lowers blood glucose, and increases working capacity.

3.6 Solutions through traditional foods

Food-based approaches focusing on dietary diversification are an active pathway for reducing micro- and macronutrient deficiencies in malnourished populations (FAO, 2010). In Bangladesh, rice is the leading cereal food consisting of two-thirds of the traditional dietary habits providing 69% of food energy although it is low in fat, essential amino acids, and micronutrients (FAO, 2007). Animal source foods, which contain high-quality protein and bioavailable iron and vitamin A, make up less than 2% of total energy intake (FPMU, 2009). Rice is accompanied by some vegetables, a little amount of pulses, and small quantities of fish. Milk and milk products and meat are consumed occasionally and in minimal amounts. Consumption of fruits is seasonal although banana and papaya are available throughout the year. The traditional dietary habits often do not meet good nutritional outcomes due to lack of inadequate nutrition information and requirement.

On the other hand, food preparation methods result in significant nutrient losses. Minerals and vitamins, especially B-complex vitamins, are lost (40% of thiamine and niacin) even during the washing of rice before cooking. Boiling rice and then discarding the water results in even more nutrient losses. The manner of washing and cooking vegetables leads to considerable losses of vitamin C and B-complex vitamins (FAO, 2007).

Dietary diversification approaches combine homestead gardening, backyard animal rearing, and pond-based aquaculture practices, which are uniquely well suited to reducing hidden hunger and malnutrition in Bangladesh. There have been many rice varieties, chicken, ducks, oxen and cows, goats, wild bulls, pigeons, rabbits, 265 species of inland fish, and more than 60 species of shrimps, lobsters, and crabs to feed the Bangladeshi population. Besides, more than 100 species of medicinal plants are available from the forest and homestead gardens (Hasan et al., 2014). All these traditionally consumed local food plants and animals contribute substantially to the local availability of nutrient-rich foods.

Most traditional foods of Bangladesh are also recognized as functional foods because of the presence of functional components such as body-healing chemicals, antioxidants, dietary fibers, and probiotics. These functional molecules help in weight management and blood sugar level balance, and they support the immunity of the body (Sarker et al., 2015). The functional properties of foods are further enhanced by processing techniques such as sprouting, malting, and fermentation (Hotz and Gibson, 2007).

The fertile alluvial soil and subtropical climate of Bangladesh make it ideal for growing a diverse range of horticultural crops and are considered a significant source of the vitamins and minerals that are essential for human nutrition. Vegetables are a substantial part of daily food intake along with rice that makes a balanced diet.

Consumption of green leafy vegetables contributes to meet the nutritional requirement and overcome micronutrient deficiency at minimum cost. *Lal shak* (Red amaranth), *kolmi shak* (Water spinach), *begoon* (brinjal), *dherosh* (Okra), and *kochu* (Taro) are now the preferred vegetables growing in the rural areas.

There is growing evidence of additional health benefits from a range of phytonutrients such as carotenoids in pumpkin, which is widely available throughout the year in Bangladesh. The carotenes help to slow the aging process, reduce the risk of certain types of cancer, improve lung function, and reduce complications associated with diabetes (Plant and Food Research, 2018). Potato is one of the mainstream crops in Bangladesh, containing higher levels of carbohydrate and provides higher energy.

Taro is a perennial, tropical plant primarily grown as a root vegetable for its edible starchy corm, and as a leaf vegetable (Fig. 3.3). In Bangladesh, taro is a popular vegetable known as *kachu*. It is usually cooked with small prawns or the ilish fish into a curry, although some dishes are cooked with dried fish. Its green leaves (*kachu pata*) and stem (*kachu*) are also eaten. Taro stolons (*kachur loti*) are favored by Bangladeshis, and are cooked with shrimps, dried fish, or the head of the ilish fish. Taro benefits include its many nutrients, including magnesium, iron, fiber, potassium, manganese, zinc, copper, and phosphorus. It contains good amounts of antioxidants, as well as vitamins A, B_6, C, and E (Li and Siddique, 2018).

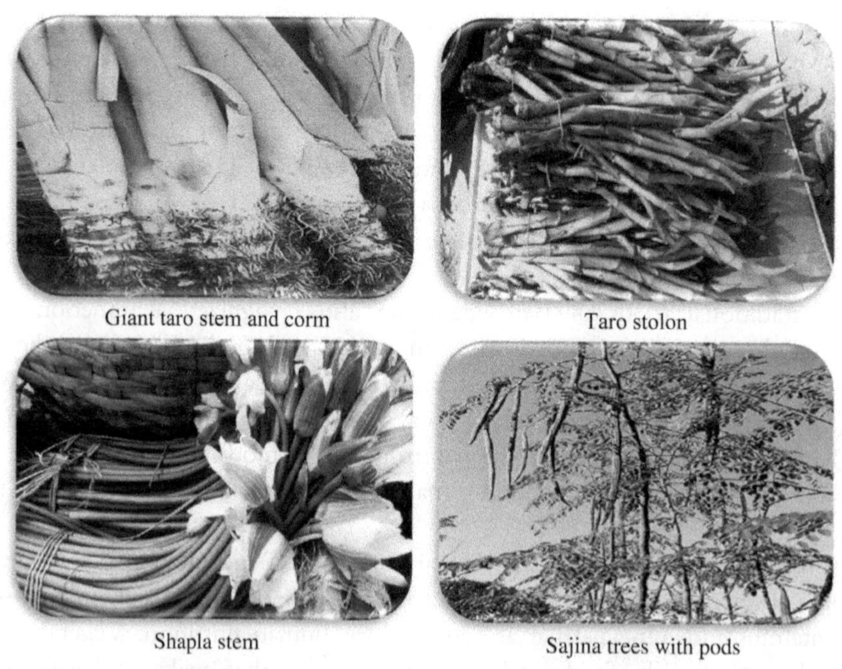

Figure 3.3 Some minor vegetables of nutrition and health benefits. *www.google.com.*

Sajina (*Moringa oleifera*) is another inexpensive, eco-friendly, and socially beneficial alternative, especially for the socially neglected population, suffering from poverty and malnutrition. This promising food source in Bangladesh is full of the leaf at the end of the dry season when other foods are typically scarce (Fig. 3.3). Sajina is universally called the "miracle plant" or "the tree of life" with enormous potentials. Various parts of the plants such as leaves, roots, seeds, barks, fruits, flowers, and immature pods attributed to multiple health effects, including cardiac and circulatory stimulants, possess antipyretic, antioxidant, antiepileptic, antiinflammatory, and antiulcer (Pal et al., 1995; Gupta et al., 2018). Sajina is said to provide 7 times more vitamin C than oranges, 10 times more vitamin A than carrots, 17 times more calcium than milk, 9 times more protein than yoghurt, 15 times more potassium than bananas, and 25 times more iron than spinach (Rockwood et al., 2013). That is why it is being called a superfood. Food and Agricultural Organization of the United Nations recognized Moringa as the September 2014 traditional crop of the month (Alegbeleye, 2018).

Many wild vegetables such as Shapla stem (*Nymphaea stellata*), Kalmishak (*Ipomoea aquatica*), and Helecha (*Enhydra fluctuans*) are traditionally consumed with staple food in both rural and urban areas in Bangladesh. These wild vegetables are rich in vital minerals such as Na, K, Ca, and Mg and essential trace elements such as Fe, Cu, and Zn, which are sufficient to fulfill the recommended dietary allowances by FAO/WHO (Satter et al., 2016).

The tropical fruits of Bangladesh are an excellent source of antioxidant vitamins such as vitamin C, β-carotene, and antioxidant minerals such as zinc, copper, and manganese iron (Shajib et al., 2013). Varieties of mangoes grown seasonally are rich sources of vitamin C, fiber, and essential minerals and provide sustainable health benefits (Ara et al., 2014).

The star gooseberry, monkey jack, pineapple, and golden apple are very rich in antioxidant vitamins and minerals; mango, blackberry, jackfruit, and carambola are also rich, whereas melon and java apple are insufficient in antioxidant vitamins and minerals.

People could meet up their vitamin C requirements with magic fruits such as amra (*Spondias mombin*), kamranga (*Averrhoa carambola*), guava (*Psidium guajva*), and amloki (*Phyllanthus emblica*), as these are available throughout the year in Bangladesh (Fig. 3.4). Amra contains twice the vitamin C contents than oranges. It is rich with antioxidant properties and makes the blood pure, prevents aging and sunburn, and manages hair fall problem. Amloki helps fight common cold and infections. Its high fiber content helps prevent constipation while various antibacterial and astringent properties help stimulate the immune system of the body (Hasin, 2018). Kamranga with its sweet and sour flavor contains pantothenic acid, potassium, and copper, which help to cure headaches and treat sore eyes. Guava, another favorite fruit, contains several vital vitamins and minerals, and the antioxidant poly-phenolic compound help to prevent cancer, antiaging, and immune booster (Hasin, 2018).

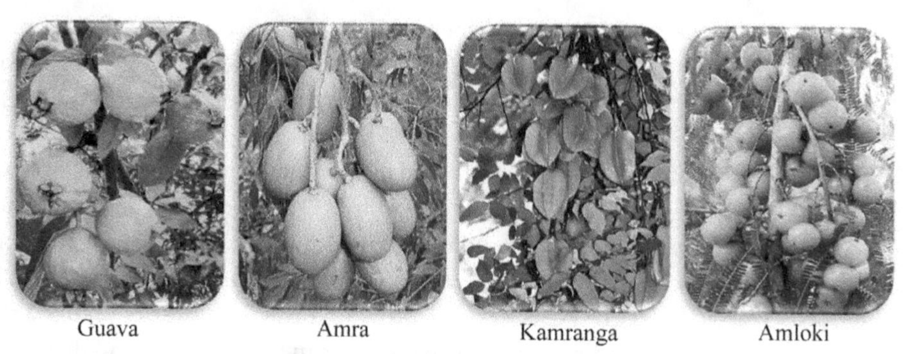

Figure 3.4 Some vitamin C rich fruits in Bangladesh. *www.pinterest.com.au.*

Underutilized or minor fruits can be used as alternative sources to combat hidden hunger such as vitamin A deficiency (Bioversity International, 2004). Nowadays, increased minor or underutilized fruits are contributing substantially to overcome the malnutrition in Bangladesh (Rahim et al., 2008). Minor fruits such as bel (*Aegle marmelous*) contains 65 mg/100 g, Kalojaam (*Syzygium cumini*) contains 25.65 mg/100 g, and Payla (*Flacourtia jangomas*) contains 25.64 mg/100 g, which are higher amounts of vitamin C than jackfruit (11 mg/100 g) and mango (*Mangifera indica*, 10.88 mg/100 g) (FAO-NFPCSP, 2010).

Micronutrient-rich small fish species are providing poor and vulnerable households in Bangladesh with a source of food and nutrition security. Mola (*Amblypharyngodon mola*), darkina (*Esomus danricus*), and dhela (*Ostreobrama cotio cotio*) have the potential to meet the nutritional needs of the Bangladeshi people (Thilsted and Wahab, 2014). Small fish, fresh or dried, are also made into *bhortas* and eaten with rice and vegetables, which are tasty, well-liked, and rich in micronutrients. Table 3.9 presents the amount of fish meat required to meet the daily requirements of vitamin A for Bangladeshi people.

People can grow these traditional food items to fight malnutrition and to achieve nutritional security compliant to the Sustainable Development Goals 2, 3, and 12 of the United Nations.

3.7 Future outlooks

Bangladesh is the largest delta on earth. Agriculture is the most important economic sector and a powerful driving force in providing foods and incomes, supporting livelihoods alleviating poverty and contributing to the overall economy. Agriculture can sustainably contribute to improving dietary diversity and nutrition outcomes. The population growth in Bangladesh is projected at 218 million by 2050 and could stabilize at around 260 million in the middle of the next century (UN, 1998). This highly

Table 3.9 Intake of vitamin A from fish meat (g/day) in the Bangladesh population.

Age group	Vitamin A requirement [a](μg RAE[b])		Required fish meat per day (g)[c]						
	Male	Female	Mola	Dhela	Taki	Koi	Ilish	Rui	Catla
Less than 1 year	375	375	15.0	40.8	269.8	127.1	1875.0	2884.6	1704.5
1–3 years	400	400	16.0	43.6	287.8	135.6	2000.0	3076.9	1818.2
4–6 years	450	450	18.0	49.0	323.7	152.5	2250.0	3461.5	2045.5
7–9 years	500	500	20.0	54.5	359.7	169.5	2500.0	3846.2	2272.7
10–18 years	600	600	24.0	65.4	431.7	203.4	3000.0	4615.4	2727.3
19–65+ years	600	600	24.0	65.4	431.7	203.4	3000.0	4615.4	2727.3
Pregnancy		800	32.0	87.1	575.5	271.2	4000.0	6153.8	3636.4
Lactation		850	34.0	92.6	611.5	288.1	4250.0	6538.5	3863.6

[a]FAO/WHO (2001) and Nahar et al. (2013).
[b]μg RAE – retinol activity equivalent.
[c]Bogard et al. (2015).

dense population will play a crucial role in constricted agricultural landscapes against all the odds of climate change vulnerabilities to augment the food production and to feed the growing population (Streatfield and Kara, 2008).

Rice continues to be the dominant crop in Bangladesh and has evolved significantly over the last 5 years, as demonstrated by Bangladesh's marked improvement in rice production and increased exports of rice and vegetables (World Bank, 2016; FTF, 2018). However, challenges to agricultural-led growth remain. The small size of farm plots, limited diversity and adaptive capacity, healthy agroecosystems, and weak local governance have made the region one of the adversely affected countries on the planet (Chowdhury, 2019).

The geopolitical situation on transboundary rivers, rising sea levels, dryness in the northern barind highlands, and increases of salinity in the southern part of Bangladesh restrict crop and fish production that requires a technological shift to alternative food production. Long-term planning is essential for facing the upcoming challenges and needs of the growing population, nutritional requirements, survival of traditional food crops and their conservation, and maintaining a sustainable consumption.

3.8 Conclusion

Inhabitants, farmers, and fishers have developed different locally adapted agricultural techniques for traditional farming and harvesting since ancient times. These traditions have resulted in a vibrant mixture of sociocultural, ecological, and economic support to humankind. Unfortunately, these agrarian practices are threatened by many influences including climate change, population pressure, pollution, invasive species, modern agricultural practices, and increased competition for harvesting natural resources that have resulted in the loss of traditional farming practices and many endemic species.

Despite having considerable progress toward reducing malnutrition in recent years, Bangladesh needs a more significant climate-smart agriculture. Diversifying farms and farming landscapes in horticulture, livestock, poultry, and fisheries together with more robust rural nonfarm enterprise development are required to foster future growth, reduce poverty, and improve food and nutrition security.

Promoting a mass awareness of nutrition education to enhance the regular intake of minor fruits and wild vegetables could help alleviate common dietary deficiency diseases from Bangladesh. Increased use of minor fruits and veggies would also help to grow imitativeness for cultivation to protect them from extinction and to maintain biodiversity.

Nationwide research is suggested to scientifically document the health benefits of traditional foods across various regions to create a database for the preservation of knowledge on food composition and dietary guidelines. This endeavor could contribute to health, nutrition, and food policy program planning for future endeavors and benefit the Bangladeshi and international communities.

References

Alegbeleye, O.O., 2018. How functional is *Moringa oleifera*? A review of its nutritive, medicinal, and socioeconomic potential. Food. Nutr. Bull. 39, 149–170.

Ahmed, F., 2000. Anaemia in Bangladesh: a review of prevalence and aetiology. Public Health Nutr. 3, 385–393. Available from: https://doi.org/10.1017/S1368980000000446.

Ahmed, T., Mahfuz, M., Ireen, S., Ahmed, A.M.S., Rahman, S., Islam, M.M., et al., 2012. Nutrition of children and women in Bangladesh: trends and directions for the future. J. Health Popul. Nutr. 30, 1–11.

Ara, R., Motalab, M., Uddin, M.N., Fakhruddin, A.N.M., Saha, B.K., 2014. Nutritional evaluation of different mango varieties available in Bangladesh. Int. Food Res. J. 21, 2169–2174.

Banik, S., Rahman, M., 2018. Prevalence of overweight and obesity in Bangladesh: a systematic review of the literature. Curr. Obes. Rep. 7, 247–253. Available from: https://doi.org/10.1007/s13679-018-0323-x.

BBS, 2016. Bangladesh Bureau of Statistics. Bangladesh Disaster-Related Statistics 2015: Climate Change and Natural Disaster Perspectives. Ministry of Planning, Government of Bangladesh, 291 pp.

BBS, 2017. Bangladesh Bureau of Statistics. Preliminary Report on Household Income and Expenditure Survey 2016. Ministry of Planning, Government of Bangladesh, 149 pp.

Biodiversity International, 2004. Banana Researchers Gather in Malaysia, Hoping to Change Lives. News Item Press Releases, News Archive for July 2004. <http://www.bioversityinternational.org/news_and_events/news/news_archives/> (accessed 09.03.19.).

BIRDEM, 2013. Bangladesh Institute of Research and Rehabilitation in Diabetes, Endocrine and Metabolic Disorders. Desirable dietary pattern for Bangladesh. National Food Policy Capacity Strengthening Programme, Dhaka, Bangladesh, 144 pp.

Bogard, J.R., Thilsted, S.H., Marks, G.C., Wahab, M.A., Hossain, M.A.R., Jakobsen, J., et al., 2015. Nutrient composition of important fish species in Bangladesh and potential contribution to recommended nutrient intakes. J. Food Compos. Anal. 42, 120–133. Available from: https://doi.org/10.1016/j.jfca.2015.03.002.

Chowdhury, M.H., 2019. Agricultural Progress and Adapting to Future Challenges for Bangladesh. The Independent. <http://www.theindependentbd.com/home/printnews/193109> (accessed 12.04.19.).

Choudhury, N., Ahmed, S.M., 2011. Maternal care practices among the ultra poor households in rural Bangladesh: a qualitative exploratory study. BMC Pregnancy Childbirth 11, 15–22. Available from: https://doi.org/10.1186/1471-2393-11-15.

EC, 2017. European Union. Country Profile on Nutrition, Bangladesh, European Commission, July 2017. <https://ec.europa.eu/europeaid/sites/devco/files/2017_country_profile_on_nutrition_-_bangladesh.pdf> (accessed 10.04.19.).

FAO, 2007. Food and Agriculture Organization. Food-Based Nutrition Strategies in Bangladesh. Department of Agriculture Extension, Government of Bangladesh and Food and Agriculture Organization (FAO) Regional Office for Asia and the Pacific, 2007, Bangkok, RAP Publication 2007/05.

FAO, 2010. Food and Agriculture Organization. Food Security Statistics. <http://www.fao.org/economic/ess/food-security-statistics/en/> (accessed 26.03.19.).

FAO, 2019. Food and Agriculture Organization. Bangladesh: Nutrition Country Profiles. Summary of the Report. <http://www.fao.org/ag/agn/nutrition/bgd_en.stm> (accessed 10.04.19.).

FAO-NFPCSP, 2010. Food and Agriculture Organization-National Food Policy Capacity Strengthening Programme. Preparation of Food Composition Database with Special Reference with Ethnic and Indigenous Foods: Report of a Joint FAO/USAID Funded Project, Ministry of Food and Disaster Management, Dhaka-1000, Bangladesh. <http://www.nfpcsp.org/Sk_Nazrul_Islam-PR11-08.pdf> (accessed 14.03.19.).

FAO/WHO, 2001. Human Vitamin and Mineral Requirements, Report of a Joint FAO/WHO Expert Consultation. Bangkok, Thailand, 286 pp. <http://www.fao.org/3/a-y2809e.pdf> (accessed 15.03.19.).

FPMU, 2009. Food Planning and Monitoring Unit. National Food Policy: Plan of Action (2008–2015). Ministry of Food and Disaster Management, Government of the People's Republic of Bangladesh. Dhaka. Monitoring Report 2009.

FTF, 2018. Feed the Future. Global Food Security Strategy: Bangladesh Country Plan 2018. <https://www.usaid.gov/documents/1867/global-food-security-strategy-gfss-bangladesh-country-plan> (accessed 04.04.19.).

Gupta, S., Jaina, R., Kachhwahab, S., Kotharic, S.L., 2018. Nutritional and medicinal applications of *Moringa oleifera* Lam. Review of current status and future possibilities. J. Herb. Med. 11, 1–11.

Hasan, M., Mahadi, S.K., Amir, H., Ali, M.A., Alamgir, A.N.M., 2014. Medicinal plant diversity in Chittagong, Bangladesh: a database of 100 medicinal plants, J. Sci. Innov. Res., 3. pp. 500–514.

Hasin, C.H., 2018. A Note on Nutrition: Country Fruits. <https://www.thedailystar.net/lifestyle/food/country-fruits-1569442> (accessed 24.03.19.).

Headey, D., Hoddinott, J., Ali, D., 2015. The other Asian enigma: explaining the rapid reduction of undernutrition in Bangladesh. World Dev. 66, 749–761.

Hotz, C., Gibson, R.S., 2007. Traditional food-processing and preparation practices to enhance the bioavailability of micronutrients in plant-based diets. J. Nutr. 137, 1097–1100.

Li, X., Siddique, K.H.M., 2018. Future Smart Food – Rediscovering Hidden Treasures of Neglected and Underutilized Species for Zero Hunger in Asia. Food and Agriculture Organization of the United Nations, Bangkok, Thailand, 242 pp.

Nahar, Q., Choudhury, S., Faruque, M.O., Sultana, S.S.S., Siddiquee, M.A., 2013. Dietary Guidelines for Bangladesh. FAO Research Grant from National Food Policy Capacity Strengthening Programme (NFPCSP) Phase II to Bangladesh Institute of Research and Rehabilitation in Diabetes, Endocrine and Metabolic Disorders (BIRDEM), Dhaka, Bangladesh, 53 pp.

Nawaz, A., 1989. *Khanar Bachan Krishi-O-Bangalee Sanskriti* (Khana's Quotes for Agricultural and Bengali Culture). Bangladesh Agricultural Research Council, Dhaka, Bangladesh, 320 pp. (in Bengali).

Nisbett, N., Davis, P., Yosef, S., Akhtar, N., 2017. Bangladesh's story of change in nutrition: strong improvements in basic and underlying determinants with an unfinished agenda for direct community level support. Glob. Food Sec. 13, 21–29.

Osmani, S.R., Ahmed, A.U., Ahmed, T., Hossain, N., Huq, S., Shahan, A., 2016. Strategic Review of Food Security and Nutrition in Bangladesh. World Food Programme, Dhaka, Bangladesh, <https://www.wfp.org/content/food-and-nutrition-security-bangladesh> (accessed 01.04.19.).

Pal, S.K., Mukherjee, P.K., Saha, B.P., 1995. Studies on the antiulcer activity of *Moringa oleifera* leaf extract on gastric ulcer models in rats. Phytother. Res. 9, 463–465.

Plant and Food Research, 2018. Annual Report 2018. <https://www.plantandfood.co.nz/file/annual-report-2018.pdf> (accessed 10.04.19.).

Rahim, M.A., Kabir, M.A., Anwar, H.R.M.M., Islam, F., Sarker, B.C., Bari, M.S., et al. (2008). ISHS Acta Horticulturae 806: International Symposium on Underutilized Plants for Food Security, Nutrition, Income and Sustainable Development. <http://www.actahort.org/books/806/806_52.htm> (accessed 27.03.19.).

Rockwood, J.L., Anderson, B.G., Casamatta, D.A., 2013. Potential uses of *Moringa oleifera* and an examination of antibiotic efficacy conferred by *M. oleifera* seed and leaf extracts using crude extraction techniques available to underserved indigenous populations. Int. J. Phytother. Res. 3, 61–71.

Sarker, P., Kumar, L.D.H., Dhumal, C., Panigrahi, S.S., Choudhary, R., 2015. Traditional and ayurvedic foods of Indian origin. J. Ethn. Foods 2, 97–109.

Shajib, M.T.I., Kawser, M., Nuruddin, M.M., Begum, P., Bhattacharjee, L., Hossain, A., et al., 2013. Nutritional composition of minor indigenous fruits: cheapest nutritional source for the rural people of Bangladesh. Food. Chem. 140, 466–470. Available from: https://doi.org/10.1016/j.foodchem.2012.11.035.

Satter, M.M.A., Khan, M.M.R.L., Jabin, S.A., Abedin, N., Islam, M.A., Shaha, B., 2016. Nutritional quality and safety aspects of wild vegetables consume in Bangladesh. Asian Pac. J. Trop. Biomed. 6, 125–131.

Sen, A., 1981. Poverty and Famines: An Essay on Entitlement and Deprivation. Oxford University Press, Reprint edition (17th impression 2011), 257 pp.

Stewart, R., Persaud, M., 2014. Adult Rates of Overweight and Obesity Rise in Bangladesh. Institute for Health Metrics and Evaluation (IHME). University of Washington, Seattle, WA, <https://www.icddrb.org/dmdocuments/Bangladesh%20obesity%20release.pdf> (accessed 10.04.19.).

Streatfield, P.K., Kara, Z.A., 2008. Population challenges for Bangladesh in the coming decades. J. Health Popul. Nutr. 26, 261–272.

Thilsted, S.H., Wahab, M.A., 2014. Nourishing Bangladesh with Micronutrient-Rich Small Fish. CGIAR Research Program on Aquatic Agricultural Systems. Penang, Malaysia. Policy Brief: AAS-2014-08. <http://www.worldfishcenter.org/resource_centre/AAS-2014-08.pdf> (accessed 14.03.19.).

UN, 1998. United Nations. Department of Economic and Social Affairs. Population Division. World Population Projections to 2150. United Nations, New York, 41 pp.

UNDP, 2019. Global Human Development Indicators. <http://hdr.undp.org/en/countries/profiles/BGD> (accessed 20.04.19.).

World Bank, 2019. Bangladesh Population Data. World Bank, <https://data.worldbank.org/country/Bangladesh> (accessed 10.04.19.).

World Bank, 2016. Dynamics of Rural Growth in Bangladesh: Sustaining Poverty Reduction. <http://documents.worldbank.org/curated/en/951091468198235153/pdf/103244-REPLACEMENT-PUBLIC-Dynamics-of-Rural-Growth-in-Bangladesh-Reformatted-conf-version-May-17.pdf> (accessed 12.04.19.).

World Data Atlas, 2018. Country Profile: Bangladesh. <https://knoema.com/atlas/Bangladesh> (accessed 25.03.18.).

WFP, 2016. World Food Programme. The Year in Review 2016. <https://docs.wfp.org/api/documents/WFP-0000019183/download/?_ga=2.158652157.675314446.1555926774-988239962.1555926774> (accessed 05.04.19.).

Yosef, S., Jones, A.D., Chakraborty, B., Gillespie, S., 2015. Agriculture and nutrition in Bangladesh: Mapping evidence to pathways. Food. Nutr. Bull. 36, 387–404.

PART 6

Food, Nutrition, and Health in Pakistan

CHAPTER 1

Introduction

Anwaar Ahmed[1], Rai Muhammad Amir[1] and Muhammad Nadeem[2]
[1]Institute of Food and Nutritional Sciences, PMAS-Arid Agriculture University, Rawalpindi, Punjab, Pakistan
[2]Department of Environmental Sciences, COMSATS University Islamabad, Vehari Campus, Vehari, Punjab, Pakistan

Contents

1.1 Introduction

Nutrition is a well-defined marker for the development of a nation. Diet plays a fundamental role in devising the nutritional status and health of a nation. Improved nutrition is a platform for advancement in health, education, employment, empowerment of women, and the reduction of poverty and inequality. Malnutrition is a worldwide issue that has been affecting most of the world's population. The unavailability of essential nutrients in the diet leads to malnutrition at any critical point in the lifecycle, from infancy to old age.

Despite sufficient food production, 3.5 billion people are facing malnutrition out of the present 7.6 billion population on the globe. Children under 5 years old face multiple burdens: 150.8 million are stunted, 50.5 million are wasted, and 38.3 million are overweight. Meanwhile, 20 million babies are born with low-birth-weight each year. Overweight and obesity among adults are at a record high level with 38.9%. Food insecurity has become one of the major national problems in Pakistan. The population is facing a high proportion of malnutrition due to nutrition insecurity, particularly children less than 5 years old are suffering from stunting, wasting, underweight, and micronutrient deficiencies. In the Pakistani diet, cereals remain the main staple food that provides 62% of total energy. Compared to other Asian countries, the level of milk consumption is significant in Pakistan, whereas the consumption of fruits and vegetables, fish, and meat remains very low. Fluctuations in the availability of important foods will probably be one of the factors responsible for the deficiency of micronutrients in Pakistan.

In Pakistan, about 19% of the population is undernourished. It is estimated that malnutrition accounts for a loss of 3% of GDP ($7.6 billion) every year. Nutrition insecurity is a challenge for Pakistan, which has resulted due to lack of nutritional awareness, high population growth, low purchasing power, price fluctuations, erratic

Nutritional and Health Aspects of Food in South Asian Countries
DOI: https://doi.org/10.1016/B978-0-12-820011-7.00027-7

food production and losses, poor quality of processed foods, inefficient marketing system, and low healthcare and hygienic services. Such unhealthy dietary practices are responsible for the increased prevalence of nutritional deficiencies and disorders, such as overweight and obesity, diabetes, hypertension, cardiovascular diseases, cancers, and other chronic diseases. Furthermore, sedentary lifestyles and lack of outdoor activities, low-quality energy-dense dietary intake, infections (due to lack of clean water, sanitation, and hygiene), especially among children and women of childbearing age, also worsen the health status of the Pakistani population.

To address all forms of malnutrition, a multisectoral program and policies are inevitable for improving diet, nutritional status of mothers and children with effective nutritional awareness, communication, coordination, collaboration, and integration across all sectors. Pakistan government is aware of the consequences. Hence, several programs have been launched like good nutrition in the first 1000 days of life (starting from the day when a woman conceives), food fortification, and biodiversifications. These have been found to be the most cost-effective and sustainable solutions to overcome micronutrient deficiencies. The economic access to minimum adapted food basket based on the desirable dietary pattern can also be an important planning tool, on the basis of which the availability and consumption trend of essential food items can be guaranteed. Hence, these set targets to undermine malnutrition can be achieved through enhanced nutrition awareness and healthy practices, institutional strengthening, and implementation of a comprehensively planned nutrition strategy.

CHAPTER 2

Food, nutrition, and health issues in Pakistan

Contents

2.1 Introduction

Food and nutrition insecurity is a major challenge for the Pakistani population. Health issues in Pakistan are increasing at an alarming stage due to nutritional deficiencies. Medical problems are causing new kinds of disorders that are difficult to treat due to the unavailability of finance and poor economic conditions (Gordon and Shaw, 1999; Moss, 2002; Wagstaff, 2002; Scheppers et al., 2006; Kapur, 2007). According to the World Health Organization (WHO), Pakistan is ranked 122 among 190 countries in terms of healthcare. Despite significant developments over the past decades, Pakistan has the third highest infant mortality rate in the world (WHO, 2000; Rasanathan et al., 2017).

Over the last decades, Pakistan has not shown much progress in the health scenario of children with disabilities. The latest National Nutrition Survey (NNS, 2011) revealed the prevalence of acute malnutrition of 15.1%, which was more than what was seen in the previous survey (13%). Moreover, the disaggregated rate of wasting in the urban and rural communities was 12.6% and 16.1%. Wasting is related to intense weight reduction demonstrated by a low weight to height ratio. This may be due to acute starvation or severe illness/disease.

In Pakistan, the nutritional status of children under the age of 5 years is extremely poor (FAO, 2010). Almost 40% of children are underweight, and about half of children are affected by stunting and around 9% by wasting (FAO, 2010). Micronutrient deficiencies are also widespread in children (Ejaz and Latif, 2010). Biochemical indices revealed a deficiency of multiple micronutrients in children under 5 years: zinc, 39.2%; vitamin D, 40.0%; iron, 43.8%; vitamin A, 54.0%; and occurrence of anemia, 61.9% (NNS, 2011). The NNS survey has given a complete nutrition profile of children in Pakistan based on daily consumption (Table 2.1).

Nutritional and Health Aspects of Food in South Asian Countries
DOI: https://doi.org/10.1016/B978-0-12-820011-7.00028-9

Table 2.1 The daily consumption of energy and nutrients by children (up to 23 months old).

Nutrients	Pakistan	Residence		Province/Region							RDA
		Rural	Urban	Punjab	Sindh	Baluchistan	KPK	GB	AJK	FATA	
Iron (mg)	3.6	3.2	4.4	3.1	3.7	5.3	6	3.2	4	5.3	11
Zinc (Zn)	1.5	1.4	1.8	1.5	1.5	2.1	1.7	1.1	1.6	1.6	3
Fats (g)	25	23	31	26	22	32	24	16	31	22	30
Protein (g)	25	23	31	26	22	32	24	16	31	22	30
Calcium (mg)	490	471	529	556	329	514	459	272	611	421	500
Phosphorus (mg)	377	356	420	394	276	427	513	246	488	461	460
Carbohydrates (g)	56	49	69	48	60	86	67	55	82	74	100
Energy (kcal)	560	492	700	523	561	808	657	423	728	602	1200

Source: The data has been extracted from NNS (National Nutrition Survey), 2011; based on reports submitted by Agha Khan University, Pakistan, Pakistan Medical Research Council (PMRC), Nutrition Wing, Ministry of Health, Pakistan. *KPK*, Khyber Pakhtunkhwa; *GB*, Gilgit Baltistan; *AJK*, Azad Jammu and Kashmir; *FATA*, Federally Administered Tribal Area; *RDA*, Recommended Dietary Allowance.

Table 2.2 Food availability per capita.

Items	Year/ units	2007–08	2008–09	2009–10	2010–11	2011–12 (E)	2012–13 (T)
Cereals	kg	158.1	160.3	158.8	158.7	159.0	160.0
Pulses	kg	7.2	5.8	6.8	6.7	6.4	6.7
Sugar	kg	30.0	25.6	26.1	26.5	30.4	31.0
Milk	L	165.4	167.2	169.1	169.8	169.0	170.0
Meat	kg	20.0	20.0	20.5	20.9	20.4	21.0
Eggs	dozen	5.5	5.6	5.8	6.0	6.0	6.0
Edible Oil	L	12.8	12.5	12.6	12.6	12.7	13.0
Calories per day	2410	2425	2415	2420	2410	2450	
Protein per day (g)	72.0	72.5	71.5	72.0	71.5	72.5	

Source: Planning Commission of Pakistan—GOP, 2018.

Food availability and consumption are indicators to assess food adequacy. According to the food balance sheet, the availability of essential food items has been an adequate level to meet national food needs. The average calories estimation through food balance sheets during the last 5 years remained above 2400 calories and protein 70 g per capita per day. During the fiscal year 2012–13, it was around 2450 calories per capita per day. The 5-year overview of food availability patterns for major food items is given in Table 2.2.

A positive relationship exists between the age of the child and the prevalence rate of stunting and underweight (NIDA-Pakistan, 2019). However, there are no gender-based differences in malnutrition (FAO, 2010). On the other hand, the mortality rate of mothers is also higher in Pakistan despite the development of the medical area. According to estimates, about 30,000 women die each year due to obstetric complications or we can say that one woman dies every 20 min (Khan et al., 2009). The disproportionately greater burden of death occurs in rural areas and urban poor neighborhoods. Anthropometric deficiencies are considerably higher in rural areas due to low living standards, poor financial status, and extremely poor or lack of access to basic health services. It is unfortunate that in recent times no food consumption survey has been conducted in Pakistan for the adequacy of food consumption and quality control. Food consumption is one of the main elements that connects and affects the nutritional status of the population (Haider and Zaidi, 2017). Other key influences can be socioeconomic factors, lack of healthcare facilities, poor financial conditions, and disease outbreak (Vorster and Kruger, 2007; Wilkinson and Marmot, 2003). Malnutrition is an imperative indicator of poverty and is closely related to the mortality of children.

About 60 million people in Pakistan are below the poverty line (Khan, 2016) and these individuals cannot meet their basic needs because of poor financial conditions.

Trends in nutrition status can be ascertained from sequential national nutrition and health surveys suggesting a negligible change in stunting and wasting rates over the last decades (Bhutta et al., 2013). Moreover, child mortality occurs as a result of respiratory and intestinal diseases in almost 50% of malnourished children under 5 years old (Caulfield et al., 2004), which is exasperating, particularly in the most populated regions (Bharmal, 2000).

Previously, Khuwaja et al. (2005) found a lag in growth among school children (6–12 years) in rural areas of southern Pakistan with 16.5% stunting. Furthermore, the sex, age, and father's occupation were found to be important risk factors for stunting growth in the children of this age group. Similarly, Asim and Nawaz (2018) reported that the most vulnerable age was 6–23 months when their diets were completely neglected. It is evident that the greater intensity of childhood malnutrition prevails in rural areas of Pakistan and is most likely due to low income, large family size, early marriages, high rates of fertility, no gap between birth spacing, and the lack of breastfeeding.

Malnutrition in a child often appears as underweight or wasting and also impairs the function of the immune system and makes the child more susceptible to infections (Waterlow, 2006). Some infections, meningitis in particular, when treated incorrectly or late, are major causes of disability (Gladstone, 2010). Another indicator of malnutrition is stunting, defined as the low height-to-age ratio. It is caused by a range of nutrition-related factors including macro- and micronutrients and has a number of negative impacts on physical and cognitive development (Grantham-McGregor, 2002). Deafness is another possible disability linked to malnutrition. It has been found that children with slight malnutrition are more likely to suffer hearing loss than infants who are not malnourished, and the risk of hearing loss is increased in infants with severe-to-profound malnutrition (Olusanya, 2010).

2.2 Maternal nutrient status in Pakistan

The nutritional status of pregnant women is not different from children (UNICEF, 2005). They produce malnourished children. These children are more susceptible to death as an infant or if they survive, they are more likely to remain malnourished and have a greater chance of getting diseases (Groce et al., 2014). The prevalence of anemia in pregnant women is the major risk factor of low-birth-weight babies (Badshah et al., 2008; Levy et al., 2005). Lone et al. (2004) investigated the relationship between maternal anemia and perinatal outcome in a group of 629 pregnant women. The study found that the risk of preterm delivery and low-birth-weight in anemic women was 4 and 1.9 times higher than the nonanemic women. In Pakistan, about 45% of people consider themselves iron deficient (Mawani et al., 2016). The prevalence of anemia in pregnant females was reported to be 29%–55% in urban areas (Khalid et al., 2017). Moreover, lack of iodine in women may also result in stillbirths, birth defects, mental retardation, and child mortality (Dunn and Delange, 2001; Zimmermann, 2012).

The importance of maternal nutrition does not end with birth. Breast milk is crucial to the growth and development of babies and contains vitamin B_{12} needed for the development of the central nervous system. Anemic mothers lack vitamin B_{12} in their milk, which leads to neurocognitive impairment (Groce et al., 2014). It has recently been found that 70% of pregnant women in Pakistan have a deficiency of iron due to the lack of vitamin B_{12} (Khalid et al., 2017).

Apart from the effect of maternal malnutrition on infants, there is a high risk of many disorders/diseases during gestation periods at different intervals, which can lead to severe dilemmas. Postpartum hemorrhage is excessive bleeding after childbirth that can lead to mortality or morbidity of the mother. In Pakistan, 27.2% of maternal deaths were caused by postpartum hemorrhage (Mir et al., 2012). Preeclampsia is another factor related to maternal mortality due to high blood pressure during pregnancy. In Pakistan, a lack of magnesium in maternal diet results in preeclampsia, which may have a severe effect on fetus growth and have a high risk of maternal mortality (Bigdeli et al., 2013).

Another emerging issue that arises with regards to malnutrition in adults is obesity. The prevalence of obesity is increasing, where it is associated with numerous metabolic and cardiac disorders and can also be associated with mortality (Bray and Bellanger, 2006). Overweight and obesity also contribute to reducing functionalities and disabilities in adults. About 50% of the population in Pakistan is obese. However, the burden of obesity is higher among women in all age groups compared to men (Tanzil and Jamali, 2016). Moreover, obesity may increase the risk of iron deficiency due to reduced absorption of nutrition associated with adiposity (Mawani et al., 2016).

Nutrition insecurity is a challenge for the Pakistani population that resulted due to lack of nutritional awareness, high population growth, low purchasing power, price fluctuations, erratic food production and losses, poor quality of processed foods, inefficient marketing system, and low healthcare and hygienic services. Such unhealthy dietary practices are responsible for the increased prevalence of nutritional deficiencies and disorders like overweight and obesity, diabetes, hypertension, cardiovascular diseases, cancers, and other chronic diseases (Singh et al., 2007; Ahmed et al., 2012; Bishwajit, 2015). Furthermore, sedentary lifestyles and lack of outdoor activities, low-quality energy-dense dietary intake, infections (due to lack of clean water, sanitation, and hygiene), especially among children and women of childbearing age, also worsen the health status of Pakistani population (Arif et al., 2012; Delisle, 2008; KhanKhattak and Shah, 2010).

2.3 Nutritional programs in Pakistan

In Pakistan, during the last few years, many nutritional programs have been initiated by the government and other nongovernmental organizations. The main focus of these programs is to raise nutritional awareness among the people while some focus on the supply of nutrients to the people of Pakistan directly or via fortification of dietary components. Although organizations are doing their best to control the malnutrition situation in Pakistan but are still far behind other countries. This may due to the reason that socioeconomic deprivation, poverty, and illiteracy is being neglected by the government (Niazi et al., 2012).

Ministry of Education, Government of Pakistan has initiated a school health program that is jointly managed by the United Nations Educational, Scientific, and Cultural Organization (UNESCO, 2019). The main component of this program is to provide relevant nutritional information to the students. This program is run on the concept that information related to nutritional interventions will also be spread among parents and relatives of the students. To eliminate the deficiencies of micronutrients such as iron, zinc, iodine, vitamin A, and folic acid, Nutrition International (NI) works with the government and the United Nations. In Pakistan, NI is working in salt iodization and flour fortification to combat micronutrient malnutrition. Their objective is to expand vitamin A supplementation to children in hard-to-reach areas, to initiate and increase complementary zinc supplementation for treatment of childhood diarrhea, to increase the production of adequately iodized salt and its use in households, to expand the use of *Sprinkles*—or multiple micronutrient powders—in the feeding of children aged 6–24 months to reduce anemia, and to increase the number of women of childbearing age consuming fortified wheat flour to enhance iron and folic acid consumption. (Nutrition International, 2019).

Ministry of Social Welfare and Special Education, Government of Pakistan initiated a program for combating malnutrition in primary school girls (Badruddin et al., 2008). The project trained women in the local community to successfully run nutrition awareness programs in their communities and provide freshly prepared meals in the afternoon to primary school girls. A few other programs include the National Program for Family Planning and Primary Healthcare, which was initiated by the government to provide primary healthcare services at doorstep in villages. The nutrition wing of the Ministry of Health, Government of Pakistan also runs the national nutrition programs that include child and maternal, infant, adolescent, adult, and elderly nutrition (GOP, 2019a,b).

In the context of the above observations, it is suggested that the malnutrition and nutrient deficiency should be considered on priority for future research being the root cause of the nutrient deficiency and the possible ways to cope with this deficiency. Various estimates and comparisons highlight that some prominent findings such as the health of the people have improved but the rate of improvement in health outcomes in some respects has been slow compared to its neighboring countries. The pace of improvement is not satisfactory due to various reasons such as resource constraints and rapid growth of population.

There is also a need for research to understand the links between malnutrition and disability in both children and adults in Pakistan. However, governments have not perceived the significance and effect of nutrition on the human health and development of the local population (Reinhardt and Fanzo, 2014). None of the studies has brought about a national intercession program for identifying the root cause of malnutrition. Additionally, some other factors are also involved in it: lack of management and nutrition research, lack of individual abilities to lead planned research, violation of laws and policies and their implementation, etc.

References

Ahmed, T., Hossain, M., Sanin, K.I., 2012. Global burden of maternal and child undernutrition and micronutrient deficiencies. Ann. Nutr. Metabol. 61, 8–17.

Arif, G.M., Nazir, S., Satti, M.N., Farooq, S., 2012. Child malnutrition in Pakistan: trends and determinants. Pak. Inst. Dev. Econ. 1–18.

Asim, M., Nawaz, Y., 2018. Child Malnutrition in Pakistan: Evidence from Literature. Children (Basel, Switzerland) 5, 60. Available from: https://doi.org/10.3390/children5050060.

Badruddin, S.H., Agha, A., Peermohamed, H., Rafique, G., Khan, K.S., Pappas, G., 2008. Tawana project-school nutrition program in Pakistan-its success, bottlenecks and lessons learned. Asia. Pac. J. Clin. Nutr. 17, 357–360.

Badshah, S., Mason, L., McKelvie, K., Payne, R., Lisboa, P.J., 2008. Risk factors for low birthweight in the public hospitals at Peshawar, NWFP-Pakistan. BMC Public Health 8, 197. Available from: https://doi.org/10.1186/1471-2458-8-197.

Bharmal, F.Y., 2000. Trends in nutrition transition: Pakistan in focus. J.-Pak. Med. Assoc. 50, 159–167.

Bhutta, Z.A., Hafeez, A., Rizvi, A., Ali, N., Khan, A., Ahmad, F., et al., 2013. Reproductive, maternal, newborn, and child health in Pakistan: challenges and opportunities. Lancet 381, 2207–2218.

Bigdeli, M., Zafar, S., Assad, H., Ghaffar, A., 2013. Health system barriers to access and use of magnesium sulfate for women with severe pre-eclampsia and eclampsia in Pakistan: evidence for policy and practice. PLoS One 8, e59158.

Bishwajit, G., 2015. Nutrition Transition in South Asia: The Emergence of Non-Communicable Chronic Diseases. F1000Research 4.

Bray, G.A., Bellanger, T., 2006. Epidemiology, trends, and morbidities of obesity and metabolic syndrome. Endocrine 29, 109–117.

Caulfield, L.E., Richard, S.A., Black, R.E., 2004. Undernutrition as an underlying cause of malaria morbidity and mortality in children less than five years old. Am. J. Trop. Med. Hyg. 71, 55–63.

Delisle, H.F., 2008. Poverty: the double burden of malnutrition in mothers and the intergenerational impact. Ann. N. Y. Acad. Sci. 1136, 172–184.

Dunn, J.T., Delange, F., 2001. Damaged reproduction: the most important consequence of iodine deficiency. J. Clin. Endocrinol. Metabol. 86, 2360–2363.

Ejaz, M.S., Latif, N., 2010. Stunting and micronutrient deficiencies in malnourished children. JPMA 60.

FAO, 2010. Food and Agriculture Organization. Nutrition and consumer protection. <http://www.fao.org/ag/agn/nutrition/pak_en.stm>.

Gladstone, M., 2010. A review of the incidence and prevalence, types and etiology of childhood cerebral palsy in resource-poor settings. Ann. Trop. Pediatr. 30, 181–196.

Gordon, D., Shaw, M., 1999. Inequalities in Health: The Evidence Presented to the Independent Inquiry Into Inequalities in Health, Chaired by Sir Donald Acheson. Policy Press.

Government of Pakistan (GOP), 2019a. Ministry of Health. National programme for family planning and primary health care. <http://www.phc.gov.pk/site/> (accessed 20.05.19.).

Government of Pakistan (GOP), 2019b. Nutrition Wing, Ministry of Health. Projects. <http://nwpk.org/projects.html/> (accessed 20.05.19.).

Grantham-McGregor, S., 2002. Linear growth retardation and cognition. Lancet 359, 542.

Groce, N., Challenger, E., Berman-Bieler, R., Farkas, A., Yilmaz, N., Schultink, W., et al., 2014. Malnutrition and disability: unexplored opportunities for collaboration. Pediatr. Int. Child Health 34, 308–314.

Haider, A., Zaidi, M., 2017. Food Consumption Patterns and Nutrition Disparity in Pakistan. <https://mpra.ub.uni-muenchen.de/83522/1/MPRA_paper_83522.pdf> (accessed 08.06.19.).

Kapur, A., 2007. Economic analysis of diabetes care. Indian J. Med. Res. 125, 473.

Khalid, N., Aslam, Z., Kausar, F., Irshad, H., Anwer, P., 2017. Maternal malnutrition and its kick on child growth: an alarming trim for Pakistan. J. Food Nutr. Popul. Health 1, 3–24.

Khan, M.Z., 2016. New poverty line makes a third of Pakistanis poor. Dawn. <https://www.dawn.com/news/1250694> (accessed 08.06.19.).

Khan, Y.P., Bhutta, S.Z., Munim, S., Bhutta, Z.A., 2009. Maternal health and survival in Pakistan: issues and options. J. Obstet. Gynecol. Can. 31, 920–929.

KhanKhattak, M.M.A., Shah, J.S.A., 2010. Malnutrition and associated risk factors in pre-school children (2–5 years) in district Swabi (NWFP)—Pakistan. J. Med. Sci. 10, 34–39.

Khuwaja, S., Selwyn, B.J., Shah, S.M., 2005. Prevalence and correlates of stunting among primary school children in rural areas of southern Pakistan. J. Trop. Pediatr. 51, 72–77.

Levy, A., Fraser, D., Katz, M., Mazor, M., Sheiner, E., 2005. Maternal anemia during pregnancy is an independent risk factor for low birthweight and preterm delivery. Eur. J. Obstet. Gynecol. Reprod. Biol. 122, 182–186.

Lone, F., Qureshi, R., Emmanuel, F., 2004. Maternal anemia and its impact on perinatal outcome in a tertiary care hospital in Pakistan. East. Mediterr. Health J. 10 (6), 801–807.

Mawani, M., Ali, S.A., Bano, G., Ali, S.A., 2016. Iron deficiency anemia among women of reproductive age, an important public health problem: situation analysis. Reprod. Syst. Sex. Disord.: Curr. Res. 5, 1.

Mir, A.M., Wajid, A., Gull, S., 2012. Helping rural women in Pakistan to prevent postpartum hemorrhage: a quasi-experimental study. BMC Pregnancy Childbirth 12, 120–120.

Moss, N.E., 2002. Gender equity and socioeconomic inequality: a framework for the patterning of women's health. Soc. Sci. Med. 54, 649–661.

Niazi, A.K., Niazi, S.K., Baber, A., 2012. Nutritional programmes in Pakistan: a review. J. Med. Nutr. Nutraceut. 12, 98–100.

NIDA-Pakistan, 2019. National Integrated Development Association. Healthy Newborn Network. <https://www.healthynewbornnetwork.org/partner/national-integrated-development-association-nida-pakistan/>.

NNS, 2011. National Nutrition Survey. Aga Khan University, Pakistan, Pakistan Medical Research Council (PMRC), Nutrition Wing, Ministry of Health, Pakistan.

Nutrition International, 2019. Pakistan Priorities. <http://www.micronutrient.org/english/view.asp?x=606> (accessed 20.05.19.).

Olusanya, B.O., 2010. Is undernutrition a risk factor for sensorineural hearing loss in early infancy? Br. J. Nutr. 103, 1296–1301.

Rasanathan, K., Bennett, S., Atkins, V., Beschel, R., Carrasquilla, G., Charles, J., et al., 2017. Governing multisectoral action for health in low-and-middle-income countries. PLoS. Med. 14, e1002285.

Reinhardt, K., Fanzo, J., 2014. Addressing chronic malnutrition through multi-sectoral, sustainable approaches: a review of the causes and consequences. Front. Nutr. 1, 13–13. Available from: https://doi.org/10.3389/fnut.2014.00013.

Scheppers, E., Van Dongen, E., Dekker, J., Geertzen, J., Dekker, J., 2006. Potential barriers to the use of health services among ethnic minorities: a review. Fam. Pract. 23, 325–348.

Singh, R.B., Pella, D., Mechirova, V., Kartikey, K., Demeester, F., Tomar, R.S., et al., 2007. Prevalence of obesity, physical inactivity, and undernutrition, a triple burden of diseases during transition in a developing economy. The Five City Study Group. Acta Cardiol. 62, 119–127.

Tanzil, S., Jamali, T., 2016. Obesity, an emerging epidemic in Pakistan—a review of evidence. J. Ayub. Med. Coll. Abbottabad 28, 597–600.

UNESCO, 2019. School Health Programme. <http://unesco.org.pk/education/documents/publications/School%20Health%20Programme.pdf> (accessed 20.05.19.).
UNICEF, 2005. Nutritional Status of Pregnant Women, Children Under 5 Years Old and School Children Aged 6–7 Years. UNICEF Representative Office in Romania.
Vorster, H., Kruger, A., 2007. Poverty, malnutrition, underdevelopment and cardiovascular disease: a South African perspective. Cardiovasc. J. Afr. 18, 321.
Wagstaff, A., 2002. Poverty and health sector inequalities. Bull. World Health Organ. 80, 97–105.
Waterlow, J., 2006. Protein-Energy Malnutrition (reprint of original 1992 version, with new supplementary material). Smith-Gordon, London.
Wilkinson, R.G., Marmot, M., 2003. Social Determinants of Health: The Solid Facts. World Health Organization.
World Health Organization, 2000. Health System Profile, Pakistan. <http://apps.who.int/medicinedocs/documents/s17305e/s17305e.pdf> (accessed 04.04.19.).
Zimmermann, M.B., 2012. The effects of iodine deficiency in pregnancy and infancy. Paediatr. Perinat. Epidemiol. 26, 108–117.

PART 7

Food, Nutrition, and Health in Iran

CHAPTER 1

Introduction

Hamid Ezzatpanah
Department of Food Science and Technology, Science and Research Branch, Islamic Azad University, Tehran, Iran

Traditional medicine, which is a mixture of skills, wisdom, knowledge, and practices, is based on experiences and beliefs of native culture. The main aspects of treatments in this kind of medicine are hygiene and nutrition. The Middle East, particularly Persia, is proud of famous medical scientists such as Avicenna, Ibn Sina (CE 980–1037), and Mohammad Ibn Zakaria Razi, Rhazes (CE 865–925), who made the country distinguished with a heritage of ancient health-promoting remedies including ethnic foods. Razi, more than 12 centuries ago, considered the nutritional effect of foods as well as the modified diet as prescribed remedial treatment. Recently, it has been revealed that the term medicinal foods in the traditional medical sciences of Iran is very close to the definition of functional foods in modern medical sciences.

Food processing practices are generally used to convert naturally available food sources to safe, wholesome, nutritious, and palatable in an efficient and economical fashion. Age-old practices such as fermentation, as an ancient nonthermal food processing method, have been utilized in rural areas of Iran to provide self-stable food products using plant and/or animal originated raw materials such as milk and cereals. Nowadays, traditional fermented Iranian foods are widely found nationally and regionally, whereas the ethnic Persian fermented dairy products have been produced at a household scale since the earliest civilizations in the Middle East from 10,000 BCE, probably when livestock domesticated and pre-Aryans invented food fermentation.

Distinctive factors such as the method of production, tradition, culture, and region are the main causes of diversity of about 500 fermented dairy products, globally. Two notable groups of fermented dairy products are ethnic and nontraditional products. For ages, Iranians used fermentation as a practical and inexpensive method of food preservation with or without heating. Among different mammal species, ovine, caprine, dromedary, bovine, buffalo, and even mare milk have been utilized to produce Persian ethnic dairy products, but their preparation procedures have remained as crude arts. The methods of preparation of these kinds of food have been passed down by word of mouth and regrettably, there is no documented reference for Iranian fermented foods.

For a long time, organoleptic attributes such as appearance, aroma, taste, texture, and flavor have played as the main crucial, basic qualitative attributes of Iranian

Nutritional and Health Aspects of Food in South Asian Countries
DOI: https://doi.org/10.1016/B978-0-12-820011-7.00029-0

fermented foods, while currently new scientific evidence revealed a wide range of hidden healthy features resulting in the consideration of traditional methods of food fermentation far above sensory or preservation goals. The increase of Iranian consumer awareness in terms of potential health-promoting effects of traditional foods led to the expansion of the ethnic functional food market in the country. These driving parameters encouraged Iranian researchers to conduct scientific investigations on these types of foods, leading to newly published articles on practices, composition, nutritional and physicochemical properties, and their potential health-promoting effects. The most interesting documented articles are related to the fermentation of dairy foods. For instance, Iranian researchers have reported antipathogenic activities, cholesterol assimilation features of lactic acid bacteria (LAB), as well as physicochemical, rheological, and sensory properties of traditional sour buttermilk, Kashk, Kashk-e Zard, Tarkhineh, and ethnic Persian cheeses such as Pot, Siamazgi, and Lighvan.

In sour Doogh or sour buttermilk, occluded and nonstarter LAB mostly the genera of *Lactobacillus* and *Pediococcus* and probably yeasts play a very critical role in terms of the shelf life elongation, creation of specific sensory attributes, and making it as a functional food. These microorganisms typically convert lactose in milk to organic acids mainly lactic acid in sour Doogh and increase the titratable acidity to 130–180 Dornic degrees and lower the pH to ranges from 3.4 to 3.9. They are also very important in other types of fermented milks such as Mast (yogurt), cheeses as well as a fermented mixture of milk–cereal products such as Kashk, Kashk-e Zard, and Tarkhineh.

Kashk and other types of milk–cereal-based fermented products have been produced traditionally in Iran to provide securely nutritious sources of protein and nutritive minerals when seasonally the availability of fresh milk products is limited. Kashk is a more dairy-based product rather than Kashk-e Zard and Tarkhined that might contain more cereals than milk. Generally, they are produced as follows:

1. Fermented full-fat ovine or ovine/caprine milk yogurt is converted to butter and sour buttermilk in a special device called Mashk.
2. Sour Doogh is boiled to concentrate and reach specific consistency and in some cases mixed with bulgar or cereal flour.
3. Semisolid fermented products are sun dried.

These nutritionally well-balanced dried fermented milk–cereal-based products are stored in ambient temperature for about 4 years.

Although, currently, more than 85% of total milk production of Iran is bovine milk, nonbovine milk mainly sheep milk has been used for producing some Iranian cheeses, while fermentation without heating and brining have been applied as two main crucial steps of cheese making from about 8000–9000 years ago. The most important types of fresh or ripened cheeses have been produced in areas around Zagros and Alborz mountain ranges. The ripening of Iranian cheeses mostly takes place in brine (e.g., Lighvan cheese), sheepskin (e.g., Siamazgi cheese), and pot (e.g., Koozeh or Pot cheese).

In the subsequent chapter, the most studied traditional fermented dairy products of Iran will be described and their tradition, practices, physicochemical and nutritional properties, as well as their health benefits will be highlighted.

CHAPTER 2

Traditional food and practices for health: Iranian dairy foods

Hamid Ezzatpanah
Department of Food Science and Technology, Science and Research Branch, Islamic Azad University, Tehran, Iran

Contents

2.1 Introduction

Middle East has been identified as the origin of yogurt, and the evolution of fermented dairy products has been referred to this part of the world (Tamime and Robinson, 2007). Various types of milk and milk products, mainly fermented types, have been produced in Iran for centuries such as yogurt, which is called Mast, sour buttermilk, Doogh, kefir, different cheeses, Kashk, Qareh-Qurut, and many others. Similar to other countries, in Iran, the request for traditional homemade foods has increased recently, resulting in the growth of protected label of the origin (PDO). PDO is applied for foods, which are produced in a defined geographical area with distinctive natural characteristics. Nowadays, PDO products, such as Tarkhineh, Doogh, Siahmazgi cheese, Lighvan cheese, dried Kashk, and many others, have been produced in Iran.

Although, in the past, ewe and goat milk were utilized as the most important raw materials, today bovine milk is the main raw material for producing these products; meanwhile, some local products are made from sheep, goat, buffalo, and even camel milk. Despite the fact that the fermentation of raw milk has been used as a nonthermal preservation method, it is also used for creating unique organoleptic properties, flavor,

Nutritional and Health Aspects of Food in South Asian Countries
DOI: https://doi.org/10.1016/B978-0-12-820011-7.00030-7

aroma, and texture in the final products. These features are applied for products produced only in specific areas of the country probably because of the particular properties of local lactic acid bacteria (LAB). Moreover, it has been demonstrated that food fermentation promotes the nutritional quality and safety of the product via improving the digestibility of food compounds as well as eliminating or decreasing the antinutritive components and toxins in the final products (Mathara et al., 2008).

2.2 The importance of lactic acid bacteria in Iranian traditional dairy foods

Several researchers have done the isolation and identification of LAB in fermented dairy foods of the country for decades to use the most suitable ones in the manufacturing of dairy products and maintaining the LAB diversity of particular areas. LAB are found in nature as well as fermented foods, for example, fermented milk and milk products. They are used as a starter culture in many types of cultured foods and present in many other fermented products as nonstarter LAB.

Fermentation process takes place using various components of milk, but LAB initially produce organic acids, mostly lactic acid by metabolizing the lactose, resulting in a reduced pH, increased titratable acidity (TA). Therefore they create unfavorable environments for both spoilage and pathogenic microorganisms (Aslim et al., 2005) also by producing a broad range of antimicrobial substances such as acetoin, bacteriocins that are antimicrobial peptides, or proteins synthesized by specific LAB strains, diacetyl, ethanol, formic acid, and hydrogen peroxide (Yang et al., 2014).

2.2.1 Lactic acid bacteria in raw milk

The presence of LAB in raw milk has been reported previously (Ortu et al., 2007; Sharma et al., 2013). Yousefi et al. (2011) investigated new strains of bacteriocin-producing LAB with antimicrobial activity in sheep and goat milk samples collected from various parts of Iran. They found that two strains of *Enterococcus* producing enterocin-like substances had a broad antibacterial activity against *Listeria monocytogenes* and *Staphylococcus aureus*. These substances with molecular weights between 24 and 29 KD were stable in a broad range of pH (3−10), maintaining their activity after 28 days of storage at refrigeration temperature, and some of them were also heat-stable (Yousefi et al., 2011).

2.3 Sour buttermilk

For centuries, sour buttermilk is produced using sheep milk in different parts of mountain ranges of Zagros and Alborz in the west and north of the country, respectively. It is the aqueous part of full-fat yogurt that remained after churning in

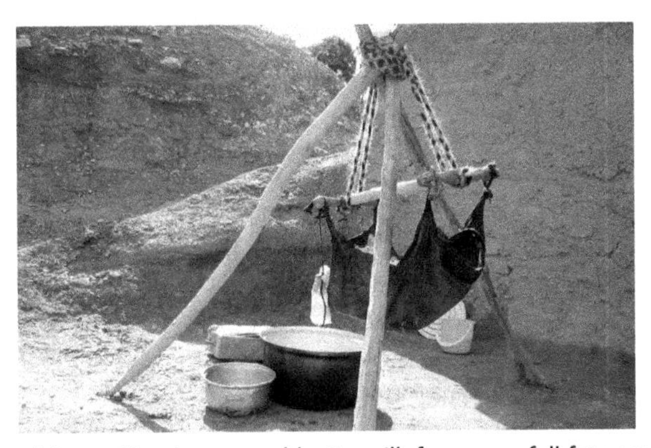

Figure 2.1 Mashk used for making butter and buttermilk from sour full-fat yogurt.

sheepskin, Mashk traditional device made from hide (Fig. 2.1) and Tulum (a traditional device made from the wood of the tree and depleted inside of tree) for butter making. As a refreshing and pleasant beverage, it is consumed in spring and summer months when ewe milk is available. Mohamadi et al. (2012) investigated the chemical composition and physical properties of samples of sour buttermilk or butter Doogh collected from the East-Azarbayejan province. The percentages of total solids (TS), crude protein (CP), lactose, ash, fat, and salt content were in the ranges of 3.51–5.47, 1.99–2.75, 0.31–0.97, 0.29–0.79, 0.16–0.45, and 0.16–0.27, respectively. The density, pH, and TA of the product were found to be in the ranges of 1.0191–1.0264 g/cm^3, 3.64–3.81 and 0.91–1 (LA%). They also demonstrated that the lactation period has a significant effect on both the chemical and physical properties of buttermilk (Mohamadi et al., 2012). Iranmanesh et al. (2012) investigated the presence of LAB in ewe milk, sour yogurt, and buttermilk produced in Mashk. *Pediococcus acidilactici* was found in both milk and buttermilk, and hence it was assumed that this isolate was able to tolerate high processing temperatures and survived in the final product (buttermilk) or might be added to the product after boiling probably originated from Mashk (Iranmanesh et al., 2012). The same researchers isolated LAB-producing bacteriocin-like inhibitory substances from milk, yogurt, and buttermilk (Fig. 2.2). The inhibitory actions of selected strains were examined against *S. aureus*, *Salmonella enteritidis*, and *L. monocytogenes*. *Lactobacillus brevis*, *Lactobacillus pentosus*, *P. acidilactici*, and *Lactobacillus paracasei* showed inhibitory action against the tested pathogens. Although their inhibitory action was completely inhibited by proteolytic enzymes, this ability remained unaffected by the action of pH neutralization and hydrogen peroxide (Iranmanesh et al., 2014). The ability of isolated strains was also characterized by cholesterol assimilation. The highest level of cholesterol reduction was found in *L. brevis*, and all the other strains were also able to reduce cholesterol to a lesser extent.

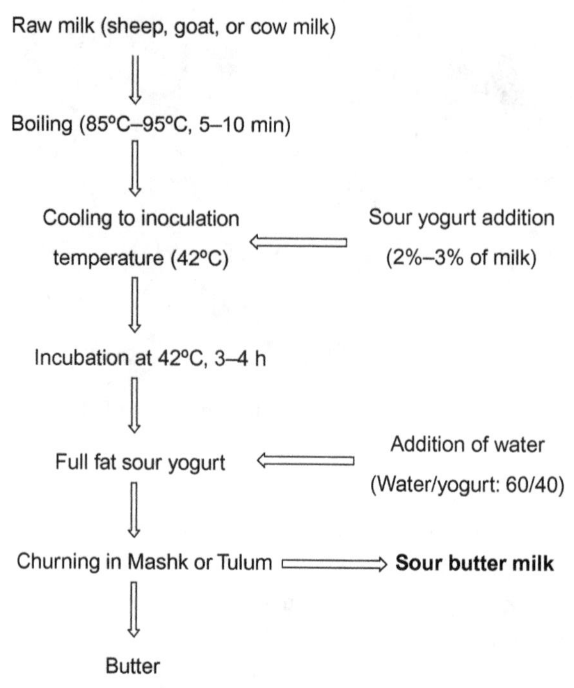

Figure 2.2 Schematic representation of sour yogurt and sour buttermilk production.

2.4 Kashk

Dried Kashk as a self-stable high protein traditional product has been produced from sour buttermilk (Fig. 2.3) in rural areas of Iran. It is a fermented/acidified, concentrated, salted, and heated product with the shelf life of 4 years at ambient temperature. The average TS, CP, NaCl, fat, and ash of dried Kashk were found to be 95.6%, 54.4%, 8.69%, 7.89%, and 3.82%, respectively, and acidity was found to be 9.05 (LA%) (Taleban and Renner, 1972). It is produced throughout the region between the eastern Mediterranean and the Indian subcontinent for centuries (Tamime et al., 2000). The name of the product differs based on used ingredients/additives, as well as the region. Tamime and Robinson (1999) reported that products containing Bulgar, parboiled cracked wheat, or flour are called as follows: Kishk in the Arab countries, Tarhana in Turkey and Greece, Chura in Tibet and Nepal, Zhum in Yemen, and Kadhi in India (Tamime and Robinson, 1999).

The main usage of dried Kashk is to prepare a kind of milk-based sauce after pulverizing and solubilizing in water (Fig. 2.4). Today, a new type of liquid Kashk is available in the market, prepared from industrially manufactured yogurt from bovine milk. However, the quality of liquid Kashk strongly depends on the type of incoming materials used, dried Kashk from ewe milk, or yogurt made from cow milk, and also

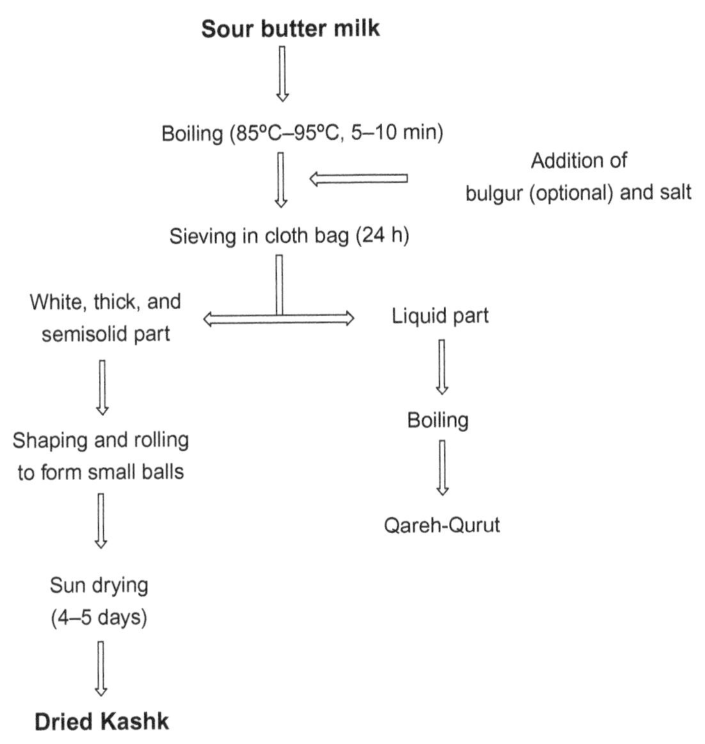

Figure 2.3 Schematic representation of dried Kashk production.

ingredients added such as Bulgur or flour. The percentages of nonfat solids, CP, NaCl, and fat in liquid Kashk are 20–25, >13, 3, and 1, respectively, and a pH less than 4.5 (Shiroodi et al., 2012).

The high-quality liquid Kashk is produced from traditional dried Kashk made from sour buttermilk and is very popular among Iranians because of its unique aroma and taste. Recently, Iranmanesh et al. (2018) characterized the volatile compounds in dried Kashk collected from various areas of Iran made from bovine or ovine milk and prepared using various production methods by producers (Fig. 2.3). Gas chromatography–mass spectrometry (GC–MS) analysis using the solid-phase microextraction detected 602 compounds in dried Kashk gathered from 11 parts of the country. They claimed that the volatile profiles of Kashk prepared using bovine or ovine raw milk were quite different. Alkanes, aldehydes, free fatty acids (FFA), esters, terpenes, sulfur compounds, ketones, alcohols, and terpenoids were the main compounds responsible for the flavor in dried Kashk. Alkenes and aldehydes were found more abundantly in samples from ovine milk than cow's milk. Higher content of aldehydes was found in samples containing bulgur or flour. A higher lipolysis rate of fat during the process of preparing sour buttermilk from sour full-fat yogurt in Mashk or Tulum is probably

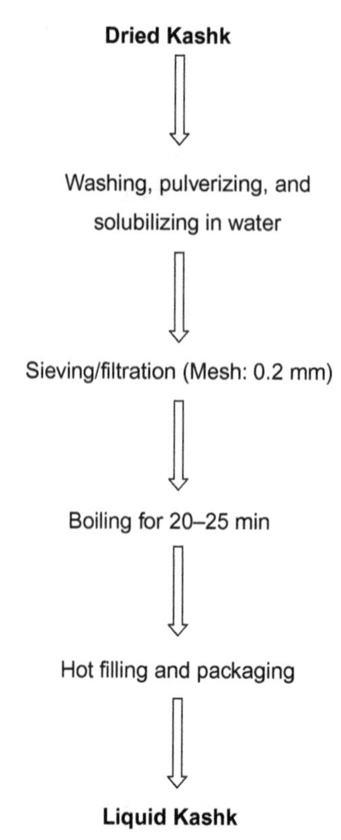

Figure 2.4 Schematic representation of liquid Kashk production.

the main reason for the high content of FFAs in Kashk samples. Higher alkenes were found in samples, which were made from ovine milk (Iranmanesh et al., 2018).

2.5 Kashk-e Zard and Tarkhineh

In the west of Iran, Hamedan, Kermanshah, and Kurdistan Provinces, Tarkhineh has been produced for centuries and it is called Tarkhowana or Doowina in Kurdish. Bulgar is soaked or boiled in sour buttermilk, followed by fermentation for 7–10 days. Ingredients such as salt, spices, and condiments are added to the semisolid product, shaped to small pieces, and sun dried.

One of the most popular fermented products in Sistan and Baluchestan Provinces is Kashk-e Zard. It is made by mixing cereal flour (mainly wheat flour), sour yogurt, salt, condiments, and spices followed by lactic and alcoholic fermentation for several days. The ratio of yogurt to cereal flour is 65/35. It is produced by two-step fermentation; first, a dough-like product is made by cereal flour followed by the addition of the first portion of yogurt and salt and kept to be fermented in a closed container in a warm place for 7 days. Then, another portion of yogurt is added and is homogenized by kneading the dough-like product. Then, spices, condiments, and garlic are added and are kept to ferment for 1 week. The fermented dough as the product is sun dried followed by grinding to granule with 1–3 mm dimensions.

Mashak et al. (2014) studied the chemical composition and microbial quality of Kashk-e Zard and Tarkhineh, as traditional Iranian cereal–dairy-based fermented foods. They gathered samples of Kashk-e Zard from household producers and market retailers of Sistan and Baluchestan Province and Tarkhineh samples from Kurdistan, Kermanshah, and Hamedan Provinces. Both products contained high TS (95%<) and carbohydrate (72%<) contents. Higher protein content was found in Tarkhineh (14.66%) compared to Kashk-e Zard (12.68%), and low-fat contents were reported in Tarkhineh (1.59%) as well as Kashk-e Zard (2.23%). pH in Tarkhineh (4.91) was higher than that in Kashk-e Zard (4.31). Although they isolated *S. aureus* from 67.5% samples of Kashk-e Zard and 77.5% samples of Tarkhineh as well as *Bacillus cereus* from all samples of Kashk-e Zard and 62.5% samples of Tarkhineh, they claimed that the levels of microbial contamination are very low and are not considered as hazards. They also recommended changing unhygienic traditional methods of production to ameliorated conditions to eliminate or reduce pathogenic microorganisms in the products (Mashak et al., 2014).

2.6 Iranian traditional cheese types

2.6.1 Pot cheese

Pot cheese is an Iranian traditional cheese that is renowned for its unique aroma and flavor (Fig. 2.5). Nonstarter LAB are the main responsible microflora of Pot cheese as no starter culture is used for producing this type of cheese. Ghaderi et al. (2013) studied the type of LAB involved in the ripening process of Pot cheese produced in Sardasht city in West Azerbaijan Province, northwest of Iran. They isolated 51 strains; the dominant genera were *Lactobacilli* (37.3%), *Enterococci* (25.5%), *Lactococci* (19.6%), *Leuconostoc* (9.8%), and *Pediococci* (7.8%). In ripened Pot cheese, dominant isolated species was *Enrococcus faecium* (8 isolates), *Lactococcus lactis* spp. *Lactis* (7 isolates), *Lactobacillus casei* spp. *casei* (4 isolates), and *P. acidilactici* (4 isolates). They assumed that these species contribute to the ripening process and development of unique aroma and flavor of the Iranian Pot cheese (Ghaderi et al., 2013).

2.6.2 Siahmazgi cheese

Siahmazgi cheese is made from ovine milk or a mixture of ovine and caprine milks in the Siahmazgi village, suburbs of Rasht, Gilan Province, and north of Iran. The curd is kept in special conditions in sheepskin during a 6 months ripening period. It has its

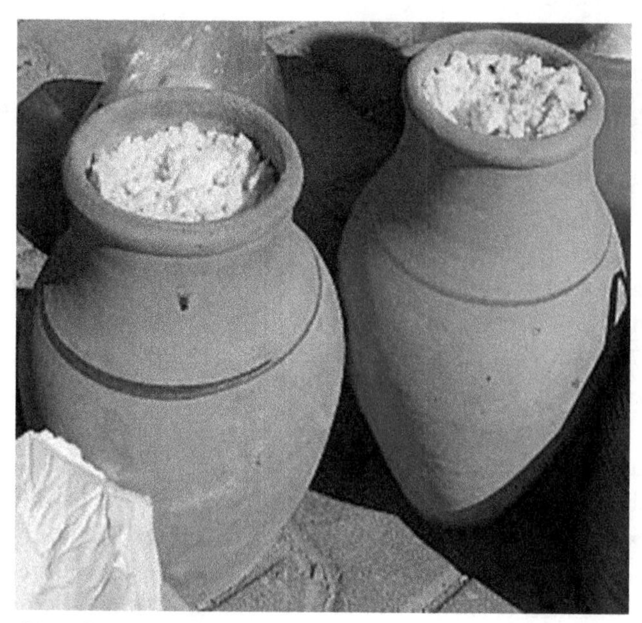

Figure 2.5 Ripened Pot cheese.

own distinct physicochemical and textural characteristics such as an extremely firm texture with some pea-sized holes, yellowish appearance and fermented taste (Farahani et al., 2014). Farahani et al. (2014) studied the effect of ripening time (6 months) on the chemical, physicochemical, rheological, and textural characteristics of Siahmazgi cheese. Rheological and textural properties were determined using a rheometer (frequency sweep) and texture analyzer (uniaxial compression). The measured values including pH, TA, TS, fat, protein, ash, salt content, water-soluble nitrogen (WSN) in total nitrogen (TN), and nonprotein-nitrogen in TN significantly increased during ripening ($P < .05$). They characterized this kind of cheese by its respectively high values of TS (59.95 ± 0.08 g/100 g), salt (5.65 ± 0.05 g/100 g), and ash (7.24 ± 0.02 g/100 g) contents and categorized it as a kind of full-fat semihard cheese. Regarding rheological and textural properties, storage modulus (G'), loss modulus (G''), fracture stress (sf), and firmness increased while loss tangent and fracture strain decreased during ripening.

Zamani (2016) isolated LAB from this type of cheese and studied the probiotic potential of isolated LAB. He reported that one strain, labeled as Lb3, showed good probiotic properties, tolerance to low pH, bile, and simulated gastrointestinal tract conditions, resistance to Streptomycin, Vancomycin, and Polymixin B, and effective antibacterial activity against two Gram-negative pathogens, lacking hemolytic activity as well as high β-galactosidase activity. The strain Lb3 was identified as *Lactobacillus plantarum* CJLP55 using biochemical characterization and *16S rRNA* sequencing assay (Zamani, 2016).

2.6.3 Lighvan cheese

Lighvan cheese, the most famous Iranian ethnic cheese, is very similar to Greek feta cheese. It has been produced for hundreds of years mainly from raw sheep milk or a mixture of sheep and goat milk in northwest of Iran, East Azerbaijan province, and Lighvan village. Every year more than 4000 tons of Lighvan cheese is produced where one fourth is exported to Japan, Canada, United States, and Malaysia. More than 200 dairies produce the artisanal Lighvan cheese in the Lighvan village with a population of about 5000 (Donnelly and Kehler, 2016). This kind of white brined cheese has a sour and salty flavor, and probably umami taste. The brittle semisoft Lighvan cheese has round shape cheese holes, which look like tears.

The TS and fat contents in sheep milk are much higher than those in bovine milk (Fox et al., 2017). Different attributes of sheep milk products, for example, Lighvan cheese are influenced by the composition of sheep milk. Table 2.1 shows the composition of sheep milk, Lighvan, and other brined cheeses.

According to Abrahamsen and Rysstad (1991), the most abundant amino acids in cow, goat, and sheep milk are glutamic acid (Glu), followed by proline (Table 2.2).

Lighvan cheese, as a sort of brined cheese, needs ripening to develop the required properties. Similar to other brined cheese, this kind of unpasteurized cheese is produced in warm climates and the usage of salt as a preservative is essential. The procedure of Lighvan cheese production starts from raw milk, mostly sheep milk and 20%–30% goat milk followed by renneting the cheese milk without the addition of starter culture. In other words, the LAB in the production of cheese originate particularly from raw milk. After curdling, fresh curd is poured in fabric baggage in triangular molds and maintained until complete drainage takes place. The triangular curds with a thickness of 20 cm are removed from the bags and cut into 3D shapes, salted with granular salt, and on the next day are transferred to tins. Although the bottom of the tins is filled with salt, this is distributed between curd cubes. Salted curds are kept at 14°C–16°C for 4–5 days followed by whey removal and filling with brine (6%–8% NaCl). Then, tins are closed and stored at 14°C–16°C. After 2 weeks, they are transferred to cold stores to start ripening. The ripening period for Lighvan cheese is usually 3–12 months. The pH value in ripened Lighvan cheese is about 4.87, whereas in other brined cheeses is 4.2–4.8. Aminifar et al. (2010) investigated the physiochemical

Table 2.1 Gross composition of sheep milk, Lighvan cheese, and brined cheese (percentage).

	Moisture	Total solids	Protein	Fat	Fat in dry matter	Salt	Salt in moisture
Sheep milk	81.5	18.5	5.15	6.82	–	–	–
Lighvan cheese	53.75	46.25	–	17.27	37.34	3.68	6.85
Brined cheese	50–58	42–50	17≤	–	45–50	–	5.5–9

Table 2.2 The amino acid contents in bovine, caprine, and ovine milk (mg amino acid/g total amino acid).

Species	*n*	Asp	Glu	Ser	Gly	His	Arg	Thr	Ala	Pro	Tyr	Val	Met	Cys	Ile	Leu	Phe	Lys
Cow	4	70.5	208.2	56.1	18.1	24.1	34.1	42.1	32.1	100.4	47.1	52.2	26.1	9.1	47.1	99.1	50.1	86.2
Goat	2	75.1	209.1	49.5	18.2	26.1	29.1	49.1	34.5	106.8	38.1	61.1	25.2	9.1	48.1	96.3	47.1	80.1
Sheep	6	75.2	203.4	52.1	18.1	26.1	34.1	41.1	40.1	102.2	47.2	57.2	29.1	8.1	49.1	90.4	48.1	83.3

characteristics, microstructure, and texture of Lighvan cheese over a 90-day ripening period. They found that the moisture content of the cheese decreased during storage and the salt-in-moisture ratio increased during this period. The most important biochemical change of the Lighvan cheese during aging was the extent of proteolysis. The WSN to TN ratio increased significantly during ripening (Aminifar et al., 2010). The volatile compounds (acids, esters, alcohols, cyclic aromatic compounds, ketones, and aldehydes) and protein profiles of Lighvan cheese over a 90-day ripening period were investigated by Aminifar et al. (2014). They used sodium dodecyl sulfate-polyacrylamide gel electrophoresis (SDS-PAGE) for the assessment of protein degradation during the ripening period. They revealed that the degradation of β- and αS-casein was higher during the initial stage of ripening (first month) of ripening than the last stages. Lavasani et al. (2012) studied the physicochemical and biochemical changes of Lighvan cheese over 90 days of ripening in brine. Acidity, pH, dry matter, fat values, lipolysis level, WSN, TN, ripening index (RI), trichloroacetic acid-soluble nitrogen (TCA-SN), and organoleptic assessments were analyzed. Dry matter and fat values decreased during ripening. Lipolysis level, RI, TCA-SN values, and salt content increased continuously until the end of the ripening period, but TN decreased throughout a 90-day storage period.

2.7 Conclusion and future perspectives

Nowadays genetics, environment, and particularly diet are the main players of human health, and increasingly health promoting and prevention of diseases have been connecting to food and food ingredients. Although, for centuries, food and food components have been considered as a remedy for treating many diseases in Persia, recently, Iranian ethnic dairy products have attracted the attention of scientists, researchers, processors, and consumers owing to their nutritional value, health-promoting, and unique organoleptic properties. Nevertheless, bovine milk products are produced these days at an industrial scale, nonbovine milk (mainly sheep milk products) have been the main traditional dairy foods such as sour buttermilk, Kashk, Kashk-e zard, Tarkhineh, Pot cheese, Siamazgi cheese, Lighvan cheese, and many other Persian ethnic dairy foods. Iranians, like other communities, are seeking safe foods containing bioactive components and/or probiotics originating from tradition or novelty, to prevent or tackle illnesses. Therefore traditional dairy foods have considered over and above short-term commercial aspects and have been the point of focus for long-term scientific investigations. Self-carbonated sour buttermilk with hypocholestrolemic properties has been consumed by consumers who regularly intake high amounts of milk fat. Within this context, self-stable Kashk has provided high calcium and protein contents for Iranians specifically children and the elderly. Adapted LAB have acted as the most important factor for therapeutic properties and self-stability of sour Doogh and various types of cheeses such as Pot, Siamazgi, and Lighvan. Additionally, they have contributed to provide distinct aroma, flavor, taste, and structure to sour buttermilk, Kashk, Kashk-e zard, Tarkhineh, Pot cheese, Siamazgi cheese, and Lighvan cheese.

Safe, functional, and traditional Iranian dairy foods, with accepted organoleptic properties for a global consumer base, are yet to be investigated. In addition, the type and the amount of bioactive components/probiotic in a particular ethnic product should be optimized based on personalized nutrition requirements. The potential of those products needs to be proved by scientifically established clinical trials. The mechanism of controlling the pathogens by LAB or other factors remains to be better understood through the systematic study of Iranian traditional dairy foods.

References

Abrahamsen, R.K., Rysstad, G., 1991. Fermentation of goats' milk with yogurt starter bacteria: a review. Cult. Dairy Prod. J. 26, 20–26.

Aminifar, M., Hamedi, M., Emam-Djomeh, Z.A.H.R.A., Mehdinia, A., 2010. Microstructural, compositional and textural properties during ripening of Lighvan cheese, a traditional raw sheep cheese. J. Texture Stud. 41 (4), 579–593.

Aminifar, M., Hamedi, M., Emam-Djomeh, Z., Mehdinia, A., 2014. Investigation on proteolysis and formation of volatile compounds of Lighvan cheese during ripening. J. Food Sci. Technol. 51 (10), 2454–2462.

Aslim, B., Yuksekdag, Z.N., Sarikaya, E., Beyatli, Y., 2005. Determination of the bacteriocin-like substances produced by some lactic acid bacteria isolated from Turkish dairy products. LWT-Food Sci. Technol. 38 (6), 691–694.

Donnelly, C., Kehler, M., 2016. The Oxford Companion to Cheese. Oxford University Press.

Farahani, G., Ezzatpanah, H., Abbasi, S., 2014. Characterization of Siahmazgi cheese, an Iranian ewe's milk variety: assessment of physico-chemical, textural and rheological specifications during ripening. LWT-Food Sci. Technol. 58 (2), 335–342.

Fox, P.F., Guinee, T.P., Cogan, T.M., McSweeney, P.L., 2017. Fundamentals of Cheese Science. Springer, Boston, MA, pp. 185–229.

Ghaderi, M., Azizi, A., Ezzatpanah, H., Hejazi, M., Hemmasi, A., 2013. Isolation and identification of lactic acid bacteria in traditional pot cheese. Iran. J. Agric. Eng. Res. 14 (3), 83–96.

Iranmanesh, M., Ezzatpanah, H., Mojgani, N., Torshizi, M.K., Aminafshar, M., Maohamadi, M., 2012. Isolation of lactic acid bacteria from ewe milk, traditional yoghurt and sour buttermilk in Iran. Eur. J. Food Res. Rev. 2 (3), 79–92.

Iranmanesh, M., Ezzatpanah, H., Mojgani, N., 2014. Antibacterial activity and cholesterol assimilation of lactic acid bacteria isolated from traditional Iranian dairy products. LWT-Food Sci. Technol. 58 (2), 355–359.

Iranmanesh, M., Ezzatpanah, H., Akbari-Adergani, B., Karimi Torshizi, M.A., 2018. SPME/GC-MS characterization of volatile compounds of Iranian traditional dried Kashk. Int. J. Food Prop. 21 (1), 1067–1079.

Lavasani, S., Ehsani, M.R., Mirdamadi, S., Ebrahim Zadeh Mousavi, M.A., 2012. Changes in physicochemical and organoleptic properties of traditional Iranian cheese Lighvan during ripening. Int. J. Dairy Technol. 65 (1), 64–70.

Mashak, Z., Sodagari, H., Mashak, B., Niknafs, S., 2014. Chemical and microbial properties of two Iranian traditional fermented cereal-dairy based foods: Kashk-e Zard and Tarkhineh. IJB 4 (12), 124–133.

Mathara, J.M., Schillinger, U., Kutima, P.M., Mbugua, S.K., Guigas, C., Franz, C., et al., 2008. Functional properties of *Lactobacillus plantarum* strains isolated from Maasai traditional fermented milk products in Kenya. Curr. Microbiol. 56 (4), 315–321.

Mohamadi, M., Ezzatpanah, H., Mahdavi, A.H., Mohammadifar, M., Aminafshar, M., 2012. The effect of lactation period on the chemical composition and physical properties of traditional Iranian bytter-milk. Iran. J. Food Technol.Nutr. 9 (2), 37–44.
Ortu, S., Felis, G.E., Marzotto, M., Deriu, A., Molicotti, P., Sechi, L.A., et al., 2007. Identification and functional characterization of *Lactobacillus* strains isolated from milk and Gioddu, a traditional Sardinian fermented milk. Int. Dairy J. 17 (11), 1312–1320.
Sharma, R., Sanodiya, B.S., Thakur, G.S., Jaiswal, P., Pal, S., Sharma, A., et al., 2013. Characterization of lactic acid bacteria from raw milk samples of cow, goat, sheep, camel and buffalo with special elucidation to lactic acid production. Microbiol. Res. J. Int. 743–752.
Shiroodi, S.G., Mohammadifar, M.A., Gorji, E.G., Ezzatpanah, H., Zohouri, N., 2012. Influence of gum tragacanth on the physicochemical and rheological properties of kashk. J. Dairy Res. 79 (1), 93–101.
Taleban, H. von, Renner, E., 1972. Untersuchungen über Kashk-ein milchprodukt in Iran. Milchwissenschaft 27, 753–756.
Tamime, A.Y., Robinson, R.K., 1999. Yoghurt: Science and Technology. Woodhead Publishing.
Tamime, A.Y., Robinson, R.K., 2007. Tamime and Robinson's Yoghurt: Science and Technology. Elsevier.
Tamime, A.Y., Muir, D.D., Khaskheli, M., Barclay, M.N.I., 2000. Effect of processing conditions and raw materials on the properties of Kishk 1. Compositional and microbiological qualities. LWT-Food Sci. Technol. 33 (6), 444–451.
Yang, S.C., Lin, C.H., Sung, C.T., Fang, J.Y., 2014. Antibacterial activities of bacteriocins: application in foods and pharmaceuticals. Front. Microbiol. 5, 241.
Yousefi, L., Ehsani, M., Fazeli, M., Mojgani, N., Ezatpanah, H., 2011. Characterization of enterocin-like substances produced by two strains of enterococci isolated from ewe's and goat's milks. Iran. J. Nutr. Sci. Food Technol. 6 (1), 33–42.
Zamani, H., 2016. Isolation of a potentially probiotic *Lactobacillus plantarum* from Siahmezgi cheese and its characterization as a potentially probiotic. Biol. J. Microorg. 4 (16), 97–108.

PART 8

Common Regulatory and Safety Issue and Future Outlook for South Asia Region

CHAPTER 1

Lifecycle stages for food safety of traditional foods

R.B. Smarta
Interlink Marketing Consultancy Pvt. Ltd., Mumbai, India; Hon. Secretary, Health Foods And Dietary Supplements Association (HADSA), Mumbai, India

Contents

1.1 Introduction

Food safety refers to the prevention of contamination and deterioration of food as well as to ensure quality food at the level of production, distribution, and consumption (Prabhakar et al., 2010). In today's world, food safety has become an important issue; yet, it is a very nascent stage of research and application. In view of population explosion in the South Asian population, if this issue is not considered in the right spirit, it may hinder achieving safe food delivery, especially of traditional foods.

South Asian countries such as Bangladesh, India, Nepal, Pakistan, and Sri Lanka have a variety of ethnic dishes that are nutrient dense. Pakistan shares common ethnic and traditional food similar to its neighbor countries such as India and Afghanistan. Indian traditional foods are relished with pungent spices such as cumin, turmeric, cardamom, pepper, and ginger. The traditional foods of India are globally accepted for their use of spices and herbs. The cooking style and authentic ingredients used in Indian traditional food vary from North to South or from East to West.

Nutritional and Health Aspects of Food in South Asian Countries
DOI: https://doi.org/10.1016/B978-0-12-820011-7.00031-9

Bangladesh, being a coastal region, has rice and fish as a staple food. The indigenous fishes such as *ilish* (Hilsa fish) and *shutki* (dried fish) are nutritious and widely consumed.

Ancient wisdom is nowadays supported and promoted by modern scientific research for its high degree of antioxidants, phytoestrogen, and vitamins. Nepal could be one of the best examples, as one of the indigenous communities from Nepal, named *Chepangs* or *Prajas*, has enormous knowledge about large numbers of plant species, which they have used for centuries (The Himalaya Times, 2018).

1.2 Food safety concerns

South Asia is renowned in the world for the legacy of the diversity of traditional foods; yet, with the increasing middle class, complex supply chain, and growing economies, this region is facing food safety challenges. In addition, after accepting the sustainable development goals to end hidden hunger, food safety must be the top priority of all South Asian countries with the treasure of traditional foods. South Asia contains almost half of the world population. Hence, developing a robust network for testing food safety is also complex. Hence, the investment done in food safety remains low due to the tropical weather conditions. Even the geographic and demographic complexities have made food safety complex in this region.

1.2.1 Food safety frameworks

Although regulations for food safety in most of the South Asian countries are getting tighter, coordination between government departments and agencies can often be time consuming and confusing and difficult for traceability and detection. Food safety does not just raise consumer safety but also raises a company or brand's reputation and revenues. Hence, elimination of food safety risks from farm to fork needs to be ensured. In addition, suppliers should manage the food safety cycle from the quality of raw materials to the export, transport, storage, packaging, and labeling.

1.3 Why food safety

An estimated three million people around the world, in developed and developing countries, die every year from food and water-borne disease, with millions more becoming sick (Food and Agriculture Organization of United States_EMPRES Food Safety). The occurrence of such diseases can easily escalate to a food safety emergency situation, which can adversely impact national economies and livelihoods through reduced availability of food. Although with the globalization of food supply people have become concerned about food safety, serious steps need to be taken to control and monitor food safety in South Asian countries.

1.3.1 Regulatory mechanisms

As every country moves from the nonregulatory phase to a regulatory phase, each has to establish its food policy and system comprehensively in tune with action points to implement and institutionalize it for better monitoring and controls.

Most of the countries such as Australia, China, India, Indonesia, Japan, Malaysia, and Thailand have developed food safety laws and programs. They also have started creating implementation agencies to enforce appropriate laws and regulations. Safety standards are defined on the basis of requirements and practices for food producers, manufacturers, handlers, processors, food supply outlets, and food consumers, especially of processed traditional foods.

This entire chain along with management of the lifecycle of food safety ensures that hygiene and health are maintained at every stage and the regulatory mechanism works through it regularly. Organic farming has been an offshoot of this process in many countries, and many countries are working on the same effectively with the ingredients being organic for the preparation of traditional foods.

Looking at the South Asian countries as an aggregate, the total food demand and the consumption right through the process of management of lifecycle stages, a nodal agency needs to be created to differentiate food safety regulatory systems for the harmonization of food safety in this region, very similar to the advisory body like CODEX especially for traditional foods.

1.3.2 Nonregulatory mechanism

Many social and even corporate houses that have a focus on food and food products can perhaps start the promotion of sustainable and safe production processes in their own capacity. Contract farming, which takes care of the entire food safety lifecycle, works out better for many corporates as a nonregulatory mechanism. Many aspects of sustainable production of safe food such as crop rotation, allowing the soil to regain fertility, controlling flooding, damage control procedures for draught, integrated pest management, promotional, and diversification of agroforestry can be a very important process of the nonregulatory mechanism. Besides infrastructure and food preservation practices, it can be training and skills development facilitated in the hospitality sectors such as hotels and catering institutions.

Hence, food safety has plenty of lifecycle stages in the chain of food production, transportation, consumption, and disposal as well as changing hands by various food handlers making it difficult to reach the target population of any area or region.

1.4 Lifecycle of food safety

As shown in Lifecycle stages of food safety (Fig. 1.1) a the production level, food safety issues emerge owing to residual aspects of contaminants. Due to inadequate

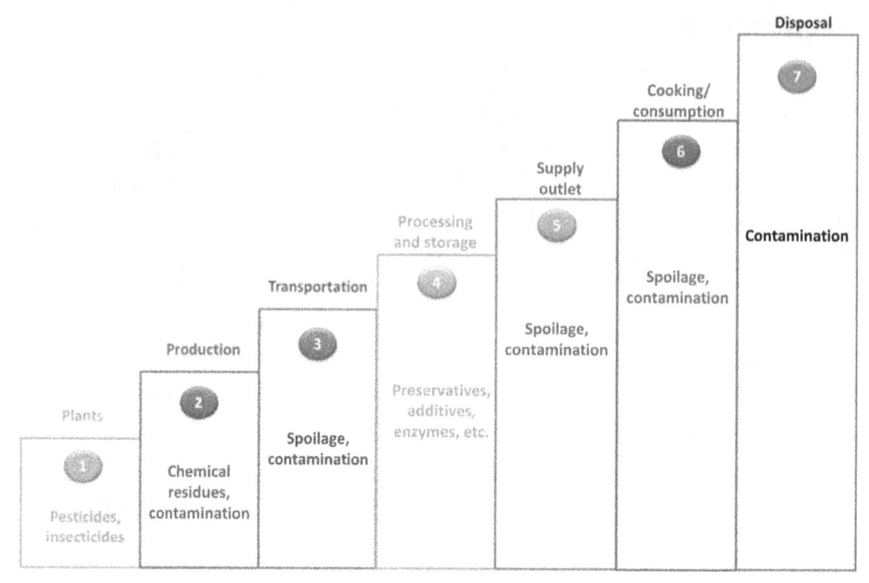

Figure 1.1 Lifecycle stages of food safety.

storage facilities and unhygienic handling of food while transportation affect the entire food safety lifecycle by the time it reaches to consumer. As a result, a single approach may not be sufficient to integrate the different stages of the lifecycle and ensure food safety. Due to this precise reason, the lifecycle approach is crucial whereby issues concerned at different stages are handled differently and yet they are integrated from one stage to another so that, in the end, food safety is the priority (Prabhakar et al., 2010).

1.5 Building stakeholder capacities

Precautions, policies, and prioritization have to be well coordinated to ensure that food safety concerns of traditional foods in the South Asian region are addressed adequately.

1.5.1 Institutional capacity

Relevant governments should create an institutional capacity among themselves to monitor and enforce safety standards in the food supply. Each country is capable of deriving safety standards on the basis of issues related to the lifecycle stages of food safety. An IT-enabled and lifecycle-based approach would provide ease to monitor and control if there is any adulteration as well as show clarity at the level of all these stages by enforcing appropriate safety standards. Trained and competent food inspectors are very vital for the execution of this entire institutionalization process.

1.5.2 Producer capacity

To get mileage and strengthen existing food producers to develop the capacity to properly handle food and manage risks that are vital to food, appropriate intervention is necessary. It has been observed that the World Bank has helped developing countries in establishing and implementing various International agreements aimed at food safety. New and modern technologies, as well as practices, would enhance good hygienic, agricultural, and manufacturing practices at small-scale food producers as well as food vendors' levels, especially for traditional foods.

1.5.3 Consumer capacity

As traditional forms of food are slowly disappearing, it is often difficult for a consumer to be aware of food safety while consuming the same in the processed form. All South Asian countries will have to start sharing information, awareness, and education among all stakeholders based on the lifecycle stages of food safety. As a result of this awareness, there will be a good holistic and integrated understanding of food safety inclusive of food labeling to improve the consumption of safe food. Food is sold at retail markets combining institutional capacity with consumer capacity. Adequate food safety that will resolve many problems of food safety starting from the stage of procurement can be ensured.

1.6 Robust approach to food safety

Each country needs to assess all lifecycle stages of food safety to identify and prioritize what needs to be done at each stage of the lifecycle. This is crucial for traditional foods too.

During the production stage, promoting sustainable production issues at higher food safety, inclusive of manure, insecticides, pesticide, and fertilizer management is needed. The next stages are basically focused on logistics and farm to fork dimensions that can be taken care by three major aspects of capacity building such as institution, producer, and consumer capacity. This will be a robust approach for the lifecycle management of food safety of traditional foods by an integrated approach for each sector.

References

Prabhakar, S.V.R.K., Sano, Daisuke, Srivastava, Nalin, 2010. Food Safety in the Asia-Pacific Region: Current Status, Policy Perspectives, and a Way Forward. Institute for Global Environmental Strategies Hayama, Japan (1).

The Himalaya Times, 2018. Wisdom of Eating: Chepangs' Food Habits <https://thehimalayantimes.com/opinion/wisdom-of-eating-chepangs-food-habits/> (accessed 15.03.19.).

Food and Agriculture Organization of United States_EMPRES Food Safety <http://www.fao.org/food/food-safety-quality/empres-food-safety/en/> (accessed 30.05.19.).

CHAPTER 2

Regulations for manufacturing traditional foods—global and regional challenges

D.B. Anantha Narayana[1] and Sudhakar T. Johnson[2]
[1]Ayurvidye Trust, and, Member, Expert Committee (Nonspecified Foods and Food Ingredients), Food Safety Standards Authority of India (FSSAI), Ministry of Health and Family Welfare, Govt. of India, Bengaluru, India
[2]Professor of Biotechnology and Center for Innovation, Incubation and Entrepreneurship, currently resides at 2-B2, Second Floor, Swarna Residency, Currency Nagar, Vijayawada - 520008, India

Contents

2.1 Descriptors and the definition of traditional foods and ethnic foods

Traditional foods (TFs) are a range of preparations or raw food commodities, the use of which is related to traditional practices experienced over centuries. Traditional foods are an integral part of the cultural heritage, history, identity, and lifestyle of a region or country (Costa et al., 2010; Trichopoulou et al., 2007). Specific eating habits also play an important role in the traditional habits of many cultures (Costa et al., 2010). Thus these foods have become part of tradition and culture. Traditional foods come with a tag of

Nutritional and Health Aspects of Food in South Asian Countries
DOI: https://doi.org/10.1016/B978-0-12-820011-7.00032-0

genuineness, minimally processed, and healthy foods. The ingredients of traditional foods are linked to local climatic and agricultural conditions that are abundantly available in addition to traditions. Due to fast-paced hectic life, lifestyle changes, and migration of rural population to nearby cities, traditional foods are rapidly disappearing from our culture (Costa et al., 2010; Trichopoulou et al., 2006). Nonetheless, there is an increased interest in traditional foods among consumers and manufacturers, as they are often perceived as having specific sensory characteristics, health benefits, and being of higher quality (Costa et al., 2010; Trichopoulou et al., 2007; Vanhonacker et al., 2010).

In most of the countries, there is currently a lack of information on the food composition of traditional foods, and it is necessary to investigate their nutrient composition by further studies (Costa et al., 2010; Trichopoulou et al., 2006). These studies are also essential for elucidating the role of such foods in the traditional dietary pattern of a population and for perpetuating the important elements of cultural inheritance (Trichopoulou et al., 2006).

Ethnic foods are regarded as unique to a particular cultural group, race, religion, nation, or heritage (Dwyer et al., 2003). "Traditional" means proven usage on the domestic market for a period that allows transmission between generations; this period is to be at least 30 years (Regulation (EU) No. 1151/2012).

A traditional food product is a product frequently consumed or associated during specific celebrations and/or seasons: for example, mass feeding during wedding and other large celebrations, in places of worship, mid-day meals served to school-going children, in institutional catering, etc. Such use does not involve prepackaging. The art and science of such TF are normally transmitted from one generation to another, and they are prepared with care in a particular way according to the gastronomic heritage, with specified processing/manipulation that is distinguished and known because of their sensory properties and associated to a certain local area, region, or country (Vanhonacker et al., 2008).

2.2 Categorization and classification of traditional food

2.2.1 Based on primary food

They may be based on primary food namely rice, wheat, pulses/lentils/legumes, cereals, corns and oats, millets, milk and milk products, vegetables and fruits, condiments and spices, oils, fats, and clarified butter. Combinations of one or more primary foods are most common to provide high sensorial and nutrition apart from promoting digestion and providing health benefits.

2.2.2 Based on process technology

A wide range of technologies is seen across categories in Asian practices. One distinctive feature enshrined perhaps by the wisdom of history of usage of TF in temperate countries of Asia is involvement of different thermal and nonthermal processes: dehydration/roasting/sun drying/salting/processing in brine or syrup base/frying in oil/cooking in water or steam, with or without fermentation or other pretreatments to provide requisite microbial quality and desired shelf life for the required duration. These technologies are used at every household or in eateries and restaurants, at varying scales of batch sizes. Shelf life of a few hours extending to even a few years (viz. pickles) are achieved by these processes. This is in contrast to many TFs in western nations that have much less of thermal processing involved and use cold processes along with high temperatures.

2.2.3 Based on prepared food forms

A wide range of food preparation forms (textural matrices) create attractiveness, add rich appeal, taste, and deliver a wow-like feeling. Forms cover the following: liquids (rasam, sambar), juices (fruit/vegetable juices), semisolids (purees, gojju, chutney/sauce), solids (with gravy, without gravy, reasonably dry-like rice preparations, vegetable curries), dried vegetables and fruits (curry leaf, seasoning herbs, dried gooseberries, almonds, cashews, grapes, and other dry fruits), powders of primary foods (chutney powder, fenugreek spice mix), herbs, spices, condiments in designated mixes to be consumed with other foods, roasted (nuts, spices), roasted and ground powders (coffee with chicory, various spice mixes referred as masalas), shallow/deep or shallow fried in oils or fats (Indian breads such as chapattis, nan, roti, samosa, savories), extruded forms both for use in dehydrated and hydrated matrices (noodles and vermicelli and their variants) as well as deep fried formats (wafers, chips, sandige, and pheni), concentrated milk and milk-based sweetened forms consumed in hot state (kheer, payasams) or in cold/frozen state (jamun, rosogulla, rasamalai, and kulfi), infusions and decoctions (tea and coffee), center-filled forms (samosa, obbattu, sandesh, modak), and cooked in steam with or without fermentation (pancake, idly, puttu, dhokla).

2.2.4 Emerging forms

The last two decades have led to the use of concentrated sources of primary foods or herbs, spices, pro- and prebiotics, and enzymes instead of consuming large proportions or morsels of food. Scientific studies have demonstrated the beneficial effects of the use of these concentrated sources taken either with food or before or immediately after food. They need to be used at specified levels in predetermined quality and concentration properties either as such or as enrichment with a primary food or a TF. Demands of lifestyle and changing scenarios are narrowing the border between food forms and drug formats. New categories of such concentrated sources of nutrients or nutritionals are also adopted for delivering drug formats such as pills, tablets, capsules, suspensions, and sweetened preparations in liquid form driven by convenience for usage and availability of unit serving sizes intended for improving compliance. These formats are intended to serve "consumers on the go." It is debatable whether 20 odd years of existence of these deserves the title of TF for such forms and concentrates.

Other forms or technologies including hybrid technologies exist in Asian nations. Examples cited earlier primarily cover India but all Asian nations would have equivalent examples to cite.

2.3 Trends in the last few decades

Traditional foods have started entering the market in a new form to suit modern trends, with long shelf life and new packing techniques. Asia has seen drastic changes in eating habits due to the influence of cross-cultural impacts, such as the blending of TF of different nations due to a desire for variety and fun in eating. Eating of TF coming from other cultures and nations either outside home or cooking and offering such foods to family and guests at home reduces cooking chores, drudgery, time and improves the convenience for both working women and men. This has led to increased use of partially processed or fully processed foods in prepackaged forms. Innovations in such foods, such as enrichment with specified nutrients, enhanced sensorial and textural properties, enhanced health benefits, and altered sweetness perception at low sugar levels are leading the trends. Packages that are microwavable and safe are emerging. The introduction of a new drug delivery format is another trend described in the preceding section. Countries such as India, Korea, Taiwan, and China are leading in providing equipment and machinery that can be partly or fully automated to produce the TF in readily packaged forms for retail distribution. Some of them are capable of operating complex steps for the effective processing of TF requiring multiple stages or processes. Newer technologies such as pasteurization, high temperature short exposure, tetra pack and Elo pack multiple laminate structure that fill and seal sterile products, nitrogen flushing, surface sterilization through ozonized or peroxide-based treatment, cryogenic processing and packing, canning, and preservation are some of the processes that assist and promote large-scale production of such prepackaged TF. Refrigerated containers, cold chain facilities, development of small-sized deep freezers, and refrigerators suitable for storing at retail levels to preserve the overall quality of packaged foods are driving these innovations. The classic example is of serving hot cooked food as part of mid-day meals packed in containers with lid in hot conditions across the cities under "Akshaya patra" (www.akshayapatra.com) in India. Foods are cooked at a central location and transported in vans or vehicles across a city to many teaching institutions for serving children as soon as it reaches the destination.

2.4 Basic regulations that apply to traditional food during manufacture, packing, and distribution

All TFs are made from/using primary foods approved in the national regulations. It is an accepted fact that using multiple ingredients and processing them as per traditional methods does not cause any concern for the safety of quality. This is true as long as the processes are adhered to and the processing is done in a clean and hygienic environment. Most nations do not have separate regulations for TF. All regulations that are applicable to foods apply to TF and if they are packaged for retail sale, then additional regulations that apply for packaging and labeling also apply. Nations normally have vertical standards defined and regulated for foods (primary). Using such primary foods, if a product is processed as described under categories in one of the sections discussed earlier, then national regulations have additional regulations set in place that most often cover the additives that are used for a particular TF/processed food. About two decades back, Codex Alimentarius developed horizontal standards recognizing the need for accepting and regulating processed foods. These horizontal standards specify the additives that can be used for a particular type of food mix or ready-to-eat food, or additives that are not permitted and the level of usage is specified. The term GMP is used in such horizontal standards, which means "an amount needed based on sound scientific and technological rationale." In certain instances these may also specify "lowest possible levels of usage to achieve the desired effect" for specified additives. Codex recognized that there is a need to provide technological requirements for making TFs safe in the regulations. Codex is normally adopted either in or with local adjustments by most nations. This approach, apt as it is, can be difficult for standardizing TF as the composition varies from region to region. The horizontal standards normally apply for the manufacturing of TF that are intended to be packed and distributed. However, years of experience have shown that in the case of TF prepared in large quantities (for mass serving in hotels/restaurants/ festivals/ mid-day meals), framing regulations and enforcing them are difficult and counterproductive. Instead of developing regulations, adopting safety audits, safety and risk assessments, and large-scale training and certification of workmen and premises for hygiene, hazard analysis critical control point (HACCP), good manufacturing practice (GMP), and good packaging practice are being advocated. The Indian Food Safety & Standards Act (FSSA) of the Ministry of Health & Family Welfare has adopted this approach. The Food Safety Standards Authority of India is aggressively pushing this route and building skills and competencies in the sector for processing and supply of quality and hygienic foods across the nation.

Although there are no specific standards/regulations available for TF in South Asia including India, all common regulations apply. Food Business Operators involved in the manufacture/packing/marketing of TF in India shall comply with different Food Safety and Standards Regulations as applicable. For example:

- License as per the Food Safety and Standards (Licensing and Registration of Food Businesses) Regulations, 2011 (Licensing, 2011, FSSA)
- Standards including additives and microbiological parameters as specified under the Food Safety and Standards (Food Product Standards and Food Additives) Regulation, 2011 (Standards, 2011, FSSA)
- Labeling as per Food Safety and Standards (Packaging and Labeling) Regulation, 2011 (Labelling, 2011, FSSA)
- Safety parameters such as heavy metals and residues as per the Food Safety and Standards (contaminants, toxins, and residues) Regulation, 2011 (Contaminants, 2011, FSSA)
- Packaging as per the Food Safety and Standards (Packaging) Regulations, 2018 (Packaging, 2011, FSSA)
- Advertisement and claims as per the Food Safety and Standards (Advertising and Claims) Regulations, 2018 (Claims, 2018, FSSA)

2.5 Proprietary foods

Regulations describe and define "proprietary food" (PF) as "means an article of food that has not been standardized under these regulations, but does not include novel foods, foods for special dietary uses, foods for special medical purposes, functional foods, nutraceuticals, and health supplements." Any deviation in quality parameters of a standardized food shall not qualify the resultant product as a proprietary food. As per regulations, proprietary food shall contain only those ingredients other than additives that are either standardized or permitted for use in the preparation of food products under the Food Safety Standards and Regulations and those food or ingredients mentioned in the Indian Food Composition Table, 2017 (IFCT, 2017). It may also contain vitamins and minerals in quantities not exceeding daily Recommended Dietary Allowance of the respective micronutrient.

There are no specific standards available for TF under FSS Act, 2006 and regulations thereof. However, under the Food Safety and Standards (Food Product Standards and Food Additives) Regulation, 2011, standards/regulations for Proprietary Food has been specified. Furthermore, the regulations also specify food additive provision for different food categories from 1 to 16.

Proprietary food shall use only such additives and at such levels, as specified for the category or subcategory under Appendix A of these regulations, to which the food belongs. Such a category or subcategory shall be clearly mentioned on the label along with the generic name, nature, and composition of the proprietary food.

Proprietary food shall comply with the microbiological requirements as specified in Appendix B of these regulations. If no microbiological standards are specified for any foods or food categories in Appendix B of these regulations, proprietary foods falling under such food categories shall not contain any pathogenic microorganism at a level that may render the food product unsafe.

The food business operator shall be fully responsible for the safety of the proprietary food with respect to human consumption, as such foods have a composition that has no specific standards in the regulations. As it is rather difficult to obtain intellectual property rights (patents), many marketers adopt this approach to make some changes in the formulations or format of the TF and classify them under PF and try to use it for marketing propositions as unique selling points.

2.6 International standards: Codex

The general standard for food additives (Codex STAN 192-19956) provides information on the food additive provisions that are acceptable for use in foods conforming to the food category 1–16. The broad categories include dairy products and analogs; fats and oils, and fat emulsions; fruits and vegetables, cereals and cereal products, bakery wares, meat, fish, snacks, prepared foods, etc. The packaged traditional food also needs to comply with the same based on the category in which it is falling. In case of prepared foods (category 16) that are not included in the other food categories (01–15), the additives in accordance with GMP (Table 3 of Codex STAN 192-1995, i.e., additives permitted for use in food in general) may be used under the conditions of good manufacturing practice (GMP) as outlined (Additives. GMP, CODEX 1995).

All Asian nations have equivalent/similar regulations for primary foods, TF and PF. All primary foods and additives used in TF need to comply with the regulations. For most of these, content claims of the ingredients and their nutritive values are permitted and normally health benefit claims are not made.

2.7 Labeling

Although normally there are no regulations that specify labeling requirements for TF that are served in hotels/restaurants/ festivals, there are detailed regulatory requirements for labeling of TF packed and supplied over retail. New developments in India are leading to asking the suppliers of TF in hotels/restaurants to label the vessels in which they are kept with basic information like calories per 100 g, and few other nutrient levels that can caution consumers and guide them to eat right (especially for sugar, salt, or fat content). The suppliers are being educated on these aspects to support healthy eating.

For all other packaged TF intended for retail selling distribution

There are detailed specific labeling requirements specified in the regulations as listed in the earlier section.

Mandatory requirements:

- Name of food and a descriptor for consumer understanding of the type of food.
- Composition in descending order of proportions of the ingredients, except those ingredients that are less than 1.0% of the composition can be given in any order.
- Presence of added permitted preservatives, colors, flavors, stabilizers, and any other additives.
- Serving sizes.
- Nutrition information giving the nutritional value (calories, contents of carbohydrate, protein, fat, trans fat, vitamins, and minerals, if added, and any other constituents important for health, such as soluble and insoluble fiber, added sugars, etc). These need to be given either per 100 g or per serving size. Those of the nutrients that come under RDA, the proportion of RDA contributed by the product per serving size or per 100 g, need to be given in the table.
- Directions for making and use.
- Storage conditions.
- Date of packing or manufacturing and best before use date.
- Other mandatory requirements like contents/weight or volume /number on the pack, price for sale, manufacturer's address and license number, consumer care number or an email ID for consumers to contact for any feedback, etc.
- The term "Proprietary Food."
- A special symbol as specified to indicate the nonvegetarian or vegetarian nature of the TF.

Nonmandatory requirements:

- Any cautionary statements
- Any advisories
- Allergen cautions
- Special instructions of any nature.

All Asian nations have equivalent/similar regulations for the labeling of TF and PF, though there may be variation in the way the nutritional composition is declared. Although some regulations specify for declarations similar to India, other representations like using traffic signal or giving sugar/salt/fat contents in the different pictorial depictions are also used. This is for easy understanding by the consumer so that he/she can decide which of these nutrients are above or at par or below recommended levels.

2.8 Good manufacturing practice aspects during manufacture

Manufacturers/repackers in India need to conform to the general hygienic and sanitary practices specified under Schedule 4 of the Food Safety and Standards (Licensing and

Registration of Food Businesses) Regulations, 2011. These are the basic-compulsory requirements for ensuring the safety of the food manufactured in any premise, and manufacturers need to continuously try to improve the sanitary and hygienic conditions at the premises with a goal of attaining HACCP standards. Details of these are not covered.

2.9 Traditional food for infants, children, and geriatrics

Most Asian nations have adopted fully or appropriately to the Codex regulations and Standards for Infant Foods of all categories (complete foods, complementary foods, weaning foods, cereal-based or noncereal-based, and other types). These provide detailed descriptions, usage, ages for infants and children, directions for use and compositions with minimum and maximum levels for various vitamins, minerals, amino acids, and other ingredients (like probiotics). Most of the categories are primarily aimed at formulated products with milk or cereals. These regulations do not necessarily cover or give guidance for TF intended to be manufactured and supplied for infants and children. Recognizing this, Indian Food Safety and Standards (Foods for Infant Nutrition) Regulations, 2017 framed standards for "Foods for Infant based on traditional food ingredients" that is in the draft stage (Infant Foods Regulations, 2017, FSSA). Foods for infants based on traditional food ingredients are products known to be prepared at home for feeding infants traditionally and have a long history of safe use. These need to be and can be processed and provided in packaged forms with specified best before use dates. These are either "Ready to Use" or to be reconstituted with a medium such as milk, water, curd/yogurt, or any other medium appropriate for an infant. Some such TF products have long been offered in some UK and European markets and India should be no exception, as it has a rich history of traditional documented knowledge. Regulations for TF for geriatric use are not common and are an area for the development of both the products and the regulations.

2.10 Developing scenario

Competition, recognition of a nation's tradition and knowledge, promoting a nation's business interests, providing personalized nutrition, age-specific/disease-specific nutrition products, products that can provide disease risk reduction, preventive healthcare foods, supplements/nutraceuticals, foods driven by ones metabolomic characteristics, *Prakruti* led nutrition/foods from Ayurveda, or Yin & Yang led nutrition/foods from traditional Chinese medicine, and parenteral nutrition are expected to develop and get into the market even before regulators would have thought about them. The challenge will be to decide whether to regulate or to train and educate the concerned business and technologists and manufacturers. This space will be driven by consumer's movement worldwide, slowly but steadily from "Illness centric (drug approach) to Wellness centric (food approach)." Challenges will be to all players in the sector. With the ever-increasing cost of innovations, there would be focus to offer TF with a history of safety and usage in packaged forms.

The regulations among Asian nations for TF are by and large on the same lines. This has made transborder trade easier. Exporters/importers of packaged TF across nations need to check specifically for compliance to local laws related to the additives used (colors, flavors, stabilizers, preservatives if any, contaminants, and their levels) before exporting consignments. There is a large variation in the contaminants to be tested and their acceptable levels, among each nation. For example, the heavy metal residues and contaminants, not only vary in the number needing testing and control, but also for the same heavy metal the acceptable levels vary, and their specified methods of analysis differ. Labeling requirements vary significantly and some nations do not permit correction by way of affixing sticker labels at the port of entry. Regulations that call for bilingual or labeling in local languages add another element of challenge. This puts a lot of challenges to manufacturers who for logistic reasons want to keep the same packaging materials and configurations across nations. However, the local production of TF for serving in hotels and restaurants, across nations may not face many challenges. Challenge for such a business would be in the event when some essential ingredients are not approved in the importing nation; therefore, regulatory approvals must be in place before starting a business, so that import of such ingredients does not face problems.

A systematic study of traditional foods and their documentation is necessary (in English as well as in regional languages). Traditional foods recipe cards containing detailed information about the recipe, ingredients, preparation process, and contents of selected nutrients need to be developed. This will help to promote them to consumers and the industry. They can be used by individuals for cooking, by schools to promote traditional foods to pupils, or by the food industry for the development of traditional products. This type of documentation has already been undertaken by Europe (Elisabeth et al., 2005).

Acknowledgments

Authors acknowledge and thank Ganesh Bhat, Technical Officer (Standards) of FSSAI for his inputs that have been used.

References

Additives. GMP, CODEX, 1995. <http://www.fao.org/gsfaonline/foods/details.html?id=268>.

Claims, 2018. FSSA, Advertisement and claims as per the Food Safety and Standards (Advertising and Claims) Regulations, 2018. <https://fssai.tk/upload/uploadfiles/files/Gazette_Notification_Advertising_Claims_27_11_2018.pdf>.

Codex STAN 192-19956, Codex STAN 192-1995. <http://www.fao.org/fao-who-codexalimentarius/sh-proxy/en/?lnk=1&url=https%253A%252F%252Fworkspace.fao.org%252Fsites%252Fcodex%252FStandards%252FCODEX%2BSTAN%2B192-1995%252FCXS_192e.pdf>.
Contaminants, 2011. FSSA, Safety parameters such as heavy metals, residues, etc. as per the Food Safety and Standards (Contaminants, Toxins and Residues) Regulation, 2011. <https://fssai.tk/upload/uploadfiles/files/Compendium_Contaminants_Regulations_20_05_2019.pdf>.
Costa, H.S., Vasilopoulou, E., Trichopoulou, A., Finglas, P., 2010. New nutritional data on traditional foods for European food composition databases. Eur. J. Clin. Nutr. 64, 73–81.
Dwyer, J., Bermudez, O.I., 2003. Encyclopedia of Food Sciences and Nutrition, second ed. <https://www.sciencedirect.com/topics/food-science/ethnic-foods>.
Dr. Elisabeth Weichselbaum and Dr. Helena 2005. Synthesis Report No 6: Traditional Foods in Europe. <http://citeseerx.ist.psu.edu/viewdoc/download?doi=10.1.1.628.5366&rep=rep1&type=pdf >.
IFCT, 2017. <http://www.ifct2017.com/frame.php?page=home>.
Infant Foods Regulations, 2017. FSSA (Foods for Infant Nutrition) Regulations, 2017 <https://fssai.tk/upload/uploadfiles/files/Draft_Notification_Infant_Nutrition_14_05_2019.pdf>.
Labelling, 2011. FSSA, Labelling as per Food Safety and Standards (Packaging and Labelling) Regulation, 2011. <https://fssai.tk/upload/uploadfiles/files/Compendium_Packaging_Labelling_Regulations_22_01_2019.pdf>.
Licensing, 2011. FSSA, License as per the Food Safety and Standards (Licensing and Registration of Food Businesses) Regulations, 2011. <https://fssai.tk/upload/uploadfiles/files/Compendium_Licensing_Regulations.pdf>.
Packaging, 2011. FSSA, Packaging as per the Food Safety and Standards (Packaging) Regulations, 2018. <https://fssai.tk/upload/uploadfiles/files/Gazette_Notification_Packaging_03_01_2019.pdf>.
Regulation (EU) No 1151/2012: Quality schemes for agricultural products and foodstuffs.
Standards, 2011. FSSA, Standards including additives and microbiological parameters as specified under the Food Safety and Standards (Food Product Standards and Food Additives) Regulation, 2011. <https://fssai.tk/upload/uploadfiles/files/Compendium_Food_Additives_Regulations_29_03_2019.pdf>.
Trichopoulou, A., Soukara, S., Vasilopoulou, E., 2007. Traditional foods: a science and society perspective. Trends Food Sci. Technol. 18, 420–427.
Trichopoulou, A., Vasilopoulou, E., Georga, K., Soukara, S., Dilis, V., 2006. Traditional foods: why and how to sustain them. Trends Food Sci. Technol. 17, 498–504.
Vanhonacker, F, et al., 2008. Consumer-based definition and general image of traditional foods in Europe. In: Perspectives of Traditional Food Supply Chains on the European Market, Proceedings of 12th Congress of the European Association of Agricultural Economists 'People, Food and Environments: Global Trends and European Strategies', 26–29 August 2008, Ghent, Belgium.
Vanhonacker, F., Lengard, V., Hersleth, M., Verbeke, W., 2010. Profiling European traditional 426 food consumers. Brit. Food J. 112 (8), 871–886.

CHAPTER 3

Marketing of traditional and functional foods for reach-out of nutrition

R.B. Smarta[1] and Dilip Ghosh[2,3,4,5,6]
[1]Interlink Marketing Consultancy Pvt. Ltd., Mumbai, India; Hon. Secretary, Health Foods And Dietary Supplements Association (HADSA), Mumbai, India
[2]Nutriconnect, Sydney, NSW, Australia
[3]Food Nutrition Partner, Auckland, New Zealand, New Zealand
[4]NICM, Western Sydney University, Sydney, NSW, Australia
[5]Health Foods and Dietary Supplements Association (HADSA), Mumbai, India
[6]Ambassador-Global Harmonization Initiatives, Vienna, Austria

Contents

3.1 Introduction

Food is associated with life processes, and the concept of the body accepting the food with the right mindset is considered as the sacred act of creating fullness in life. Foods can be classified in various ways, as ethnic, traditional, functional, contemporary, etc.; yet, the major role they play in the life of human beings is to create sufficient energy and satisfy the body, mind, and soul. In Indian tradition, the saying goes, "While

Nutritional and Health Aspects of Food in South Asian Countries
DOI: https://doi.org/10.1016/B978-0-12-820011-7.00033-2

taking the first morsel, chant the name of the Creator, which provides for easy digestion and eating does not remain merely an act of fulfilling the stomach but a sacred act of consuming a healthy meal and assimilating essential nutrients from a wholesome meal. So, be humble and be satisfied with the food."

Heritage foods of each country are sometimes not known outside the geographic regions, and the origin of such food is difficult to trace. Sometimes they evolve locally depending on the availability of raw ingredients and the environmental practices. Cultural issues and local food habits evolved through changing times have always impacted traditional foods. Philosophical and religious overtones played a prominent role in society and its evolvement, as in India, these overtones created several philosophies and religions that grew from these philosophies, interacted with each other, and made their impact on Indian traditional food cultures.

Diets were created by our ancestors originally to meet their survival needs. People of various Indian cultures gradually enriched them through long empirical experience using a variety of primary food materials, especially the locally available food grains and vegetables that nutritionally complement and supplement each other. This contributed to better health, better immunity, good digestibility, resistance to health disorders, and increased longevity.

3.2 South Asian overview

Among the South Asian countries, Sri Lanka has a variety of ethnic dishes that are nutrient dense. If we look at the example of the most popular plate known as *Pescatarian*, it is a plant-based recipe blended with good fats derived from coconuts and 100% grass-fed cow/buffalo ghee. The ingredients used to prepare this plate have medicinal properties of reducing inflammatory processes in the body. Additionally, the authentic spices used in this cuisine take it to a higher level of taste and nutrition (Gulf News Asia, 2019). There are some traditional foods ingredients that are widely used in Sri Lanka, such as *kathuru murunga*, leaves of the hummingbird tree (source of vitamin and minerals), horse gram (high protein and calcium), tamarind, and spices (source of antioxidants) (Weerasekara et al., 2018).

In the case of Afghanistan, the cuisine is majorly influenced by Iran, Mongolia, and India. Although it has been influenced by neighboring countries, it has its own cuisine style. If we look at the climatic conditions of Afghanistan, then the use of fatty fishes is considered to be an important fuel in the freezing winters. Universally, Afghanistan is also considered to be one of the best countries for a variety of dry fruits, and the inclusion of these dry fruits is also an important aspect of their food habits. Pakistan, the neighboring country of India, shares common ethnic and traditional food. The food items that are listed under the Halal law specify what foods are allowed, and how the food must be prepared. This law is universally accepted and followed by food operators and pharmaceutical manufacturers.

Bangladesh, being a coastal region, has rice and fish as their staple food. The indigenous fishes such as *ilish* (Hilsa fish) and *shutki* (dried fish) are widely consumed for its nutrient content. In Bhutan, the locals have rice as their staple food. Red rice cultivated in Bhutan is considered to be healthy for losing weight and for diabetics. The national dish of Bhutan is *Ema Datshi*, which is a blend of a spicy mix of chilies and local cheese known as *Datshi*. It is considered as a nutrient-dense cuisine. In addition, bamboo shoots are considered to be one of the delicacies in this region. The preparation for bamboo shoots involves stock and soups and these are also pickled for long time use. They are considered to be nutrient dense (mainly proteins, carbohydrates, and minerals) and have a low-fat content. Bamboo shoots are widely researched all over the globe for their phytosterols and a high amount of fiber that have cholesterol-lowering and anticarcinogenic activity and hence can be used as an ingredient for nutraceutical formulations. (Dahal et al., 2007).

The ancient wisdom of traditional foods is nowadays supported and promoted by modern scientific studies of its high degree of antioxidants, phytoestrogen, and vitamins. Nepal could be the best example as one of the indigenous communities from Nepal, named *Chepangs* or *Prajas*, has enormous knowledge about large numbers of plant species on which they have been dependent for centuries (The Himalaya Times, 2018). The plants such as aerial yam, wild edible yam, and deltoid yam have been found to contain five times more protein than potatoes and sweet potatoes. In addition, they are rich in dietary fibers and certain micronutrients that are recognized to combat cancer, diabetes, and heart diseases. Hence, these are considered to be potent "functional foods."

3.3 Traditional food and nutrients

One of the best examples of cereals grown in the Indian subcontinent is finger millet or *Ragi*. It has been grown since ages for its health benefits. Modern research has shown that finger millet has a high amount of calcium (344 mg%) and potassium (408 mg%). The study also revealed that it has higher dietary fiber, minerals, and sulfur-containing amino acids (Shobana et al., 2013). The fermented batter of various cereals and whole grains is considered to be nutrient-rich as it provides amino acids like lysine.

The gastrointestinal microflora in humans plays a key role in nutrition and health. The *Lactobacillus* in *Dahi* (Indian yogurt) is considered to be good bacteria that provide protection from colon cancer and increase overall immune-modulatory action. Various pickles are also considered to be a good source of vitamin C, minerals, and antioxidant components (Srinivasan, 2010). The North East region of India is well known for its meat-based delicacies. A survey conducted has shown that the recipes made by all three tribes of Meghalaya, namely *Khasi, Jaintia,* and *Garo* are healthy and highly nutritive in macro and micronutrients (Govindasamy et al., 2018).

Mango, grown from ancient times, is considered to be the king of all fruits by natives. It is a rich source of bioactive-like phenols and carotenoids, isoquercetin, ellagic acid, and β-glucogallin. The fruits such as gooseberry, tamarind, and *kokum* (*Garcinia indica*) are commonly used in Indian subcontinental cuisine to impart a desirable sour taste to certain food preparations. These fruits are rich in vitamin C and polyphenols. The dried fruit rinds of kokum commonly known as "*Malabar tamarind,*" are liberally used in the coastal regions of India as a traditional food acidulant in culinary practices. The dark red fruit of *Garcinia indica* is valued for its nutritive value and outstanding medicinal properties. This fruit is known to reduce obesity and to beneficially regulate blood lipid chemistry.

The fresh green leaves of Betel vine, locally known as *Paan*, is traditionally used as a mouth freshener and for a digestive stimulating effect. The southern part of India is famous for spices. The spices such as *chilli*, ginger, turmeric, and garlic are considered to have high antioxidant properties with functional constituents such as curcumin, capsaicin, flavonoids, and essential oils.

In summary, with the heritage of traditional and functional foods, South Asian countries need clarity and understanding of its nutritional composition and effectiveness for fulfilling specific nutritional needs.

3.4 Status of nutrition of South Asian countries and health issues

Being home to a population of almost one-fifth of the world, South Asia is a vibrant, dynamic, and fast-growing region. Still, the region of strategic importance, South Asia, faces public health challenges. The core health issues of maternal and child health, infectious diseases, and access to health are still relevant. Globally, 2.6 million newborns died in 2016 and about 1 million (39%) of the world's newborn deaths occurred in the South Asia countries (UNICEF, 2016). The region has witnessed rapid urbanization with a concurrent rise in noncommunicable diseases, smoking, mental illnesses, injuries, conflicts, natural disasters, and infectious disease that has stalled progress on health indicators (BMJ, 2017). The region is under the stage of transition demographically, epidemiologically, environmentally, and economically. Food plays an important role in this situation. This transition has impacted the lifestyle of the population in such a way that physical activity and consumption of a calorie-dense diet have increased the risk of noncommunicable diseases.

The study conducted by the World Bank in the 52 countries all over the world has shown India, Nepal, Pakistan, Sri Lanka, and Bangladesh, to have adverse health conditions at an early age. These countries have a population that is at a high risk of getting their first heart attack at younger ages and also has high levels of other risk factors, such as diabetes, cardiovascular diseases, and early onset of cancers. Food based on tradition can make a big difference in combating these health issues (The Hindu, 2016). Studies conducted in this region have indicated that there is a high prevalence of noncommunicable diseases such as hypertension, cardiovascular diseases, psychosocial stress, and diabetes in the population. In addition, the age-standardized blood pressure and cholesterol levels have increased in South Asia over the past decades.

The incidences of communicable diseases such as tuberculosis and HIV/AIDS are second only to those of sub-Saharan Africa. Urban areas in these countries can at least receive timely primary healthcare, whereas rural areas do worse in life expectancy, immunization rates, maternal health, and malaria incidences.

With as many as 194.6 million (almost 15% of the total population) starving people, the country has been ranked as the most undernourished in the world by the Food and Agriculture Organization. As we have seen earlier, the undernourished population impacts a nation's economy adversely. An undernourished population suffers from numerous health disorders. Although child undernourishment rates have declined since 2006, this development is still well below to achieve global nutrition targets adopted by the World Health Assembly. The major risk among newborns and their mothers in India is loss of life. As India is second lowest in taking folic acid supplements during pregnancy, it leads to severe birth defects every year. With respect to children under 5 years old, it is noted that a large number of deaths (50%) occur mainly due to poor nutrition (TOI, 2015); moreover, those who manage to survive experience serious health problems in their adulthood. As shown in Fig. 3.1, in India, 39% of children above 5 years are stunted (low height for age) and 15% are wasted (low weight for height). As children grow into adolescence, problems of overweight (11%) and obesity (2%) are observed (Global Nutrition Report, 2018). Anemia is also prevalent with 56% of young girls and 30% of young boys in the age group 15–19 years (Fig. 3.1).

Hence, we can clearly see that entire South Asia is at a crossroads with economic disparity, access to quality and safe food, education, a growing share of unhealthy youth as well as the aging population, and health systems that are failing to adjust to people.

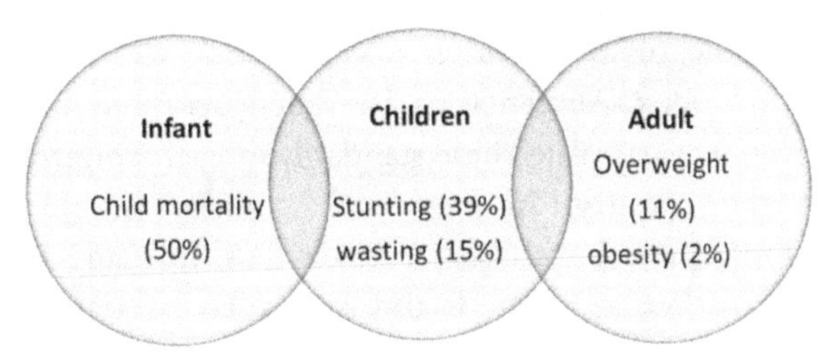

Figure 3.1 Indian health status.

As there are disparities and differences in nutritional status, there is a need to create awareness among the population, and there are countrywise preferences depending on agricultural and economic progress to promote traditional foods, and certain marketing issues have cropped up. Can traditional foods, their nutrition, and affordability offer any solution to these issues?

3.5 Marketing issues

To start the process of achieving benchmark targets and to reach out for the nutritional requirements, many countries take action on social marketing or other marketing methods. Before coming up with specific marketing strategies, based on the strengths and weaknesses of each country, there are core marketing issues that crop up. After analyzing South Asian countries and predominantly moving around India, following are the major issues that need attention before deciding a specific marketing strategy:

3.5.1 Demographic, health, and food variables

To advocate specific benefits of traditional foods and functional foods, it is very important to gather status and existing food habits of each country along with their socioeconomic, political, regulatory, and technological conditions. It is also equally important to look at certain deep-rooted beliefs and will to invest in social welfare, per capita food production, and food distribution issues as well as their concern for importing certain traditional foods. Besides these aspects, it is essential to arrive at existing disease burdens of the country that provides another point of view to work on required nutrition for a specific country.

3.5.2 Regulatory and other food policies for marketing and promotions

From a regulatory point of view, India comes first as enforcement has been fully achieved at the beginning of 2018 and it is considering to take the next steps for global harmonization. Codex Alimentarius has been accepted universally and in a proper way, it is pertinent to escalate these standards in each country provided there is no objection from the country. In fact, each country should welcome Codex Alimentarius regulations as it is beneficial for its citizens. In many Asian countries like the rest of the world, marketing methods and routes have certain laws and specifications such as for advertising, labels, Weights and Measures Act, and Magic Remedies Act that will enable or otherwise provide direction to marketing and promotional practices.

3.5.3 Proposal promise and credibility of marketing

Understanding fundamental deep-rooted beliefs and faith in certain foods, whether originated within the country, traditional foods, or widely available as functional foods, is of prime importance. On the basis of this, understanding whatever marketing strategy is adopted would either be accepted or totally rejected. Obviously, the right promotion with the right media selection will have to develop its promise in nutritional value and the basic strategic platform depending on the country's mindset.

To address these issues and to find out ways of marketing functional and traditional food to reach out nutrition, the marketing team has to undergo a few challenges in each country and South Asia is no exception.

3.6 Marketing challenges in traditional foods

Several challenges need to be considered by each country depending on its intensity. These ought to be considered concomitantly with the strategy, and marketing plan for each processed traditional food.

3.6.1 Knowledge and use of traditional foods in modern society

It is obvious that although there is a common platform of marketing at a strategic level, marketing in each country will be further customized on the basis of knowledge and usage as well as attitudes of citizens for existing traditional and functional foods and also modern functional foods that have taken an adequate shape through nutraceuticals in the world. In nutraceuticals, traditional ingredients are used as fortifying elements to make food as functional or fortified. There is a challenge in this, as individual countries may have different levels of attitudes, knowledge, usages, and conviction for each traditional or functional food. This insight can be generalized for a specific country on the basis of its demographics dependent on variables such as education, income, food habits, occupation, and per capita income.

3.6.2 Trust and evidence of the perceived quality of traditional and functional foods

When it comes to beliefs and faith, the best way to touch this delicate aspect is through scientific support for all traditional and functional foods. Hence, evidence-based perceived quality needs to be channeled in such a way that an old paradigm can resolve or evolve to a new paradigm without losing its essence or years of tradition and wisdom in food practices.

3.6.3 The challenge of food safety

Countries at different developmental stages of health and economy evolve from the acute phase to the prevention, growth, and developmental stage. There are a few countries where different levels of development are seen in different parts; hence, it is observed that unless a common factor such as food safety gets evolved, countries do not climb from one stage of development to the next. When many developmental stages are present concurrently in one country, there is bound to be an inequality in income, sanitation, as well as nutrition. This challenge has to be taken upfront with private–public participation (PPP) where the concern of the country is seen and understood by all citizens.

3.6.4 The research and development with the adaptation of technology

Conversion of traditional food products, as well as functional foods, is usually supported by new product development through R&D and also adding a technology edge for a delivery mechanism to ensure that tracking and tracing of claimed nutrition content are feasible at the level of consumer. This challenge influences each country's attitude toward R&D efforts of certain institutes and to provide concessional tariffs as they need such products for their citizens.

3.6.5 The challenge of communicating the holistic nature of traditional food

This challenge percolates to communication and messaging patterns that are different for each language and country. It needs to address the right target customer, probably a decision-maker in each family with their requirements so that its holistic nature is communicated and understood.

3.6.6 Personalized nutrition

To ensure that these foods are relevant and of utility to the society, adequate distribution outlets, as well as awareness camps, are essential besides communication and messages. Personalized nutrition would leverage relevance and utility and ensure that each individual is benefited once a belief level in every family is reached. This is typically a very difficult step unless there are active participation and a reasonable economic resource available to the family. If the food itself is scarce along with its socioeconomical aspects, it can take secondary consideration. In such a case, food is cooked for the entire family and would not become individualistic at all.

3.6.7 Regulatory in terms of products, labels, claims, and promotions

Some countries have fewer regulations with respect to traditional foods. To make food safe and healthy for each consumer, each country will have to evolve regulatory reforms and harmonization processes to deliver nutrition from traditional food through a consultative process. Although this process is time consuming, it will bring the benefits of traditional foods on a common platform.

3.7 The marketing platform for traditional foods

As there cannot be any individualistic marketing model for each country, based on a basic hypothesis on the South Asian region, it is possible to evolve a new holistic traditional functional food platform considering the issues of these countries. The platform would look like as shown in Fig. 3.2.

It is a conceptual model, and if adequately validated, it has possibilities and power to become a major platform on which marketing models will play.

One of the major cornerstones of this platform is to ensure that the wisdom and goodness of traditional and functional foods with their health benefits are communicated well. The second cornerstone is built upon the contribution of foods of different varieties for transferring the goodness of traditional foods to maintain the right nutritional balance and provide accessibility and diversity.

The third cornerstone is a customized one where it adds value to individual transactions and thereby facilitates the wisdom and goodness of traditional and functional foods coupled with the communication of nutritional value at the individual level. As it is a subjective and customized cornerstone for an individual country, it all depends on who takes part in this facilitation, for example, government and public sectors can take part in social marketing. Social marketing of milk, eggs, vaccines, etc. have been totally successful. Creatives and media options are open to private as well as public

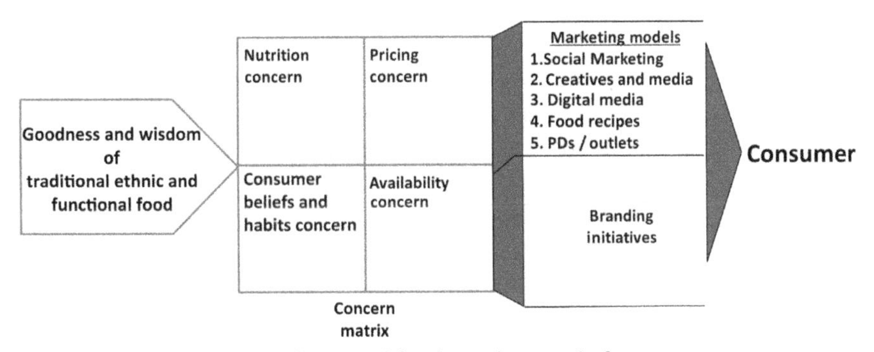

Figure 3.2 Holistic traditional and functional foods marketing platform.

sector organizations whereby they can reach individuals through digital marketing with the selection of the right media. Its accessibility can be further advanced by the overall creativity of promoting traditional foods and its nutrition.

For many countries, food security and food safety are important issues at the government level; hence, they have designed certain ways of public distribution systems and ensured that food is not scarce and available to everyone through specialized outlets. Specialized food packages are also prepared and distributed for the needy to correct severe imbalances, and it is in this area that traditional foods can play a very big role. Once it is done, it can be further supported by providing creative recipes and also personalized nutrition through the diversity of foods.

Branding is a level where traditional and functional foods get lifted from commodities to brand level once the same consumer starts getting value either through a convenient form, safety and trust of a brand owner and overall continuous reminder of the same along with its promise and performance. All these initiatives need to be taken to brand-specific solutions for increasing the consumption of traditional and functional foods at each country level.

3.8 Commercial marketing models

Based on holistic traditional and functional foods marketing platform, individual marketing models can be developed. Fig. 3.3 is a model that is adapted by Dr. R.B. Smarta (Interlink) from the consumer behavior model of Howard and Sheth.

This model has unique features in its different facets, and each facet is useful for a marketer to consider for its marketing ways, strategies, and tactics (Fig. 3.3).

This model is focused on consumers as a marketing platform and can be adopted for the marketing of traditional foods.

Once the consumer has access to information or gets influenced, his basic choice satisfies him for the promised claim and his needs. Thereon repeat transaction of his usage and purchase with his satisfaction helps to build brand consciousness. This process helps marketers to build brands.

As suggested, once marketing platforms and marketing models are operative, an evolution of traditional foods and functional foods to its newer form is observed. This is accepted by present-day consumers to bridge the gap of nutritional imbalance. This evolution could be quick-paced in a few countries, and it could be redefined as a revolution.

In conclusion, when it comes to heritage foods, food culture has become so diversified with numerous traditional and ethnic food preparations that over a period of time different dietary patterns have evolved. At the root of the miracle of biodiversity and agriculture, lies the customs, practices, and what is grown in that region sustainably.

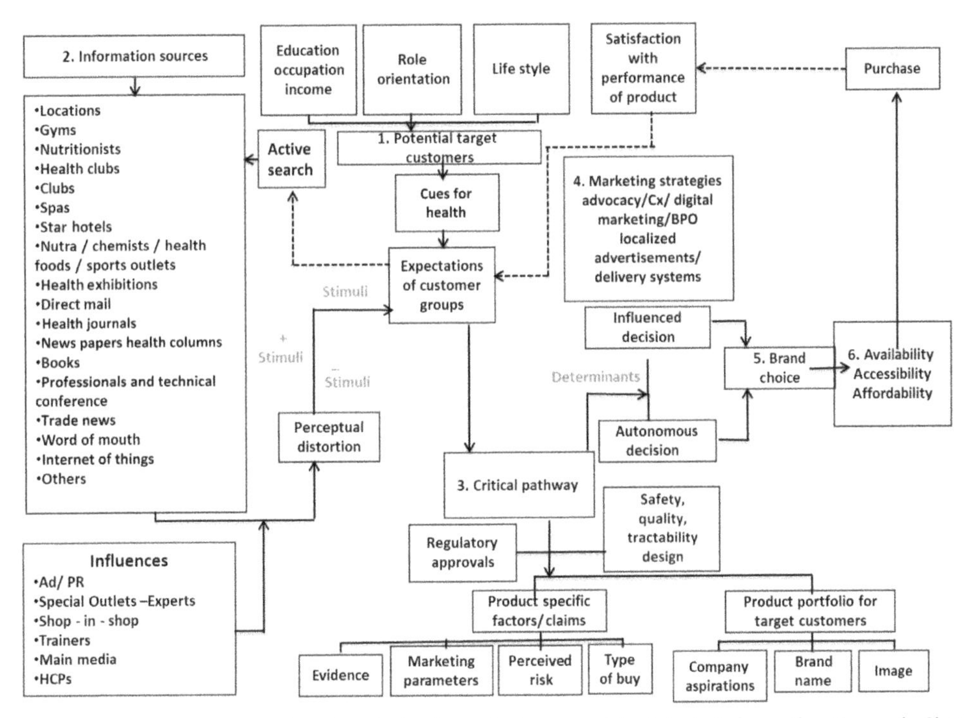

Figure 3.3 Traditional and functional food marketing model. *Adapted from the Howard–Sheth model of consumer behavior.*

References

BMJ, 2017. Health research priorities and gaps in South Asia_ BMJ (accessed 25.03.19.).

Dahal, N.R., Karki, T.B., Swamylingappa, B., Li, Q., Gu, G., 2007. Traditional Foods and Beverages of Nepal—A Review. Taylor and Francis.

Global Nutrition Report, 2018. <https://globalnutritionreport.org/reports/global-nutrition-report-2018/> (accessed 25.03.19.).

Govindasamy, K., Banerjee, B.B., Arun, A., Milton, P., Katiyar, R., Meitei, S., 2018. Meat-based ethnic delicacies of Meghalaya state in Eastern Himalaya: preparation methods and significance. J. Ethnic Foods 5.

Gulf News Asia, 2019. Why Sri Lankan food is one of the healthiest ways of eating. <https://gulfnews.com/world/asia/why-sri-lankan-food-is-one-of-the-healthiest-ways-of-eating-1.1549195011610> (accessed 15.03.19.).

Shobana, S., Krishnaswamy, K., Sudha, V., Malleshi, N.G., Anjana, R.M., Palaniappan, L., et al., 2013. Finger Millet (Ragi, *Eleusine coracana* L.). A Review of Its Nutritional Properties, Processing, and Plausible Health Benefits. Elsevier.

Srinivasan, K., 2010. Traditional Indian Functional Foods.

The Himalaya Times, 2018. Wisdom of eating: Chepangs' food habits <https://thehimalayantimes.com/opinion/wisdom-of-eating-chepangs-food-habits/> (accessed 15.03.19.).

The Hindu, 2016. South Asian countries facing "health crisis": World Bank. The Hindu, <https://www.thehindu.com/sci-tech/health/South-Asian-countries-facing-ldquohealth-crisisrdquo-World-Bank/article15293137.ece> (accessed 15.03.19.).

TOI, 2015. India has highest number of deaths of children under five years of age. TOI, <https://timesofindia.indiatimes.com/india/India-has-highest-number-of-deaths-of-children-under-five-years-of-age/articleshow/46722307.cms> Accessed 25.03.19.

UNICEF, 2016. The UNICEF Progress Report-Save Newborns. <http://www.unicefrosaprogressreport.org/savenewborns.html> (accessed 25.03.19.).

Weerasekara, P.C., Withanachchi, C.R., Ginigaddara, G.A.S., Ploeger, A., 2018. Nutrition Transition and Traditional Food Cultural Changes in Sri Lanka During Colonization and Post-Colonization. Foods.

Index

Note: Page numbers followed by "*f*" and "*t*" refer to figures and tables, respectively.

C

D

J

M

Q

R

CPSIA information can be obtained
at www.ICGtesting.com
Printed in the USA
LVHW010208020523
745849LV00011B/322